Essentials of Primary Care Sports Medicine

Gregory L. Landry, MD
David T. Bernhardt, MD

University of Wisconsin

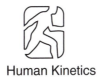

Human Kinetics

Library of Congress Cataloging-in-Publication Data

Landry, Gregory L., 1953-
    Essentials of primary care sports medicine / Gregory L. Landry, David
T.
Bernhardt.
        p. ; cm.
Includes bibliographical references and index.
    ISBN 0-7360-0323-1 (hard cover)
    1. Primary care (Medicine)--Handbooks, manuals, etc.   2. Sports
medicine--Handbooks, manuals, etc.
    [DNLM: 1. Athletic Injuries.   2. Sports Medicine.   QT 261 L262e
2003]   I.
Bernhardt, David T., 1962- II. Title.
    RC55.L26 2003
    617.1′027--dc21

                                                    2003004106

ISBN-10: 0-7360-0323-1
ISBN-13: 978-0-7360-0323-0

The Web addresses cited in this text were current as of March 2003, unless otherwise noted.

Acquisitions Editor: Loarn D. Robertson, PhD; **Developmental Editor:** Elaine H. Mustain; **Assistant Editors:** Kathleen Bernard, Derek Campbell, and Maggie Schwarzentraub; **Writer:** Brian C. Mustain; **Copyeditor:** Barbara Walsh; **Proofreader:** Erin Cler; **Indexer:** Gerry Lynn Messner; **Permission Manager:** Dalene Reeder; **Graphic Designer:** Andrew Tietz; **Graphic Artist:** Kathleen Boudreau-Fuoss; **Photo Manager:** Kareema McLendon; **Cover Designer:** Andrea Souflee; **Photographer (cover):** © Empics; **Photographer (interior):** Gregory L. Landry (figures 2.2, 2.3, 5.2, and 5.15), David T. Bernhardt (figures 6.3, 8.3, and 8.4), and © Human Kinetics unless otherwise noted; **Art Manager:** Kelly Hendren; **Illustrator:** Jason McAlexander of Interactive Composition Corporation (medical art) and Mic Greenburg; **Printer:** Sheridan Books

Printed in the United States of America   10   9   8   7   6   5   4   3

The paper in this book is certified under a sustainable forestry program.

Human Kinetics
Web site: www.HumanKinetics.com

United States: Human Kinetics
P.O. Box 5076, Champaign, IL 61825-5076
800-747-4457
e-mail: humank@hkusa.com

Canada: Human Kinetics
475 Devonshire Road Unit 100, Windsor, ON N8Y 2L5
800-465-7301 (in Canada only)
e-mail: info@hkcanada.com

Europe: Human Kinetics
107 Bradford Road, Stanningley, Leeds LS28 6AT, United Kingdom
+44 (0) 113 255 5665
e-mail: hk@hkeurope.com

Australia: Human Kinetics, 57A Price Avenue, Lower Mitcham, South Australia 5062
08 8372 0999
e-mail: info@hkaustralia.com

New Zealand: Human Kinetics, Division of Sports Distributors NZ Ltd.
P.O. Box 300 226 Albany, North Shore City, Auckland
0064 9 448 1207
e-mail: info@humankinetics.co.nz

We would like to dedicate this book
to our families.
To Ann, Kerry, and Megan Landry
and to Colleen Clark Bernhardt
and Alex, Ryan, and Spencer Bernhardt
we express our gratitude
for your patience, love, and support.

CONTENTS

PART IV　SPECIAL ISSUES

PREFACE

Essentials of Primary Care Sports Medicine covers fundamental medical issues as they relate to exercise and participation in sports. The topics and organization of this book sprang from the syllabus of a course titled "Medical Aspects of Exercise and Sports" at the University of Wisconsin–Madison that we have taught for the past 12 years. Although we designed the course for undergraduates studying to become athletic trainers, it has attracted a variety of professionals including teachers, coaches, dietitians, nurses, and emergency medical personnel who work with athletes. The students universally have found the information in this course useful in their work with athletes. They also have told us that the subject matter was not taught in any other course.

Unlike most books on sports medicine, this book does *not* address traumatic or musculoskeletal aspects of sports medicine. Instead, we focus on a myriad of health problems—from asthma to amenorrhea, from folliculitis to pharyngitis, from tachycardia to tinnitus—that you may confront in your work with athletes. In fact, you may be the first person to note the symptoms of some problems mentioned in this book. Whether you are an athletic or personal trainer, a school nurse, a physical therapist or kinesiotherapist, or perhaps even a clinical exercise physiologist, you are often on the front lines of many health-care issues simply because of your frequent contact with athletes. It's fine for you to know how to take care of a sprained ankle. But what if an athlete comes to you having an elevated temperature, looking pale, and complaining of dizziness after an intense workout? Is the athlete in the first throes of heatstroke? Is he simply dehydrated? Could his workout have interacted with a prescription drug he is taking? Or what if a young woman is missing menstrual periods: Should you immediately refer her to a gynecologist, or should you ask her to cut back on the intensity of her workouts? If she's also been losing weight, should you refer her to a counselor to screen for anorexia, or should you simply talk with her about her diet? What if the young man in your fitness center has gained 30 lb of lean body mass over the past 2 months and his friends are concerned because he is isolating himself and seems depressed? How would you approach him? Does he need to see a psychotherapist?

This book covers the large majority of pathologies you will see as you work with athletes. Some topics occur almost exclusively in the athletic environment—such as hyperthermia, sudden cardiac death, and exercise-induced asthma. And although others are just as common among nonathletes as among athletes, their manifestations in the athletic setting tend to be unique—for example, the effects of eating prior to competition, or the issue of permitting individuals with mononucleosis to return to normal activities. And many topics, from sunburn to vitamin deficiencies to peritonitis, have almost nothing to do with athletics; we discuss them here solely because you may be the first person to recognize that an athlete has a problem and needs treatment; and you also need to be aware of how these problems affect an athlete's ability to return to play.

Although knowledge of human anatomy and physiology is helpful in understanding the material in this textbook, we have written it for people who have little background in these areas. Our focus is on symptoms and how they affect athletes, not on theoretical understanding of what's happening on the cellular level. We want to help you understand how to deal with athletes who have various problems—how to recognize a multitude of common medical disorders, what questions to ask in taking medical histories, and how to know when to refer athletes to a physician. We have tried to make it clear when you should consult a physician or a subspecialist. We have discussed some procedures with the expectation that only a physician will perform them. We hope this information will help other health providers counsel the athlete before and after the consultation with the physician.

The appendix discusses the development of sports medicine as a specialty and outlines the specialized training a sports medicine physician must undergo. Athletic trainers and other allied health professionals in sports settings who work closely with sports medicine physicians will find this background information useful.

By increasing the knowledge base of professionals who work with athletes, we hope this book in the long run will lead to healthier athletes.

ACKNOWLEDGMENTS

The authors are most grateful to the University of Wisconsin–Madison undergraduate students enrolled in "Medical Aspects of Exercise and Sport" for their feedback and constructive criticisms, which ultimately helped to shape the content of this book. Dr. Andrew Winterstein provided assistance at a critical time in the editorial process. His experience as an educator of athletic training students and his candid comments on our chapters were extremely valuable to us.

We would like to thank the following individuals: Loarn Robertson, for his willingness to allow us to embark on a unique project with his staff; Brian Mustain, for getting us started; and Elaine Mustain, our editor, for her patience, persistence, and attention to detail.

Finally, we would like to thank all of our patients who allowed us to provide medical care for them both in the athletic setting and the primary care setting. It is our privilege to provide medical care for so many individuals and families.

PART I

SYSTEM DISORDERS

CHAPTER 1

Sudden Cardiac Death

OBJECTIVES

Upon completion of this chapter the reader will be able to do the following:

1. Describe the causes of sudden cardiac death

2. Discuss the guidelines for screening athletes for cardiovascular conditions

3. Explain the Bethesda guidelines for identifying individuals whom you should not allow to engage in vigorous sports

4. Identify common signs and symptoms to determine which athletes should be referred for further cardiovascular testing

Most people assume that well-trained athletes are exceptionally healthy. When a young athlete dies suddenly, without warning, the tragedy can devastate the athlete's family, community, and medical team. "When you lose a child, you lose your future," says Dianna Havick, whose 14-yr-old son died suddenly while playing basketball ("Working through their grief: Son's death still a mystery to the Havicks" 1996).

The untimely deaths of famous athletes such as Pete Maravich, Hank Gathers, Reggie Lewis, and Sergei Grinkov have led to significant public and medical scrutiny of sudden unexpected cardiac death. It is no simple matter, however, to detect the rare conditions that may lead to sudden death, or even to determine who needs further diagnostic testing or cardiovascular evaluation.

Case Study

An 18-yr-old male basketball player passes out during preseason conditioning. As the athletic trainer covering the event, you recognize the potential serious consequences of this, monitor his vital signs, and contact your team physician. The athlete denies any history of similar events, chest pain associated with this or any other previous event, or history of similar problems in any family members; this is the first time he has ever passed out. He also reports no history of sudden, unexpected death caused by known or unknown causes in any family members. His physical exam shows only a very soft systolic murmur at the left lower sternal border. His blood pressure (BP), pulse, and femoral pulses are all normal. He has no other physical stigmata of any other genetic syndrome. The team physician refers the patient to a cardiologist for further workup. Diagnostic testing reveals hypertrophic cardiomyopathy. Treatment recommendations include refraining from any competitive sporting activity and placement of an implantable defibrillator.

SUDDEN CARDIAC DEATH—BASIC CONCEPTS AND INCIDENCE

Sudden cardiac death related to exercise is caused by cardiac arrest that occurs instantaneously with an abrupt change in an individual's preexisting clinical state or within a few minutes of that change (Van Camp 1992) and is by definition associated with exercise. This definition does *not* include drug-related sudden death.

Fortunately, sudden unexpected cardiac death is extremely rare, especially among athletes <35 yr. The incidence in the United States is estimated to be 1 to 2 cases per 200,000 athletes per year (Epstein and Maron 1986). From 1985 through 1995, the most prevalent cause of the 158 sudden unexpected deaths among U.S. athletes was hypertrophic cardiomyopathy (36%), followed by aberrant coronary arteries (13%), unexplained increase in cardiac mass (10%), "other" coronary anomalies (6%), ruptured aortic root presumably secondary to Marfan's syndrome (5%), tunneled left anterior descending (LAD) coronary artery (5%), aortic stenosis (4%), myocarditis (3%), idiopathic dilated cardiomyopathy (3%), arrhythmogenic right ventricular dysplasia (ARVD) (3%), idiopathic myocardial scarring (3%), mitral valve prolapse (2%), and atherosclerotic coronary artery disease (2%); less frequent causes included other congenital heart diseases (1.5%), long QT syndrome (0.5%), sarcoidosis (0.5%), and sickle cell trait (0.5%). Interestingly, 2% had a normal heart without a cause for the sudden death (Maron, Shirani et al. 1996) (figure 1.1).

Among athletes over 35 yr, the most common cause of sudden death is atherosclerotic coronary artery disease. A study of joggers in Rhode Island estimated the annual incidence of death during jogging for men aged 30 to 64 yr as 1 per 7,620

Terms and Definitions

auscultation—The act of listening with a stethoscope.

electrocardiogram (ECG)—An electrical study of the heart.

hypertrophic cardiomyopathy (HCM)—Abnormal enlargement of diseased heart muscle.

hypertrophy—Abnormal growth or enlargement resulting from enlargement of cells.

ischemia—Lack of oxygen in a specific area of tissue caused by inadequate blood flow.

long QT syndrome—A genetic condition in which the heart's ability to repolarize, or electrically recharge itself, is abnormal. The QT interval is the time between the start of the heart being polarized to contract the muscle and when the heart is completely repolarized.

scoliosis—Lateral curvature of the spine.

stenosis—Narrowing.

syncope—Loss of consciousness caused by inadequate blood flow to the brain; fainting.

Valsalva maneuver or event—An effort to forcibly expel air while intentionally blocking the exit of air from mouth and nostrils (as is often done when trying to clear the eustachian tubes during air travel).

(Thompson et al. 1982). Before seeking an exercise prescription, athletes over 35 should consult a physician if they have a risk profile of hypertension, hypercholesterolemia, or smoking, or a family history of premature coronary artery disease. Premature atherosclerotic coronary artery disease in the second or third decade of life is usually secondary to a congenital cholesterol metabolism problem.

YOUNG ATHLETES—CAUSES OF SUDDEN DEATH

Sudden cardiac death in younger athletes generally traces not to atherosclerosis but to several much rarer conditions that, unfortunately, may remain undiagnosed until the occurrence of sudden death.

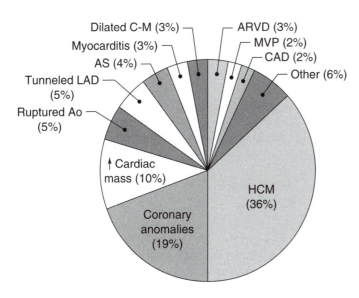

■ **Figure 1.1** Causes of sudden cardiac death in young competitive athletes based on systematic tracking of 158 athletes in the United States.

Data from Maron et al., 1996.

Hypertrophic Cardiomyopathy

Hypertrophic cardiomyopathy (HCM) is characterized by asymmetric **hypertrophy** of the left ventricle in the absence of other cardiac or systemic disease (figure 1.2). Other common names for this condition used in the past include *asymmetric septal hypertrophy, hypertrophic obstructive cardiomyopathy,* and *idiopathic hypertrophic subaortic stenosis.*

Dynamic left ventricular outflow obstruction is present in 20% to 30% of HCM patients at rest. The obstruction increases during a **Valsalva event,** after exercise, or when the individual rises to a standing position. Diastolic dysfunction (abnormalities during cardiac relaxation) occurs in 80% of patients with HCM. The diastolic dysfunction may relate to the myofibrillar disorganization commonly seen in such people but is not

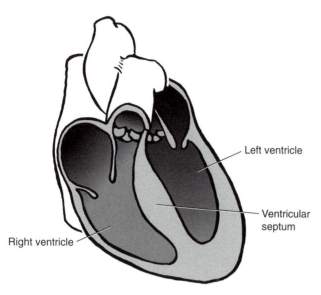

■ **Figure 1.2** Asymmetric hypertrophy of the left ventricle. Hypertrophic cardiomyopathy is characterized by asymmetric thickening of the ventricular septum without an increase in chamber size. The diseased septal muscle independent of left ventricular outflow obstruction characterizes the disease and predisposes the afflicted athlete to sudden death.

necessarily correlated with systolic obstruction or with the severity of the hypertrophy.

HCM often leads to sudden unexpected death with no previous symptoms. In some cases, however, athletes with or without obstruction of left ventricular outflow may experience **syncope,** shortness of breath, fatigue, or chest pain. Physical examination findings may vary with the degree of obstruction. A patient with significant obstruction may present with a systolic ejection murmur (an abnormal vibratory sound between the first and second heart sounds) at the left sternal border; the murmur may increase with standing or with Valsalva. When no obstruction is present, there is either no murmur or at most a soft murmur. Most patients with symptoms develop those symptoms in adulthood.

Although **electrocardiogram (ECG)** testing may reveal nonspecific changes and is abnormal in more than 90% of patients with HCM, the ECG does not reliably detect the presence of obstruction or predict risk of sudden death. Echocardiography (an ultrasound test of the heart that defines the anatomy of the heart better than an ECG does) is the most effective test for diagnosing HCM. Echocardiographic findings include a thickened septum with or without left ventricular outflow obstruction, along with evidence of diastolic dysfunction.

For people with HCM, the natural history of sudden cardiac death is unpredictable in terms of the clinical course and patient outcome and is not necessarily related to the presence of left ventricular outflow obstruction. Sudden death appears to be secondary to an arrhythmia, with most patients asymptomatic prior to death. Among patients with known HCM, the annual mortality rate is between 2% and 6%.

The 26th Bethesda Conference recommended that athletes with known HCM not participate in most competitive sports—with the possible exception of low-intensity sports (billiards, bowling, golf, curling) (Maron and Mitchell 1994). These recommendations apply whether or not athletes have symptoms or obstructed left ventricular outflow. Further treatment may involve the placement of an implantable defibrillator in those athletes thought to be at high risk for a life-threatening arrhythmia.

Research into the genetics of HCM is too complex for this chapter to detail. About half of all cases reveal an inheritance pattern in which other family members have the same problem; an identifiable genetic link exists. The other half are thought to result from a new mutation. Future investigation into the genetics of this disorder may help identify people at higher risk for sudden death.

Aberrant Coronary Arteries

Anomalous origin of the coronary arteries is rare. The two most common types of aberrant patterns associated with sudden death are aberrant origin of the left coronary artery from the right sinus and origin of the right coronary from the left sinus, with the anomalous artery coursing between the aorta and the pulmonary artery (figure 1.3).

Although athletes with aberrant coronary arteries are usually asymptomatic, occasionally they exhibit symptoms of coronary **ischemia** typical of older athletes with atherosclerosis. They may report anginal chest pain or **syncope** associated with exercise. Physical examination is generally quite normal, with no detectable

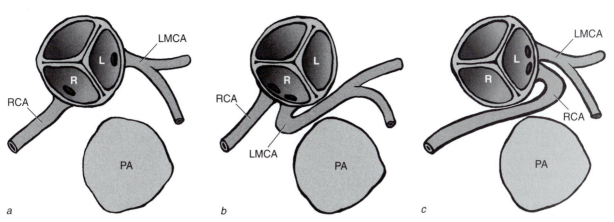

■ **Figure 1.3**   Aberrant coronary arteries. *(a)* Normal anatomy. *(b)* Left coronary artery (LMCA) originating from the right aortic sinus (R). *(c)* Right coronary artery (RCA) originating from the left aortic sinus (L). Note the severe construction of the anomalous arteries between the aorta and the pulmonary artery (PA) in *(b)* and *(c)*. Compression of one of the coronary arteries between the two major vessels causes ischemia and possibly myocardial infarction.

murmur unless there is an independent congenital cardiac abnormality. This condition is extremely difficult to diagnose. An exercise stress test may detect ischemic changes to the myocardium. Echocardiography sometimes can detect the aberrant origin of the artery. *Only cardiac catheterization can provide a definitive diagnosis of aberrant coronary arteries.* An athlete diagnosed with this disorder should be cleared for continued exercise only after her condition has been surgically corrected and a cardiologist has approved participation.

Marfan's Syndrome and Aortic Rupture

A genetic condition that affects about 5 to 8 of every 100,000 people, Marfan's syndrome manifests a constellation of symptoms. The disorder causes abnormal collagen synthesis, resulting in abnormal connective tissue throughout the body—especially in the musculoskeletal, cardiovascular, and ocular systems. The predominant physical features include tall stature, spiderlike fingers (arachnodactyly), superior dislocation of the lens, **scoliosis,** pectus excavatum (a concave deformity of the sternum), mitral valve prolapse, and aortic root dilation (see *Signs of Marfan's Syndrome,* page 8).

Although the constellation of physical findings may be obvious, in some patients the signs may be more subtle. Suspicion of Marfan's syndrome should lead to consultation with a team physician, who will likely need help from a geneticist and a cardiologist for a more thorough evaluation. Sudden cardiac death in Marfan's patients usually results from aortic rupture due to the abnormal collagen. The 26th Bethesda guidelines recommend only low-intensity sports for any athlete with Marfan's syndrome who demonstrates dilation of the aortic root on an echocardiogram; athletes may engage in more moderate activity (classes IA [low static, low dynamic] and IIA [moderate static, low dynamic]) only if they have no evidence of aortic root dilation and no family history of sudden death (Maron and Mitchell 1994) (table 1.1). Echocardiographic measurements of the aortic root should be repeated every 6 months to monitor any aortic changes.

Aortic Stenosis

One of the most common forms of congenital heart disease, aortic stenosis describes any lesion that results in obstruction near the aortic valve. Athletes with only mild **stenosis** may be asymptomatic; more severe lesions can cause syncope, chest pain, and shortness of breath. The classic sign is a harsh systolic murmur that

Signs of Marfan's Syndrome

Musculoskeletal
- Arachnodactyly
- Sternal deformity
- High narrow palate
- Tall stature
- Hyperextensible joints
- Scoliosis
- Pes planus (flat feet)

Cardiovascular
- Mitral valve prolapse
- Aortic root dilation

Ocular
- Superior dislocation of the lens
- Nearsightedness (myopia)
- Retinal detachment

Table 1.1 Classification of Sports

High to moderate dynamic and static demands	High to moderate dynamic and low static demands	High to moderate static and low dynamic demands	Low intensity (low dynamic and low static demands)
Boxing	Badminton	Archery	Bowling
Crew or rowing	Baseball	Auto racing	Cricket
Cross-country skiing	Basketball	Diving	Curling
Cycling	Field hockey	Field events (throwing)	Golf
Downhill skiing	Lacrosse	Gymnastics	Riflery
Fencing	Racewalking	Horseback riding (jumping)	
Football	Racquetball	Karate or judo	
Ice hockey	Soccer	Motorcycling	
Rugby	Squash	Rodeo	
Running (sprinting)	Swimming	Sailing	
Speed skating	Table tennis	Ski jumping	
Water polo	Tennis	Waterskiing	
Wrestling	Volleyball	Weightlifting	

Reprinted from *Journal of American College of Cardiology,* vol. 24, B.J. Maron et al., "Recommendations for determining eligibility for athletes with cardiovascular abnormalities," pp. 845-899, © 1994, with permission from American College of Cardiology Foundation.

is loudest at the upper right sternal border; the murmur often radiates to the carotid arteries. Most people with this condition have normal growth, development, and vital signs. Echocardiography confirms the diagnosis.

Bethesda recommendations vary with the degree of stenosis. Mild stenosis should not limit athletes as long as they remain asymptomatic. Athletes with severe stenosis, or symptomatic patients with moderate stenosis, should not engage in any highly active sports (Maron and Mitchell 1994).

Unknown Etiology, Arrhythmias, and Long QT Syndrome

An 11-yr study by Maron and colleagues (Maron, Shirani et al. 1996) suggested that increased left ventricular mass was a cause of sudden death in a significant percentage of athletes. Yet many athletes have increased left ventricular mass as a result of their conditioning. So-called "athlete's heart" exhibits symmetric hypertrophy of the left ventricle, no significant disarray of the myofibrils, no abnormal arteries, and no genetic history of left ventricular hypertrophy. It therefore is not clear whether the cause of death among athletes in Maron's article was unambiguously related to left ventricular mass.

Some arrhythmias whose etiology is otherwise unknown may be the cause of death in some patients. One potentially underlying cause of the arrhythmia is **long QT syndrome,** an uncommon condition with a recognizable ECG pattern that is evident on baseline ECG (figure 1.4). Long QT is a genetic condition in which the heart's ability to repolarize, or electrically recharge itself, is abnormal. Long QT refers to an abnormal lengthening of the QT interval on the ECG. Patients with this condition are predisposed to syncope and fatal ventricular arrhythmias, sometimes in response to sudden frightful, noxious, or emotionally or physically stressful stimuli. Because they are at risk of sudden death with activity, individuals with long QT syndrome should be restricted from all active sports (Maron and Mitchell 1994). Unfortunately, long QT syndrome cannot be diagnosed as a cause of sudden death unless a baseline ECG is obtained before the individual's death (however, researchers are working on genetic tests that may someday directly reveal the existence of this syndrome).

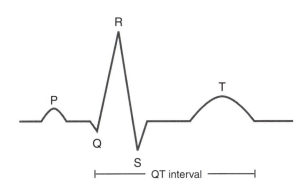

■ **Figure 1.4**   Normal ECG. P wave = atrial polarization/contraction; QRS wave = ventricular polarization/contraction; T wave = ventricular repolarization.

SCREENING AND REFERRALS FOR CARDIAC EVALUATION

The American Heart Association recommends preparticipation cardiovascular screening for high school and college athletes. Screening should include a thorough cardiac history and physical examination (see chapter 19). Because neither invasive nor noninvasive cardiac testing is cost-effective as a mass-screening tool for such rare disorders, screening procedures should comprise thorough medical and family histories from athletes and their parents.

The history should include the following:

- Any history of exertional chest pain or discomfort
- Any history of exertional syncope or near syncope
- Any history of excessive, unexplained shortness of breath
- A history of a heart murmur
- A history of hypertension
- A family history of cardiovascular disease or premature death before the age of 50
- A family history of significant disability secondary to a cardiac event or etiology (including hypertrophic cardiomyopathy, Marfan's syndrome, long QT syndrome, arrhythmias, or premature coronary artery disease)

A detailed physical examination should also be performed by a primary care provider who can reliably obtain a cardiac history, perform a physical examination,

For Further Information

Print Resources

Estes, N.A.M., D.N. Salem, and P.J. Wang. 1998. *Sudden cardiac death in the athlete.* Armonk, NY: Futura. Received good review by Steinbeck, G. 1999. *New England Journal of Medicine* 340(9): 740.

Web Resources

National Heart, Lung, and Blood Institute
www.nhlbi.nih.gov/index.htm
The National Heart, Lung, and Blood Institute (NHLBI) Web site is searchable and provides information and health facts on a variety of cardiac conditions. The NHLBI is part of the National Institutes of Health (NIH).

National Institutes of Health and National Library of Medicine
www.nlm.nih.gov/medlineplus/
A searchable Web site sponsored by the National Institutes of Health and National Library of Medicine. Extensive information available on a variety of cardiac conditions.

American Heart Association
www.americanheart.org
Web home of the American Heart Association that includes publications and facts about all aspects of heart disease. Search feature allows a user to look for specific information about sudden cardiac death and heart attacks.

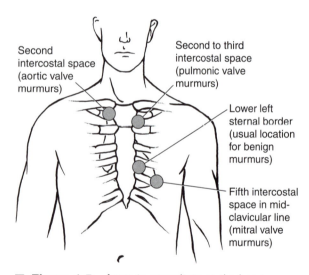

■ Figure 1.5   Areas to auscultate on the heart.

and recognize heart disease. The physical exam should include inspection for any systemic signs of heart failure, such as increased respiratory rate. A displaced point of maximal cardiac impulse may indicate left ventricular outflow obstruction with hypertrophy or heart failure. The exam should include palpation to locate the point of maximal impulse, palpation of femoral pulses, and measurement of blood pressure in both upper and lower extremities. The absence of femoral pulses, or lower-extremity blood pressure that is significantly less than the upper-extremity blood pressure, indicates congenital narrowing (coarctation) of the aorta. Evidence of hypertension warrants further investigation, especially in young athletes. Finally, **auscultation** of the heart in both the supine and standing positions is necessary to evaluate a possible murmur (figure 1.5).

Primary care physicians should refer to a cardiologist any athlete with a new or loud murmur, a diastolic murmur, tachycardia or irregular heart rhythm, hypertension, findings suggestive of Marfan's syndrome, or a positive medical or family history as noted in the previous list.

SUMMARY

1. *Describe the causes of sudden cardiac death.*

Sudden cardiac death related to exercise is caused by cardiac arrest that occurs instantaneously with an abrupt change in an individual's preexisting clinical state or within a few minutes of that change and is by definition associated with exercise. This definition does *not* include drug-related sudden death.

Sudden cardiac death is extremely rare. The most common causes include hypertrophic cardiomyopathy, congenital aberrant coronary arteries, and unexplained increases in cardiac mass. In most instances, unfortunately, no significant history would have led to discovery of the condition. Even if a condition is discovered, it is often impossible to determine the exact risk of sudden death. Heightened awareness, comprehensive history questionnaires, and detailed physical examinations performed by qualified medical providers can help prevent possible life-threatening events for some at-risk athletes.

2. *Discuss the guidelines for screening athletes for cardiovascular conditions.*

The American Heart Association recommends preparticipation cardiovascular screening for high school and college athletes. Screening should include a thorough cardiac history and physical examination (see chapter 19). Because neither invasive nor noninvasive cardiac testing is cost-effective as a mass-screening tool for such rare disorders, screening procedures should comprise thorough medical and family histories from athletes and their parents. A detailed physical examination should also be performed by a primary care provider who can reliably obtain a cardiac history, perform a physical examination, and recognize heart disease.

3. *Explain the Bethesda guidelines for identifying individuals whom you should not allow to engage in vigorous sports.*

The 26th Bethesda Conference established recommendations for athletic participation based on the nature of the underlying cardiac pathologies. Athletes with known hypertrophic cardiomyopathy (HCM) should not participate in most competitive sports—with the possible exception of low-intensity sports (billiards, bowling, golf, curling). Athletes with aberrant coronary arteries should be cleared for continued exercise only after their conditions have been surgically corrected and a cardiologist has approved their participation.

The guidelines recommend only low-intensity sports for any athlete with Marfan's syndrome who demonstrates dilation of the aortic root on an echocardiogram; athletes may engage in more moderate activity (classes IA and IIA) only if they have no evidence of aortic root dilation and no family history of sudden death. Echocardiographic measurements of the aortic root should be repeated every 6 months to monitor any aortic changes.

The recommendations for athletes with aortic stenosis vary with the degree of stenosis. Mild stenosis should not limit athletes as long as they remain asymptomatic. Athletes with severe stenosis, or symptomatic patients with moderate stenosis, should not engage in any highly active sports.

4. *Identify common signs and symptoms to determine which athletes should be referred for further cardiovascular testing.*

Any athlete with episodes of syncope, hypertension, or changes in heart rhythm should be referred immediately to a physician. Further referral to a cardiologist should be made for any athlete with a new or loud murmur, a diastolic murmur, tachycardia or irregular heart rhythm, hypertension, findings suggestive of Marfan's syndrome, or a positive medical or family history.

CHAPTER 2

Gastroenterological Pathologies

OBJECTIVES

Upon completion of this chapter the reader will be able to do the following:

1. Demonstrate a proper assessment of the abdomen

2. Identify the signs and symptoms of irritable bowel syndrome

3. Recognize and manage acute abdominal trauma

Because of the complexity of disorders that can cause abdominal pain, even experienced physicians can find it difficult to evaluate such symptoms. Abdominal pain may be secondary to a nonabdominal disorder (e.g., streptococcal pharyngitis, pneumonia). Moreover, the severity of the pain may not indicate the seriousness of the disorder: Viral gastroenteritis may cause severe, cramping abdominal pain, for example, but is usually not a serious threat; whereas a person with appendicitis, which is dangerous and usually requires surgery, may feel only mild abdominal pain. This chapter discusses the initial evaluation of abdominal pain, specific conditions that may cause abdominal pain, and finally the management of abdominal pain associated with abdominal trauma.

Case Study

A 16-yr-old softball player comes to you with a 4-month history of what she calls a "nervous stomach." In the past, her physician has given her a diagnosis of irritable bowel syndrome due to the intermittent diarrhea, gas, and constipation associated with her problem. She reports a relatively recent symptom of intermittent bloody diarrhea, and a 10-lb (4.5-kg) weight loss associated with malaise and fatigue. As the athletic trainer you weigh the patient and document the 10-lb (4.5-kg) weight loss. Your abdominal exam reveals no tenderness or abnormalities. You are concerned about possible infectious causes of this problem or even the chance of an inflammatory bowel disorder and refer the patient back to her primary physician for further evaluation. Stool cultures turn out to be negative. Based on further testing the patient is ultimately diagnosed with Crohn's disease.

HISTORY

The history is the most important aspect of evaluating the nonspecific symptom of abdominal pain. Always record as much information as you can about the individual's problem—especially the nature, character, and time course of abdominal pain; its location; and any associated symptoms.

Note the nature of abdominal pain as acute or chronic, intermittent or constant. Both acute and chronic pain can be secondary to a specific organic cause, such as appendicitis, or to a "functional" cause (a euphemism for unclear etiology). Severe abdominal pain with abrupt onset may indicate a serious disorder such as perforation of a visceral organ, aortic rupture, or renal colic. A more gradual onset with less severity may indicate an inflammatory condition such as appendicitis.

The character of the pain can also be revealing. The pain may be **colicky** (characterized by fluctuations of pain), *constant, burning,* or *stabbing.* Colicky pain may occur in people with a small bowel obstruction, gallstones, or kidney stones—but it can also accompany appendicitis. The severity of the pain can be quite subjective and is often not useful in determining etiology. Young people with constipation or gastroenteritis may experience much greater pain than those with much more dangerous appendicitis or cancer.

The location of abdominal pain can help reveal its cause. Diffuse pain early in the course of the presentation may become more localized with time. For appendicitis, the classic presentation is central abdominal discomfort that later moves to the lower right quadrant.

You can help differentiate the etiology of abdominal pain by looking at other symptoms associated with it, as well as factors that aggravate or relieve it. For example, appendicitis is often associated with anorexia and low-grade fever.

Terms and Definitions

colicky—Characterized by fluctuations in degree of pain.

computerized axial tomography (CT or CAT scan)—X-ray beams are converted to electronic impulses and processed by a computer to display the body in cross-section.

dysuria—Pain with urination.

fecolith—Small piece of stool sometimes stuck in appendiceal lumen (opening).

gastroesophageal reflux—Movement of stomach acid into the lower esophagus.

gastrointestinal (GI)—Pertaining to the stomach and intestine.

hematuria—The finding of blood in the urine.

hypotension—Abnormally low blood pressure.

hypovolemia—Abnormally low volume of blood plasma in the body.

ileus—Lack of peristalsis, or quiet intestine.

irritable bowel syndrome (IBS)—A common disorder of the intestines that leads to crampy pain, gassiness, bloating, and changes in bowel habits.

muscle guarding—Muscle spasm in an attempt to protect the painful area.

obstipation—Intractable constipation.

orthostatic hypotension—Decreased blood pressure and concomitant increased heart rate a person experiences when rising from supine to standing or sitting position.

peritoneum—The membrane that lines the cavity of the abdomen.

peritonitis—Inflammation or infection of the abdominal lining.

periumbilical—Around the navel or the central region of the abdomen.

rebound tenderness—Abdominal pain that hurts more when the hand is suddenly released from palpation; a sign of possible peritonitis.

tachycardia—Abnormally rapid heartbeat.

Esophagitis is characterized by a burning substernal pain exacerbated by lying down and relieved by antacids. Peptic ulcer disease may cause pain that is worse with an empty stomach and relieved by eating or by taking antacids. **Obstipation** (intractable constipation) is associated with a bowel obstruction. Poorly localized pain, associated with alternation between diarrhea and constipation, may suggest irritable bowel syndrome. Frequent urinating (frequency) or **dysuria** may stem from a urinary tract infection.

In addition to reviewing the pain history, always review the athlete's current and past medical and surgical history. Use of salicylates (e.g., aspirin) or nonsteroidal anti-inflammatories (e.g., ibuprofen) can cause abdominal discomfort secondary to gastritis or peptic ulcer disease. Previous abdominal surgery increases the likelihood of a small bowel obstruction secondary to adhesions or scar tissue. A thorough review of a female athlete's menstrual, obstetric, and gynecologic history is imperative since pregnancy, ovarian cysts, menstrual cramping, endometriosis, and sexually transmitted diseases all can cause abdominal discomfort.

PHYSICAL EXAMINATION

To avoid missing an extra-abdominal cause of pain, always see that athletes have a thorough physical exam when they complain of chronic intestinal discomfort or of extreme acute pain. If you are an athletic trainer, coach, or other nonphysician, be sure to follow through with the athlete to make sure that he or she sees a physician (for high school athletes, it's best to talk with parents about this—teens are highly unlikely to be enthusiastic about seeing a doctor!). Be sure to check for all possible etiologies as described in the next few paragraphs. A detailed abdominal exam may then further localize the etiology of the abdominal discomfort, assuming that an extra-abdominal cause of the patient's discomfort is not found.

Checking Abdominal Problems

In checking vital signs, note that **tachycardia** (rapid heartbeat), **hypotension** (abnormally low blood pressure), or **orthostatic hypotension** (significant decline of blood pressure when the person stands) can indicate acute blood loss or dehydration.

Auscultation for bowel sounds can be helpful. The examiner should listen for several minutes. The examiner also should be experienced—preferably a practitioner familiar with abdominal problems—since both the quiet abdomen of an ileus and the high-pitched, "tinny" bowel sound of an obstruction can be difficult for an inexperienced examiner to detect.

Finally, palpation to determine the point of maximal tenderness may help focus diagnostic possibilities (see figure 2.1). Functional abdominal pain usually results in maximal tenderness over the periumbilical area. In addition, palpation can detect **muscle guarding** and **rebound tenderness** that indicate peritoneal irritation. Signs indicative of an inflamed appendix include the obturator and psoas signs (figures 2.2 and 2.3): An inflamed appendix irritates the psoas and obturator muscles, causing pain in the lower right quadrant when these muscles are stretched.

The athlete's general appearance may help reveal the seriousness of an abdominal disorder. Paleness, distress, or little or no body movement are all worrisome signs of a serious illness such as a perforated ulcer or pancreatitis. Peritoneal irritation also causes patients to remain quite still. Look for a gross deformity, distension, or scars that may be related to the pain.

COMMON DISORDERS

Athletes often exhibit motility disorders affecting both the upper and lower **gastrointestinal (GI)** tract. Nausea, vomiting, and heartburn are commonly associated with upper GI disorders. Diarrhea (increased frequency and looser consistency), cramping, and urgency, however, point to the lower GI tract. The most common cause of diarrhea is gastroenteritis, usually caused by a virus. Treatment consisting of supportive care; fluids; and constipating foods such as bananas, rice, applesauce, and toast (BRAT diet) is recommended initially.

Exercise can affect upper GI motility. Neufer showed that increasing the intensity of exercise tends to delay gastric emptying, leading to symptoms such as nausea, vomiting, and anorexia (Neufer et al. 1989). Exercise can also cause **gastroesophageal reflux,** leading to exertional heartburn. The most obvious treatment for abdominal discomfort associated with exercise is to decrease the intensity of exercise—but few athletes will follow this recommendation. They can decrease the likelihood and intensity of symptoms by avoiding high-fat, high-calorie meals before exercise (such foods empty slowly from the stomach). Various types of prescription and nonprescription antacids may decrease the degree of discomfort associated with reflux. If the usual nonprescription antacids such as calcium carbonate (in the most common chewable antacids) or ranitidine (Zantac®) do not

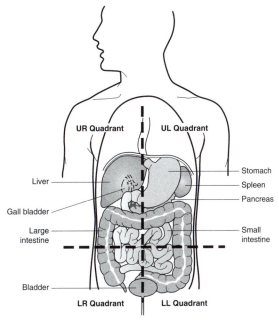

Diagnostic possibilities based on area of maximal tenderness

Epigastric	RUQ	LUQ	RLQ	LLQ	Suprapubic
Peptic ulcer disease GE reflux	Liver Gall bladder UTI	Spleen Gastric ulcer	Appendicitis	Constipation Meckel's diverticulum	UTI STD

■ **Figure 2.1**   Abdominal quadrants: Generalized pain occurs in two or more sections of the abdomen.

Reprinted, by permission, from S.J. Shultz, P.A. Houglum, and D.H. Perrin, 2000, *Assessment of athletic injuries* (Champaign, IL: Human Kinetics), 391.

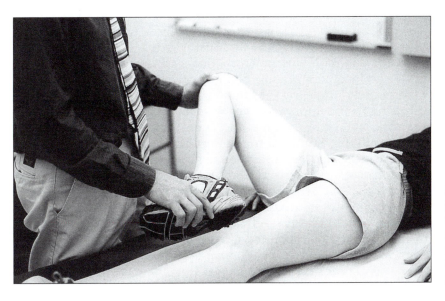

■ **Figure 2.2**   Obturator sign—with the patient supine, the hip is flexed to 90°. External rotation of the hip will elicit pain due to stretching of an irritated obturator muscle. The sign is positive if it elicits pain.

result in significant relief, referral to a physician for further evaluation and treatment is required.

Diarrhea associated with running is commonly termed "runner's trots." Many of the symptoms associated with lower GI motility can be attributed to **irritable**

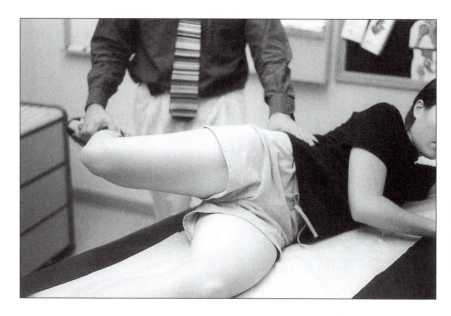

■ **Figure 2.3** Psoas sign—with the patient on her side, painful side up, the hip is extended with the knee flexed to stretch the iliopsoas muscle. The sign is positive if this maneuver elicits pain.

bowel syndrome (IBS). A person with IBS complains of intermittent crampy pain, gassiness, bloating, and changes in bowel habits. The etiology is unknown. Most people are able to control their symptoms with dietary management, stress reduction, and sometimes medication. Keeping a journal to document the foods that seem to worsen symptoms may be helpful. Dietary management includes increasing dietary fiber, avoiding caffeine (a GI motility stimulant), and avoiding eating immediately before exercise. Eating several hours prior to exercise can help stimulate the gastrocolic reflex, which results in initiating a bowel movement and potentially avoiding problems later during competition or practice. Note that fever, bloody stools, weight loss, and severe pain are *not* associated with IBS—the presence of any of these symptoms warrants evaluation for more serious disorders such as inflammatory bowel disease (Crohn's disease or ulcerative colitis) or infectious causes.

Athletic trainers traveling with a team occasionally encounter an athlete with acute abdominal pain. Appendicitis, of course, is the greatest immediate concern—it is the most common surgical condition of the abdomen. The peak incidence of this condition occurs among people between 10 and 30 yr of age. Obstruction of the narrowed appendiceal lumen initiates the condition, with the obstruction often arising from lymphoid hyperplasia or from a **fecolith.** Common symptoms include abdominal pain, nausea, and anorexia. In about half of people with appendicitis, the pain migrates from the **periumbilical** area to the right lower quadrant of the abdomen. Typically, the pain worsens and is unrelieved by vomiting or having a bowel movement. A physical exam usually finds tenderness over the lower right quadrant with associated rebound as well as guarding and obturator and psoas signs (see *Checking Abdominal Problems*, page 16). But note that in many cases, appendicitis does not have a classic presentation. A graduate student at a northeastern university once consulted a resident at the university medical service. The student was doubled over in agonizing pain. The young doctor said, "I don't know what this *is*, but I can tell you what it isn't—it *isn't* appendicitis." Yet the more experienced doctor to whom the student was referred examined the student for about 60 s before rushing him to the operating room for an emergency appendectomy. Because appendicitis is *not easy* to diagnose, all health-care providers—from athletic trainers to primary care physicians—must maintain a high index of suspicion and be quick to refer people with potential symptoms of appendicitis to general surgeons for further evaluation. Such caution can help prevent the complications of rupture, including secondary **peritonitis** (inflammation of the **peritoneum**), abscess formation, and infertility.

ABDOMINAL TRAUMA

Blunt abdominal trauma can result in a life-threatening condition. The abdomen's large surface area without bony protection makes it susceptible to blunt trauma in sports that involve contact or collision. Most such sports do not require padding of the abdominal area, making the area susceptible to injury. Fortunately, the incidence of injury to abdominal structures is low. Structures susceptible to injury include the spleen, liver, kidneys, pancreas, duodenum, and ileum. Initial presentation may vary from mild abdominal discomfort to severe abdominal pain. Initial evaluation should include basic ABCs (airway, breathing, circulation), including orthostatic blood pressure measurement. **Ileus,** revealed by the absence of bowel sounds, indicates a severe injury. Severe pain sometimes makes palpation impractical. Delayed presentation makes repeat examination imperative. *Serial*

Injury to Abdominal Organs

The spleen is the most frequently injured solid organ. Splenic injury results in rapid bleeding with signs of **hypovolemia** (decreased blood volume), including hypotension and tachycardia. Tenderness in the upper left quadrant may be seen along with referred pain to the left shoulder from diaphragmatic irritation (Kehr sign). Referral to an emergency department for surgical consultation is necessary if this injury is suspected. **Computerized axial tomography (CT or CAT scan)** is the imaging study of choice when abdominal trauma results in persistent pain or when the presentation arouses suspicion. Although splenectomy used to be the treatment of choice for splenic injury, today the more routine treatment is conservative management with intense observation, careful monitoring of vital signs, and serial hematocrits.

Although sports injuries occasionally lead to liver, pancreas, or intestinal trauma, the incidence is much less frequent than injury to the spleen. Kidney trauma presents with diffuse pain associated with **hematuria** (blood in the urine). Conservative (nonoperative) management with intense monitoring of vital signs and serial blood counts is again the treatment of choice unless the bleeding is life threatening. Any patient with increasing abdominal pain following blunt trauma to the abdomen should be referred for further evaluation so as not to miss a potentially serious, life-threatening condition.

examinations may need to be done hourly until the clinician is convinced the athlete has no evidence of injury. Because of the severity of the complications associated with some of these injuries, a low threshold for referral and diagnostic testing is required.

SUMMARY

1. *Demonstrate a proper assessment of the abdomen.*

Abdominal pain can be difficult to diagnose, one reason being that the severity of abdominal pain is not necessarily correlated with the severity of a disorder. Most athletes' abdominal discomfort results from an underlying medical problem as opposed to a specific trauma.

The most important aspect of evaluating abdominal pain is obtaining a detailed history of the pain. Athletic trainers must have a low threshold for referral when dealing with abdominal pain. Athletes should be referred to their primary care physicians any time there is chronic abdominal discomfort, including pain, diarrhea, dysuria, nausea, or heartburn. Allied health and support personnel must ensure that athletes are referred to a physician (for high school athletes, it's best to talk with parents about this—teens are highly unlikely to be enthusiastic about seeing a doctor!). Any athlete who has acute abdominal pain with rebound tenderness, or who experiences severe abdominal pain following a trauma, should be sent to the emergency room.

2. *Identify the signs and symptoms of irritable bowel syndrome.*

Often, the symptoms associated with lower gastrointestinal motility can be attributed to irritable bowel syndrome (IBS). IBS presents with intermittent crampy pain, gassiness, bloating, and changes in bowel habits. The etiology is unknown. Most people are able to control their symptoms with dietary management, stress reduction, and sometimes medication. Dietary management includes increasing dietary fiber, avoiding caffeine (a gastrointestinal motility stimulant), and avoiding eating immediately before exercise.

3. *Recognize and manage acute abdominal trauma.*

The abdomen's large surface area without bony protection makes it susceptible to blunt trauma in contact or collision sports. Structures susceptible to injury include the spleen, liver, kidneys, pancreas, duodenum, and ileum. Initial presentation may vary from mild abdominal discomfort to severe abdominal pain. Initial evaluation should include basic ABCs (airway, breathing, circulation), including orthostatic blood pressure measurement. Ileus, revealed by the absence of bowel sounds, indicates a severe injury. Severe pain sometimes makes palpation impractical. Delayed presentation makes repeat examination imperative. *Serial examinations may need to be done hourly until the clinician is convinced the athlete has no evidence of injury.* Because of the severity of the complications associated with some of these injuries, a low threshold for referral and diagnostic testing is required.

The spleen is the most frequently injured solid organ. Referral to an emergency department for surgical consultation is necessary if this injury is suspected. CT (computerized tomography) is the imaging study of choice when abdominal trauma results in persistent pain or when the presentation arouses suspicion. Although sports injuries occasionally lead to liver, pancreas, or intestinal trauma, the incidence is much less frequent than injury to the spleen. Kidney trauma presents with diffuse pain associated with hematuria (blood in the urine). Conservative (nonoperative) management with intense monitoring of vital signs and serial blood counts is again the treatment of choice unless the bleeding is life threatening.

CHAPTER 3

Neurological Pathologies

OBJECTIVES

Upon completion of this chapter the reader will be able to do the following:

1. Discuss mild traumatic brain injuries (concussions), including recognition, diagnosis, and return-to-play criteria

2. Recognize signs and symptoms of serious head injuries, including subdural and epidural hematomas, second impact syndrome, and postconcussive syndrome

3. Demonstrate proper management techniques for the seizing athlete

4. Differentiate between meningitis and encephalitis

5. Recognize the variety of headaches that active participants might experience

Anyone who works in either training or caring for athletes is likely at some point to encounter a young person with a neurological problem, whether it is caused by a sport injury or is an ongoing disorder completely unrelated to the individual's athletic efforts. Deciding how to evaluate and treat such problems can be a challenge; mismanagement of concussions and seizure disorders in an acute setting can result in significant morbidity or even mortality. Moreover, repeated blows to the head, even if they appear minor, may result in long-term neurological changes so subtle that neither examiner nor patient may be able to detect each incremental change. Taken together over a length of time, however, they may result in a significant neurological change. Athletic trainers may also confront other neurological problems that can affect an athlete's ability to compete. These disorders include the common but often debilitating migraine headache and the rarer but very serious infections that result in meningitis or encephalitis. This chapter focuses on acute management and return-to-play decisions involving concussions and seizure disorders along with infectious disorders and headaches.

RETURN-TO-PLAY DECISIONS

The issue of allowing an athlete to return to play is not as straightforward as you might think. The Americans With Disabilities Act gives players with a disability or medical condition the right to participate in sports regardless of their disability. This means that the professional cannot legally forbid an athlete to play but can only recommend strongly that the athlete not participate. On the other hand, the possibility exists that if the professional does not make the dangers of play clear to the athlete—and in the case of minor athletes, to their families—and the athlete therefore plays and is injured or dies, the professional might face a lawsuit for negligence.

Most athletes, of course, are happy to abide by the recommendations of those entrusted with their care. If an athlete balks, however, your first step should be to involve her family in the decision to play or not to play. Be sure that you present in writing to all parties the dangers of play. If she still insists on participation, it may be helpful to have the athlete (and her family, if she is a minor) sign an informed consent form that spells out the dangers and makes it clear in writing that the athlete and those responsible for her are making the decision to play with full understanding of the risks. It is our strong recommendation that you follow this procedure. An athletic trainer should follow this advice with regard to the cardiac

Case Study

A 20-yr-old soccer player collides with her opponent, sustaining a direct blow to her right temple. She loses consciousness for approximately 45 s. Upon regaining consciousness, she appears somewhat groggy—but she has no evidence of changes in mental status and a completely **nonfocal neurological examination.** Assuming she completely clears and becomes asymptomatic within 10 to 15 min, you will have to decide immediately whether to refer her to the nearest emergency facility. Later you will have to deal with the possibilities of both short- and long-term complications, and when she may return to play.

Let's complicate the scenario even more. What if this player has been previously diagnosed with epilepsy and the traumatic blow to her head leads to a seizure that lasts about 7 min? If no one else with greater medical expertise is present, you may be the one responsible for the initial management of this situation on the playing field.

Terms and Definitions

antegrade amnesia—Inability to remember events occurring *after* a traumatic incident.

ataxia—Inability to coordinate muscular movements.

brain herniation—Shift of the intracranial contents through the cranial foramen with increasing intracranial pressure.

concussion—Traumatically induced alteration in mental status, with or without loss of consciousness.

dura mater—The outer, tough membrane that covers the brain and spinal cord.

epidural hematoma—Clot caused by bleeding between the skull and the dura mater.

focal neurological examination—Specific finding on a neurological exam that localizes a neurological injury (or tumor) to one area of the brain.

hyperacusis—Sensitivity to loud noise.

magnetic resonance imaging (MRI)—Exposure of human tissue to a magnetic field causes molecules in the tissue to generate different frequencies of vibration. These frequencies are detected by a coil and converted into images that show the body part in cross-section.

mass effect—Pressure on and movement of brain tissue that results from swelling and bleeding.

mild traumatic brain injury (MTBI)—See **concussion.**

nonfocal neurological examination—Completely normal neurological exam that finds nothing to indicate a localizing process such as unilateral weakness, sensory changes, or coordination difficulty.

photophobia—Abnormal visual intolerance to light.

postconcussive syndrome (PCS)—When symptoms from a concussion persist beyond the first few days of the injury.

post-ictal phase—Phase of a seizure that follows convulsing; characterized by increased somnolence and sometimes confusion.

retrograde amnesia—Inability to remember events occurring immediately *before* a traumatic incident.

subdural hematoma—Clot caused by bleeding under the dura mater but outside of the brain surface.

tinnitus—Ringing or roaring in the ears.

tonic-clonic seizure—Disorganized electrical brain activity that leads to loss of consciousness and generalized muscle contractions; may be associated with urinary incontinence and biting of the tongue. A post-ictal state generally follows the seizure.

problems discussed in the case study in chapter 1 as well, although you will not face that situation nearly as often as you will the question of returning to play after injury—particularly head injury.

CONCUSSIONS

Concussion, or **mild traumatic brain injury (MTBI),** is defined as a traumatically induced alteration in mental status, with or without loss of consciousness. A more complete definition used at the 2001 Vienna Symposium on Concussion in Sport describes a complex pathophysiological process affecting the brain, induced by traumatic biomechanical forces (Aubry et al. 2002). It is common in most sports that involve contact and collision, with the incidence varying by sport. Professional boxing has the highest incidence of concussion, with many of the bouts

Table 3.1   Incidence of Concussion by Sport (per 1,000 Athletic Exposures)

Sport	Incidence
Football	0.59
Wrestling	0.25
Soccer	0.18 (boys), 0.23 (girls)
Basketball	0.11 (boys), 0.16 (girls)
Field hockey	0.09 (girls)

Adapted, by permission, from J.W. Powell and F.K. Barber, 1999, "Traumatic brain injury in high school athletes," *Journal of the American Medical Association* 282: 958-963.

ending in a technical knockout (i.e., concussion); in fact, at least in professional boxing, the primary goal of the sport is to create a concussion in your opponent! Traditional high school sports with a high incidence of concussion include football, wrestling, and soccer (table 3.1). The incidence of concussion appears to increase with age: In a study of ice hockey players, the frequency of mild head injuries increased with age and level of play (Stuart and Smith 1995).

Memory is the cognitive function most susceptible to impairment from concussion. The sequence of alterations in memory following a closed head injury usually begins with a very brief period (seconds) of **retrograde amnesia** (memory loss of the period immediately *before* the injury). Loss of consciousness may ensue, followed by a more variable degree of post-traumatic amnesia, or **antegrade amnesia** (inability to remember events that occur *after* the injury).

Several schemes are available for classifying the severity of concussion. The most recently published and accepted guidelines from the American Academy of Neurology (1997) describe *mild* or *grade 1 concussion* as transient confusion followed by <15 min of related symptoms, *moderate* or *grade 2 concussion* as transient confusion with symptoms lasting >15 min, and *severe* or *grade 3 concussion* as including loss of consciousness (table 3.2). According to the same guidelines, the severity of the concussion determines return to play: A longer period of inactivity is recommended for increasing severity of injury (Kelly and Rosenberg 1997). The cardinal rule is that *no athlete should return to practice or competition until he or she is completely asymptomatic.*

Recent studies have questioned the significance of loss of consciousness in predicting long-term neuropsychological consequences. In the neuropsychological parameters examined by Lovell et al. (1999), subjects who experienced loss of consciousness showed no more dramatic decline than those who remained conscious but exhibited similar mental status after the trauma.

Table 3.2   Classification of Concussions

Grade 1 (mild)	Grade 2 (moderate)	Grade 3 (severe)
Transient confusion	Transient confusion	Loss of consciousness
Concussion symptoms < 15 min	Concussion symptoms > 15 min	
Remove from game	Remove from game	Remove from game
Examine every 5 min	Examine on sidelines, looking for signs of increasing intracranial pressure	Transport to local ER if athlete has prolonged period of unconsciousness or if worrisome signs are detected
May return if no symptoms within 15 min	No practice or return to play for 1 week after symptom-free	

Reprinted, by permission, from M. McCrea et al., 1997, "Standardized assessment of concussion in football players," *Neurology* 48: 586-588.

Evaluating the athlete at the event can be a formidable task. A useful tool in this regard is the standardized assessment of concussion (SAC) (figure 3.1), which can help you evaluate an athlete's orientation, concentration, and immediate and delayed recall. However, an examiner unfamiliar with an athlete's baseline score or neuropsychological status cannot know what is normal or abnormal with this tool: Neither the SAC nor any other neuropsychometric assessment tool is reliable unless one knows an athlete's baseline (i.e., pre-trauma) abilities. Yet such issues as

- which baseline tests are the most sensitive,
- who will pay for the baseline evaluations, and
- the degree of fairness involved in administering such tests (e.g., do only those athletes whose families can afford to pay receive the evaluation?)

make the question of whether to obtain such data on each athlete a controversial one. Thus, most programs—particularly on the high school level—must make do without baseline information. Keep in mind that even so-called "simple" serial 7s (i.e., counting backward from 100 by increments of 7) is difficult for 50% of high school athletes *without* a history of head injury (Young et al. 1997). Stating the months in reverse is a more specific test when evaluating head injuries in the high school population and is therefore included in the SAC.

Orientation

Month: _____ 0 1
Date: _____ 0 1
Day of week: _____ 0 1
Year: _____ 0 1
Time (within 1 hr): _____ 0 1
Orientation total score: _____ /5

Concentration

Digits backward
(If correct, go to next string length. If incorrect, read trial 2. Stop if both incorrect.)
4-9-3 6-2-9 _____ 0 1
3-8-1-4 3-2-7-9 _____ 0 1
1-5-2-8-6 _____ 0 1
7-1-8-4-6-2 5-9-1-4-8 _____ 0 1
Months in reverse order (entire sequence correct for 1 pt)
Dec. → Jan. _____ 0 1
Concentration total score _____ /5

Immediate memory (All three trials are complete regardless of score on trials 1 and 2; total score equals sum across all three trials.)

List	Trial 1	Trial 2	Trial 3	
Word 1	0 1	0 1	0 1	Exertional maneuvers
Word 2	0 1	0 1	0 1	Coordination
Word 3	0 1	0 1	0 1	Strength
Word 4	0 1	0 1	0 1	Sensation
Word 5	0 1	0 1	0 1	Recall of injury
Immediate memory total score _____ /15				Total

Delayed recall

Word 1 0 1
Word 2 0 1
Word 3 0 1
Word 4 0 1
Word 5 0 1
Delayed recall total score _____ /5
Summary of total scores _____ /30

■ **Figure 3.1** Standardized assessment of concussion (SAC).

When you are caring for an athlete with a head injury, your goal is to detect and prevent both acute and long-term complications. Even when the injury appears confined to the head, it is important to follow the basic principles of all injuries. Most important, evaluate the airway, breathing, and circulation (ABCs) of any significant trauma. Always assume that an athlete with an altered mental status, including one who is unconscious, has an injury to the cervical spine, and immobilize the cervical spine until radiographic evaluation can be obtained. This procedure is necessary for the following reasons:

- Although a cervical spine injury does not cause the altered mental state, the mental deficit may impede the athlete's ability to describe problems arising from the cervical injury.
- The mechanism of axial load for cervical spine injury is often the same as for head injury.

Remember: Do not remove the helmets of hockey players or football players who are experiencing altered mental states, who are unconscious, or in whom you have the slightest suspicion of injured cervical spine. To establish an airway, the face mask will need to be removed by a cutter device or, for the newer football helmets, even a power screwdriver (see figure 3.2).

Situations *rarely* occur in which you need to remove an injured athlete's helmet to give him proper care. When those unusual situations arise, you must use utmost care in removing the helmet *without any movement of the spine.* Figure 3.3 illustrates the proper procedure. Study it carefully and know the steps that can help prevent further injury to the athlete. If you must remove the helmet, remember that the athlete's head will tip back to the surface on which he is lying unless you take appropriate precautions. Without these precautions, the neck will be placed in extension, leading to possible further damage. The simplest way to avoid neck extension is to have a pad (e.g., a folded-up towel) ready to slip under the athlete's head as the helmet is removed to maintain proper alignment of the head and neck (figure 3.3e).

Not every mild traumatic brain injury results in a concussion. The following symptoms often suggest increased intracranial pressure resulting from bleeding:

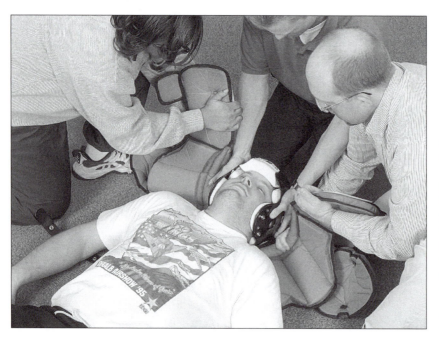

■ **Figure 3.2** Face mask–removal procedures. To remove a helmet face mask, either cut the plastic retaining pieces on both sides of the helmet, or use a power screwdriver, depending on the design of the helmet. Swing the face mask up to gain access to the athlete's face.

Reprinted, by permission, from L.A. Cartwright and W.A. Pitney, 1999, *Athletic training for student assistants* (Champaign, IL: Human Kinetics), 60.

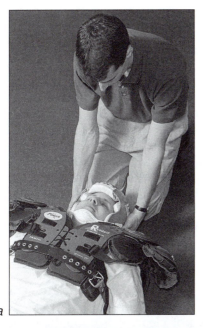

a

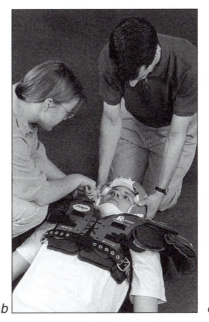

b

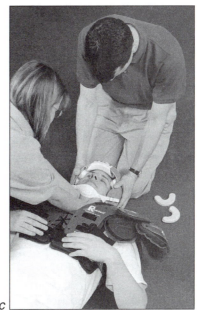

c

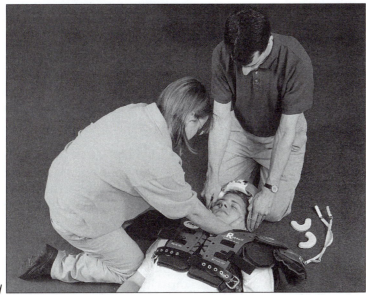

d

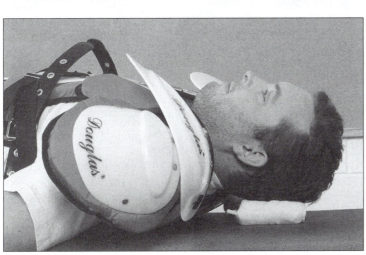

e

■ Figure 3.3 Safe helmet removal. Safe helmet removal requires the athletic trainer, one assistant trained in first aid, and a second assistant to slip a pad beneath the athlete's head as the helmet is removed. Here are the steps to follow: *(a)* The athletic trainer firmly holds the helmet to ensure that the athlete's head does not move during the next step. *(b)* The first assistant loosens and removes the cheek pads and unfastens the chin strap. *(c)* The first assistant firmly holds the athlete's head from inside the helmet to ensure that the athlete's head does not move during the next step. *(d)* The athletic trainer holds the helmet by the ear holes, widens it as much as possible, and pulls it off gently from the top. *(e)* As the athletic trainer pulls the helmet off, a second assistant slips a pad that has been prepared ahead of time beneath the athlete's head to ensure that the neck does not extend as the helmet is removed.

Reprinted, by permission, from L.A. Cartwright and W.A. Pitney, 1999, *Athletic training for student assistants* (Champaign, IL: Human Kinetics), 61.

worsening headache, recurrent vomiting, worsening disorientation, changing levels of consciousness, and increasing blood pressure associated with a decreased pulse rate. Serious head injuries may cause dilation of one or both pupils because of herniation resulting from increased intracranial pressure; other signs of herniation, however (including unresponsiveness), make examination of pupils of little use with an *acute* head injury in a conscious patient. **Subdural hematoma**—an area of bleeding under the **dura mater** but outside of the brain surface—carries a high mortality rate and is usually evidenced by a dramatic worsening state of consciousness, increased intracranial pressure, **mass effect** (pressure and movement of brain tissue resulting from swelling and bleeding), and **brain herniation.** **Epidural hematoma** usually occurs when a temporal skull fracture tears the middle meningeal artery, resulting in an area of bleeding between the skull and the dura mater. The athlete classically presents with a lucid period followed by a precipitous loss of consciousness; coma; and, if not evacuated immediately at an emergency hospital facility, death.

Second impact syndrome can occur in an athlete who sustains a second head injury before symptoms of a prior head injury have cleared. A second, sometimes minor, collision results in sudden collapse and rapid deterioration of the athlete's condition—including dilated pupils, loss of eye movements, and respiratory failure. The pathophysiology of this condition is not clear; it is thought to be secondary to loss of autoregulation of cerebral blood flow, resulting in massive engorgement of the blood vessels to the brain with subsequent cerebral swelling, cerebral herniation, and often death. Immediate recognition and treatment with intubation, hyperventilation, and osmotic diuretics are essential to prevent death. Thus it is imperative that you get the athlete immediately to emergency facilities if you suspect this condition. Thirty confirmed cases of second impact syndrome were reported to the National Center for Catastrophic Sports Injury Research between 1980 and 1991 (Cantu 1992). According to McCrory and Berkovic (1998), all the athletes reported with this condition have been <20 yr of age, suggesting that the developing brain may be particularly susceptible to such injury. Although second impact syndrome is rare and some even question the syndrome's existence (McCrory 2001), its enormous risks may provide you with a compelling argument to persuade a player who continues to be symptomatic (or her family or coach) to withdraw from competition.

Postconcussive syndrome (PCS) can occur even after a mild head injury and includes headache, dizziness, and changes in attentiveness or personality (Evans 1992) (see *Manifestations of Postconcussive Syndrome,* page 29). Headaches, the most common manifestation, can be of any type—muscle contraction, vascular, temporomandibular, and so on. Neuropsychological testing may reveal cognitive impairment, especially involving tasks that require speed of performance and complex decision making. You may note decreased vigilance and increased distractibility. Although the pathogenesis of PCS is not well understood, it probably involves a combination of organic and psychological factors. Most manifestations of PCS are temporary and brief; long-term disability is rare, although occasionally the symptoms may last for months. Treatment may require a team approach involving a primary care provider, an athletic trainer, and a psychologist. Detailed neuropsychological testing may be required to document any cognitive deficits and to help the athlete develop adaptive coping strategies.

The surest route to preventing or detecting serious complications would be to scan all athletes who have had an acute head injury; clearly, however, this is not a cost-effective solution. We suggest a general rule: Refer to the emergency room for further evaluation—including, possibly, a CT scan—any athlete with a focal neurological examination, worsening headache or mental status, or signs of increased intracranial pressure. The choice for an acute injury is CT, because it can

Manifestations of Postconcussive Syndrome

- Recurrent headaches
- Dizziness
- Memory impairment
- Difficulty concentrating
- Depression
- Loss of libido
- **Tinnitus**
- **Ataxia**
- Alcohol intolerance
- Anxiety
- **Hyperacusis**
- **Photophobia**

usually be done quickly and provides a straightforward way to detect acute bleeding.

The question of whether an athlete should play after experiencing repetitive concussions is quite contentious. It is generally better to be conservative than to entertain the risk of an athlete's dying or being permanently disabled. Always note whether postconcussive symptoms are increasing in duration or in severity. When baseline data are available, compare athletes' symptoms to baselines of previous neuropsychological testing; this information can provide a powerful argument in convincing athletes that participating in contact or collision sports is no longer in their best interest. The ability to compare such data provides another good reason to recommend baseline neuropsychological testing for every athlete (see earlier discussion).

Case Study

Our 20-yr-old soccer player has a headache that initially resolves. Her headache symptoms worsen over the next hour, however, and she appears somewhat confused. Because of her worsening symptoms, you appropriately refer her to an emergency facility, where a CT scan is normal. She returns to you and for 2-3 weeks continues to have persistent headache, dizziness, depression, and problems focusing on school. Although her focus and dizziness improve, her recurrent headaches persist for 3 months. She has never had headaches before this injury. She sees the team primary care physician, who diagnoses her with postconcussive syndrome. A mutual decision between the athlete and the team physician is made that she take 1 yr away from soccer and reevaluate returning to play at the end of that time based on her symptoms.

SEIZURES

Seizures are the result of electrical neuronal brain dysfunction. Most seizures you see probably will result from preexisting epilepsy, a recurrent seizure disorder that is either genetic or acquired. Seizures can also be a rare complication of a head injury, and you should be prepared for them on the field and should understand how they affect decisions about playability. Of the several different types of seizures, we focus here on generalized **tonic-clonic seizures,** as these cause the most worry for both athlete and practitioner.

The first priority during a seizure is to protect the individual from injury. The next is to turn the athlete onto his side to prevent aspiration. Never place anything in a convulsing person's mouth. During the **post-ictal phase** (the time of lethargy, among other symptoms, after the convulsions), protect the airway. Most generalized seizures are brief, lasting no more than 5 min. If any seizure lasts more than 5 min, see that the individual obtains emergency medical treatment to check for possible etiologies including brain injury, tumor, or metabolic disorder. Those experiencing first-time seizures, even if brief, should be referred to a medical provider for similar reasons. Note that prolonged seizures may cause brain damage if not controlled by anticonvulsant medication.

Do not be too quick to deny clearance to play to a person who has experienced seizures or has a seizure disorder, since the physical and psychological benefits of sports are just as real to such athletes as to anyone else. Exercise per se poses little risk to an athlete with epilepsy, and exercise does not affect dosing of anticonvulsant medications. When considering whether to clear an athlete for a sport, consider a broad range of factors: the athlete's motivation, the frequency of seizures, the intrinsic risks of the activity for someone who might have a seizure, and the potential level of supervision for the athlete. Always determine eligibility on an individual basis. The most important factor is how well the seizures can be controlled—that is, how frequently they occur. Because trauma by itself has not been proven to increase the risk of seizures, people with epilepsy generally may participate in sports such as football and soccer with no problems. In fact, you generally can allow an athlete with good control (no seizures in the last year) to participate in almost any sport except for one in which a seizure might be *inherently* dangerous, such as any water sport (including crew), where a seizure could lead to drowning; any sport where an athlete must operate machinery or equipment (e.g., auto racing, hang gliding); or any activity in which a seizure could lead to a life-threatening fall (e.g., rock climbing, parachuting). For reasons not only of safety but also of legal liability, do not entrust the supervision of a person with epilepsy to teammates or coaches, especially at the high school and college levels.

Do not allow an athlete who has had a seizure at practice or during an athletic contest to return to play until he has been cleared by his primary care giver. Athletes with poorly controlled epilepsy should consult with their primary care physician or neurologist for evaluation of whether they can return to play.

The primary care physician should coordinate long-term management of a seizure disorder and carefully monitor and prescribe any anticonvulsant medications, since many of these have significant side effects.

INFECTIOUS BRAIN DISEASES

Meningitis and encephalitis are serious infections that can involve the brain and surrounding tissue. They are serious because they can lead to brain damage and even death.

Meningitis

Meningitis is an inflammation of the lining of the brain or spinal cord (meninges) and spinal fluid. It can be caused by bacteria, viruses, or fungi. Viral meningitis is more common than bacterial meningitis; it can be caused by a wide variety of viruses and is usually considered the less serious of the two. Bacterial meningitis is a much more serious problem because it is more likely to cause brain damage or death. Diagnosis is based on the results of spinal fluid testing obtained by a spinal tap.

The signs and symptoms of meningitis can often be confused with those of other ailments, with a flulike illness often characterizing the initial presentation. Fever, severe headache, vomiting, photophobia, and stiff neck are classic symptoms; other associated symptoms may include myalgias, diarrhea, and coldlike symptoms. Physical exam findings include a nuchal rigidity (the inability to flex the neck due to involuntary muscle spasm) along with positive Kernig and Brudzinski signs (see figure 3.4). Kernig sign is produced with the patient supine and passively flexing the hip to 90° while the knee is flexed to 90°. Attempts to extend the knee

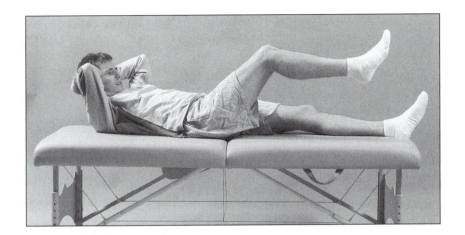

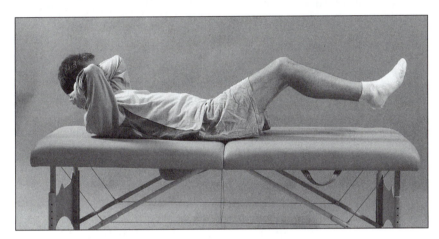

■ **Figure 3.4** Kernig-Brudzinski test.

Reprinted, by permission, from F.J. Cerny and H.W. Burton, 2001, *Exercise physiology for health care professionals* (Champaign, IL: Human Kinetics), 107.

produce pain in the hamstrings and resistance to further extension. Brudzinski sign occurs with the patient supine. The examiner passively flexes the neck. The sign is positive when this maneuver produces flexion at the hips.

Bacterial meningitis in school-age children along with high school and college students is usually caused by *Neisseria meningitidis*. Otherwise known as meningococcus, these bacteria can be carried in the nasopharynx for months in otherwise healthy individuals. Rarely, they can overwhelm the body's defense mechanisms (weakened by other infections, overtraining, lack of sleep, or poor nutrition) and cause serious infection of the blood or central nervous system. Infection of the blood, or septicemia, causes a classic rash that is characteristic of menigicoccal infection but can be seen in other serious bacterial blood infections as well. The rash is characterized by tiny red spots that look like pinpricks and larger lesions that look like clusters of blood just under the skin. The rash may or may not appear with meningococcal disease.

Suspicion of the bacterial disease, with or without the rash, requires immediate referral to a physician because early diagnosis and treatment are important. Early recognition, referral, and treatment with appropriate intravenous (IV) antibiotics have resulted in a mortality rate of approximately 10%. Infected persons are not considered contagious after 24 hours of appropriate antibiotic therapy. After hospitalization, they pose no risk to classmates and may return to school. Students who have been exposed to oral secretions of an infected classmate, such as occurs during kissing or sharing of food and drink, should receive chemoprophylaxis—antibiotics to decrease the risk of infection. For other students with less-direct contact, close observation for fever and other associated symptoms is recommended.

Immunization of collegiate student athletes who may be at increased risk for meningococcal infection as a result of their living in close quarters with each other has been controversial. The American College Health Association recommends immunization of college students. Athletic trainers and primary care physicians should educate students and parents about the risk of meningococcal disease and the existence of a safe and effective vaccine.

Encephalitis

Whereas meningitis is caused by an infection of the meninges and spinal fluid, encephalitis is characterized by inflammation and infection of the brain tissue itself. The predominant feature of encephalitis is a change in mental status, manifested by confusion, delirium, stupor, coma, convulsions, aphasia (inability to talk), hallucinations, and change in personality. Other signs and symptoms are similar in presentation to those of meningitis, including fever, headache, stiff neck, and photophobia. Encephalitis is usually caused by one of a number of viruses, only some of which can be treated with antiviral medications. Diagnosis is usually based on spinal fluid results, with **magnetic resonance imaging (MRI)** possibly providing additional information as to which areas of the brain may be affected. The prognosis of encephalitis is variable; some illnesses are self-limited and short-term and others cause permanent sequelae, including memory loss, confusion, and even death.

HEADACHES

Some athletes are prone to headaches associated with exertion. Exercise-induced headaches may be mild or may be severe enough to interfere with competition. Finally, exercise-induced headaches may have a serious origin such as tumors, infection, or blood clots. The athletic trainer must be aware of the different types of headaches and know when to refer (see *Types of Headaches in Athletes*, page 33).

Intracerebral hemorrhage into the brain substance or subarachnoid hemorrhage from rupture of blood vessels near the brain surface is usually caused by an aneurysm (balloonlike outpouching of a blood vessel), arteriovenous malformations, or severe hypertension. A large bleed of either type can be catastrophic, resulting in death, whereas smaller bleeds may present with severe headaches, nausea, blurry vision, photophobia, aphasia, and neck stiffness. Suspicion of this bleeding from any cause warrants referral to the emergency room for diagnostic imaging and immediate treatment. This diagnosis is unusual in athletes under the age of 35 yr, and therefore younger athletes with severe headaches and no other associated symptoms can be observed for other symptoms and improvement in clinical course before you refer them for further testing.

Case Study

A 26-yr-old professional basketball player reports to you 60 min before the game that he has a severe, pounding, throbbing headache. He denies any drug use. He has had similar headaches many times in the past. As usual, he has significant photophobia and some mild nausea but no vomiting. His primary care physician has diagnosed migraines in the past and prescribed sumatriptan (Imitrex®) intranasally. He does not have any medication with him. On examination, he has no fever. A neurological exam is normal. There are no signs of meningitis or encephalitis. As the athletic trainer, you contact the team physician, who calls in a prescription to the nearest pharmacy. He clears the athlete to play if he is able because there is no associated head trauma.

Types of Headaches in Athletes

- Intracranial hemorrhage (bleeding)
- Meningitis/encephalitis
- Tumor
- Hypertension
- Infection

- Vascular (migraines and migraine variants)
- Tension
- Post-traumatic (with or without concussion)
- Benign exertional
- Altitude

Tumor presentation can be somewhat vague initially, with the report of only a dull headache that waxes and wanes. Over time, the athlete will generally develop worsening headaches, focal neurological abnormalities, and headache on waking. It is unusual for patients with a tumor to report headaches provoked by exercise as their only symptom.

Vascular headaches include migraines and a number of migraine variants such as cluster headaches and exertional headaches. Migraines in general affect between 5% and 10% of the general population. A family history is positive in approximately 90% of migraine sufferers. Migraines are characterized by a unilateral, often severe, throbbing headache associated with photophobia, hypersensitivity

For Further Information

Print Resources

American Academy of Neurology. 1997. Practice parameter: The management of concussion in sports (summary statement). *Neurology* 48: 581-85.

Evans, R.W. 1992. The post-concussion syndrome and the sequelae of mild head injury. *Neurology Clinics of North America* 10: 815-47.

McCrory, P.R., and S.F. Berkovic. 1998. Second impact syndrome. *Neurology* 50: 677-83.

Powell, J.W., and F.K. Barber. 1999. Traumatic brain injury in high school athletes. *JAMA* 282: 958-63.

Web Resources

Pashby Sports Safety Fund Concussion Site
www.concussionsafety.com
A privately funded Web site that has been peer reviewed by the Canadian Academy of Sports Medicine.

Centers for Disease Control and Prevention
www.cdc.gov/ncidod/dbmd/diseaseinfo/
A helpful government site sponsored by the U.S. Department of Heath and Human Services; information regarding neurological disorders, infectious disease, health bulletins on various topics, and current funding and research projects.

National Institute of Naurological Disorders and Stroke
www.ninds.nih.gov/health_and_medical/disorders/encmenin_doc.htm
The National Institute of Neurological Disorders and Stroke (NINDS) is the National Institutes of Health organization for research on encephalitis and meningitis. This site is the NINDS information page for encephalitis and meningitis.

National Institutes of Health and National Library of Medicine
www.nlm.nih.gov/medlineplus/encephalitis.html
The National Library of Medicine and National Institutes of Health maintain this searchable Web site. Information is available on a number of encephalitis-related issues.

to loud noise, nausea, and sometimes vomiting. In some migraine patients, an aura or prodrome consisting of visual symptoms precedes the onset of the headache and is thought to be caused by vascular constriction. Other forms of aura have been described, including aphasia, ataxia, weakness, paresthesias, and syncope. Treatment of migraine headaches requires referral to a physician for medications to abort the symptoms. Nonsteroidal anti-inflammatory agents are often used as the initial treatment; stronger medications, which may have more side effects, may be prescribed based on the patient's response to the initial medication.

Tension headaches are usually not as severe as migraine headaches and are often located bilaterally in the temple area. These headaches usually respond to over-the-counter pain medications, and they do not usually interfere with an athlete's function or ability to play.

Benign exertional headaches are characterized as headaches that occur with exertion and without any evidence of a space-occupying lesion such as a tumor or bleed within the brain. An exertional headache is specifically brought on by exercise, is usually bilateral, is throbbing in nature, and can last from 5 min to 24 h. The neurological examination is normal. Recurrent exertional headaches deserve investigation because they can result from tumor (rarely), trauma, bleeding, or cervical spinal cord abnormalities. Therapy can include the use of nonsteroidal anti-inflammatory medications and activity modification, depending on the type of activity that produces the headache.

SUMMARY

1. *Discuss mild traumatic brain injuries (concussions), including recognition, diagnosis, and return-to-play criteria.*

Concussion is common in contact sports, with the incidence appearing to increase with age. The question of whether loss of consciousness is a good predictor of long-term problems is controversial. The most useful tool for evaluating the severity of a concussion is probably the standard assessment of concussion, or SAC. The following symptoms should lead to immediate transfer of an individual to an emergency department: worsening headache, recurrent vomiting, worsening disorientation, changing levels of consciousness, or increasing blood pressure associated with a decreased pulse rate, or if the athlete exhibits an initial lucid period followed by a precipitous loss of consciousness. Athletes should return to practice or to play only when completely free of symptoms.

2. *Recognize signs and symptoms of serious head injuries, including subdural and epidural hematomas, second impact syndrome, and postconcussive syndrome.*

A subdural hematoma is an area of bleeding under the dura mater but outside of the brain surface. It carries a high mortality rate and is usually evidenced by a dramatically worsening state of consciousness, increased intracranial pressure, mass effect (pressure and movement of brain tissue resulting from swelling and bleeding), and brain herniation. An epidural hematoma usually occurs when a temporal skull fracture tears the middle meningeal artery, resulting in an area of bleeding between the skull and the dura mater. This injury typically presents with a lucid period followed by a precipitous loss of consciousness, coma, and, if not evacuated immediately to emergency hospital facilities, death.

Second impact syndrome can occur in an athlete who sustains a second head injury before symptoms of an earlier head injury have cleared. This condition has catastrophic consequences and must be recognized and treated immediately to prevent death. Although second impact syndrome is rare, the enormous risks may provide you with a compelling argument to persuade a player who continues to be symptomatic (or his family or coach) to withdraw from competition.

Persistent symptoms following concussion have been classified as postconcussive syndrome (PCS). PCS can occur even after a mild head injury, and its symptoms include headache, dizziness, and changes in attentiveness or personality. Most manifestations of PCS are temporary and brief; long-term disability is rare, although occasionally the symptoms may last for months. Treatment may require a team approach involving a primary care provider, an athletic trainer, and a psychologist. Neuropsychological testing may be required to document any cognitive deficits and to help the athlete develop adaptive coping strategies.

3. *Demonstrate proper management techniques for the seizing athlete.*

The first priority during a seizure is to protect the individual from injury. The next priority is to turn the athlete onto her side to prevent aspiration. Never place anything in a convulsing person's mouth. During the post-ictal phase (the time of lethargy, among other symptoms, after the convulsions), protect the airway. Seizures are rare and generally last <5 min. Any athlete whose seizure lasts >5 min should receive immediate emergency medical care. Athletes with epilepsy generally can play any sport, even more violent sports such as football or rugby, as long as they have been free of seizures for at least a year.

4. *Differentiate between meningitis and encephalitis.*

Serious infections of the meninges and spinal fluid, the brain, or both can have serious sequelae that may be prevented through proper recognition, referral, and treatment. The athletic trainer should be able to recognize the common signs and symptoms of these diseases in hopes of preventing serious long-term complications.

Meningitis and encephalitis are serious infections that involve the brain and surrounding tissue. Meningitis by definition is inflammation of the lining of the brain and can be caused by bacteria, viruses, or fungi. Viral meningitis, which is more common than bacterial, is caused by a wide variety of viruses and is usually thought to be less serious. Bacterial meningitis is less common but a much more serious problem. Diagnosis is based on spinal fluid results. If not recognized and treated, it can be fatal.

Encephalitis is usually caused by one of a number of viruses, only some of which can be treated with antiviral medications. Diagnosis is usually based on spinal fluid results, with magnetic resonance imaging (MRI) possibly providing additional information as to which areas of the brain may be affected. The prognosis of encephalitis is variable; some illnesses are self-limited and short-term, whereas others cause permanent sequelae such as memory loss, confusion, and even death.

5. *Recognize the variety of headaches that active participants might experience.*

Headaches result from a variety of causes, including hypertension, trauma, tumor, migraines, and exercise (exertional headaches). The athletic trainer must know which headaches may have a serious origin and must be prepared to refer accordingly.

CHAPTER 4

Diabetes Mellitus

OBJECTIVES

Upon completion of this chapter the reader will be able to do the following:

1. Identify the signs and symptoms of type 1 (insulin-dependent) and type 2 (non-insulin-dependent) diabetes

2. Discuss the diagnosis and treatment of type 1 and type 2 diabetes

3. Explain the importance of monitoring glucose levels when designing a treatment plan

4. Describe the role exercise plays in improving the quality of life and reducing the morbidity associated with diabetes

5. Explain the need for adequate caloric intake for the active patient with diabetes and recognize the symptoms and treatment for hypoglycemia and hyperglycemia

Asthma and diabetes are the two life-threatening diseases you will encounter most often among athletes. As with asthma, the large majority of diabetes cases can be controlled so that individuals can participate fully in their choice of sports. Many highly successful, even world-class, athletes have diabetes.

You should be aware, however, of the potential complications that can occur with diabetes. And you should be aware of basic strategies of control so that you can help athletes treat their disease in ways that will maximally enhance their health as well as their athletic performance. This chapter provides valuable information for precisely that purpose.

Diabetes mellitus is characterized by a deficiency of the hormone **insulin** or by the inability of the body to use insulin. Without insulin or the ability to utilize it, cells cannot metabolize glucose to produce energy. *Type 1 diabetes,* also called *insulin-dependent diabetes mellitus* or *juvenile-onset diabetes,* is an autoimmune disorder that destroys the insulin-producing islet cells in the pancreas. Without insulin, blood sugar rises to dangerous levels and the body begins to produce ketones and a variety of organic acids. We discuss this condition (diabetic ketoacidosis) later in the

Case Study

Seventeen-yr-old Mark just moved to your school district and reports to football camp. He says he was diagnosed with diabetes mellitus 18 months ago and reports no problems while playing football at his previous school. His doctor has recommended two shots of insulin per day. Although he says that he is under good control, he cannot recall his glycosylated hemoglobin levels and does not have a written record of his blood sugars. When you check the memory in his glucometer, you see several measurements in the 200 to 250 range and two recordings over 300. He reports that he takes 22 units of NPH insulin and 3 units of regular insulin in the morning and 17 units of NPH and 6 to 10 units of regular insulin in the afternoon. Mark does not change his doses very often and reports one episode of hypoglycemia per week, which he treats with soda pop and candy. You insist that he meet with the team physician before starting football camp.

The team physician orders a glycosylated hemoglobin test, which is 12.8% (normal is 4-8%)—indicating that his diabetes is not under very good control. The physician insists that Mark keep a log of his blood sugar and that he test his blood sugar in the training room. The physician anticipates that the athlete's insulin requirements will decrease during twice-a-day football practices, and that careful monitoring will be necessary to prevent hypoglycemia. The physician also informs Mark that his "honeymoon period" (the time when his pancreas is still making small amounts of insulin) may be over, and that he may now find it more challenging to control his diabetes. The physician recommends that Mark have prepractice blood sugars above 180 mg/dl to prevent hypoglycemia, and that sports drink and some fruit be available in case he experiences low blood sugar, along with keeping glucagons available for severe cases of hypoglycemia.

On the first day of practice, Mark's blood sugar is 190 mg/dl in the morning, and he takes his regular doses of insulin. After the second practice in the afternoon, he comes into the training room angry and very edgy. You insist that he check his blood sugar, and after some arguing he does so; it is 52 mg/dl. After consuming a sports drink and some apple and orange quarters, he begins to act like himself. You instruct Mark to consult the team physician about decreasing his evening insulin doses to avoid hypoglycemia. The physician's recommendation is to decrease both the evening and the morning doses.

This scenario repeats several more times in the first week of practice, by which time Mark's insulin requirements have decreased to 80% of the daily dose he was taking at the onset of the season. His insulin requirement gradually increased, however, when the team changed from two practices a day to only one a day. Mark continues to need coaching on how to adjust his doses according to his blood sugar levels.

Terms and Definitions

adenosine triphosphate (ATP)—A nucleotide compound occurring in all cells where it represents energy storage in the form of phosphate bonds. To release energy, it is hydrolyzed to adenosine diphosphate (ADP) and a phosphate group.

cortisol—A hormone secreted by the adrenal gland resulting in protein breakdown, fatty acid breakdown, and an increase in blood glucose concentration.

diabetic ketoacidosis (DKA)—Serious metabolic condition resulting from gross insulin deficiency leading to severe hyperglycemia, dehydration, and electrolyte abnormalities.

epinephrine—A hormone secreted by the adrenal gland. Actions include counterbalancing the effects of insulin and reacting to stress by increasing metabolism, blood pressure, heart rate, and blood flow to muscles.

free fatty acids (FFA)—The body's primary energy source in the blood.

glucagon—A hormone produced by the pancreas; released in response to decreased glucose levels.

gluconeogenesis—Synthesis of glucose, mainly in the liver, from noncarbohydrate precursors such as lactate and pyruvate; occurs primarily as a response to intense exercise.

glucose tolerance test (GTT)—Screening test for diabetes wherein the patient drinks a prescribed fluid with high sugar content. In diabetics, blood sugars rise higher than normal after drinking this solution.

glycogen—A storage carbohydrate found mainly in the liver but also in muscle cells; consists of long chains of glucose. It is broken down during high-intensity exercise to provide glucose for energy.

glycosuria—The presence of sugar (glucose) in the urine, generally defined as 1 g or more in a 24-h period.

glycosylated hemoglobin (GHgb)—Hemoglobin in the blood that is bound to glucose. Everyone has a small percentage of GHgb, and it increases if blood sugar levels are elevated.

growth hormone—Hormone released by the pituitary gland.

hypercholesterolemia—An excess of cholesterol in the blood, usually more than 200 mg/dl in an adult.

hypertriglyceridemia—An excess of triglycerides in the blood. The upper limit of normal rises with increasing age.

insulin—A hormone produced by the pancreas; released in response to elevated glucose levels.

ketoacidosis—Elevation of ketones and various organic acids in the blood; results from high levels of blood sugar.

norepinephrine—A hormone similar in action to epinephrine. Also secreted by the adrenal gland.

chapter. The blood sugar of nondiabetic people stays within a fairly wide range of 70 to 110 mg/dl. Anything above or below this range can produce unpleasant and dangerous symptoms (discussed later). Death may result from blood sugars that dip or remain too low or rise or remain too high, and permanent damage to many body systems results from poorly controlled fluctuations in blood sugar levels.

Type 1 diabetes usually begins in childhood; though it can develop at any age, the incidence peaks in early to middle puberty. It affects perhaps 1 in 500 children younger than 18 yr. It occurs equally in males and females worldwide, in all ethnic groups.

There is no single "diabetes gene"; rather, numerous genes are associated with diabetes. Inheritance of certain antigens on lymphocytes is associated with an increased risk of type 1 diabetes. It is thought that some external or environmental trigger such as an infection initiates an autoimmune process that begins to destroy the beta cells of the pancreas. At least 80% of the cells must be destroyed for a person to develop symptoms of diabetes. This destructive process generally takes months, and occasionally years.

Type 2 diabetes—also known as *non-insulin-dependent diabetes mellitus* or *adult-onset diabetes*—usually develops in adults over age 40 and is most common in people over age 55. It is increasing in prevalence worldwide. Recent data suggest that it can begin developing early in overweight adolescents. Type 2 diabetes is characterized not by a lack of insulin but rather by resistance to the action of insulin—which leads the body to produce higher insulin levels than it normally would. Because insulin resistance causes glucose to remain in the blood instead of getting into the cells to be metabolized, blood glucose levels rise. While this results in high blood sugar, **ketoacidosis** is rare. Type 2 diabetes is thought to affect about 20 million Americans over the age of 20. About 80% of people with type 2 diabetes are overweight; a significant genetic component also appears to exist in that individuals are more likely to have the disease if other members of their family have it.

DIAGNOSIS

Symptoms of type 1 diabetes include excessive hunger, excessive thirst, abnormally frequent urination (polyuria), and weight loss. A random blood glucose level greater than 200 mg/dl usually confirms the diagnosis, which rarely needs to be verified with a **glucose tolerance test (GTT).** If the person is asymptomatic, such as usually occurs with type 2 diabetes, diabetes is diagnosed when the fasting blood sugar is more than 126 mg/dl, or the 2-h blood glucose in an oral GTT is greater than 200 mg/dl. The younger the child, the more difficult it is to make the diagnosis before the onset of ketoacidosis (see next paragraph). Any child with new-onset bedwetting or who often leaves the classroom to go to the bathroom should be checked for type 1 diabetes. A simple dipstick test of the urine for glucose can effectively rule out type 1 diabetes since glucose appears in the urine whenever the blood sugar is above 200 mg/dl.

Many young children and adolescents with undiagnosed type 1 diabetes develop potentially life-threatening complications as their first clinical presentation of the disease. Lacking insulin to facilitate glucose metabolism, and with elevations of the counter-regulatory hormones that drive glucose levels even higher, the body tries to keep up with energy requirements by metabolizing fat—and the by-product of such metabolism is ketones and acids in the blood: **diabetic ketoacidosis (DKA).** The urine excretes excessive glucose from the blood, causing excessive loss of not only water but also sodium and potassium. By definition, DKA is present when blood glucose is 250 mg/dl or higher, serum pH is <7.3 (normal is 7.4), and serum bicarbonate is 15 meq/L or less (normal is 22-26 meq/L). In most cases, ketones are present in both the blood and the urine. DKA is often associated with muscle weakness and a rapid respiratory rate, the latter being the body's effort to remove acid from the body by expiring more carbon dioxide than normal (when CO_2 is dissolved in the blood, it forms carbonic acid). Ketones are also expired, producing a fruity odor in the breath. DKA eventually produces nausea and vomiting, which worsens the metabolic abnormalities in a vicious cycle. Eventually the metabolic anomalies and dehydration affect consciousness and lead to coma. If untreated, the individual will die.

DKA usually requires hospitalization and intensive care for treatment of the metabolic abnormalities. If blood glucose is corrected too quickly with insulin, metabolic changes can produce seizures and heart rhythm abnormalities. DKA occurs most often in people with newly diagnosed type 1 diabetes, diabetics who stop taking insulin, and diabetics who are ill with an infection and are not taking enough insulin and consuming sufficient calories to fight the infection.

High blood sugar increases the amount of glucose that is bound to other chemicals in the body (this is called *glycosylation*). Hemoglobin takes up glucose in the blood to form **glycosylated hemoglobin (GHgb).** A small percentage of the hemoglobin molecules, in the range of 4.0% to 8.0%, are glycosylated in healthy people with normal blood sugar levels. In people with poorly controlled diabetes, GHgb is significantly elevated. A newer test looks only at glycosylation of a major subfraction of the hemoglobin called hemoglobin A1C, with normal percentages in the range of 4.3% to 6.0%. Either of these measures of glycosylation reflects the control of diabetes over the past 2 to 3 months.

INSULIN TREATMENT

Before the discovery of insulin, exercise and diet were the only treatments for diabetes. In 1919, researchers demonstrated that exercise lowers blood sugar; later, exercise was shown to potentiate the hypoglycemic effect of insulin. Exercise is an important component of treatment for people with type 2 diabetes because it increases insulin sensitivity. While exercise can also be an important adjunct therapy for type 1 diabetes, it is not nearly as important as optimal management of insulin. We discuss exercise in detail a bit later in this chapter.

The mainstay of treatment for type 1 diabetes is insulin, which is injected subcutaneously. Several types of insulin are available (see table 4.1):

- Regular insulin is rapid acting; it is the insulin used to rapidly treat hyperglycemia and DKA.
- Insulin lispro (brand name Humalog®) is a biosynthetic analog of regular insulin that acts even faster than the natural hormone; it is both absorbed and cleared from the system more rapidly than regular insulin.
- Semilente is another short-acting insulin.
- Lente and neutral protamine Hagedorn (NPH) are intermediate in peak and duration of action.
- Ultralente is a long-acting insulin with duration of more than 24 to 36 h.

Insulin is given intravenously to people hospitalized with DKA and subcutaneously once the patient is stable. Most people with type 1 diabetes require at least

Table 4.1   Comparison of Insulin Types

Insulin name	Action	Initial onset*	Peak time*	Duration*
Insulin lispro (LP; e.g., Humalog)	Rapid-acting insulin	5-15 min	1-2 hr	4-5 hr
Regular (R)	Short-acting insulin	30 min	2-4 hr	6-8 hr
NPH (N)	Intermediate-acting insulin	1-3 hr	5-7 hr	13-18 hr
Lente (L)	Intermediate-acting insulin	1-3 hr	4-8 hr	13-20 hr
Ultralente (U)	Long-acting insulin	2-4 hr	8-14 hr	20-24 hr
Premixed 70/30 NPH and regular	Short-acting and intermediate-acting insulin mix	30 min	7-12 hr	16-24 hr

* = Onset, peak time, and duration are given as ranges because individuals differ in their responses to the various insulins available for treating type 1 diabetes.

Reprinted, by permission, from F.J. Cerny and H.W. Burton, 2001, *Exercise physiology for health care professionals* (Champaign, IL: Human Kinetics), 62.

two injections per day, each consisting of a dose of short-acting and a dose of long-acting insulin. Injections are usually given before breakfast and dinner. For the first year or more, when there are still some islet cells producing insulin, the person might be able to manage with only one injection per day. Blood sugar is usually much easier to control during this "honeymoon" period.

Frequent glucose monitoring is important to help people adjust insulin dosing for dietary changes and changes in exercise. Glucose monitors are now small, very portable, and very accurate. (See *Checking Blood Sugar With a Blood-Glucose Meter,* page 46.) If the morning fasting glucose level is high, for example, the evening long-acting insulin dose should be increased. During the honeymoon period, an individual may require a daily insulin dose of less than 0.5 unit/kg body weight (0.23 unit/lb). Once all the islet cells are gone, most children require 0.75 to 1.0 unit/kg (0.34-0.45 unit/lb) body weight per day. Adolescents typically need 1.0 to 1.2 units/kg (0.45-0.54 unit/lb) per day to achieve good metabolic control. All people with diabetes should keep careful records of blood glucose and insulin doses. Review of the written records can reveal the degree of metabolic control and stabilization of blood sugar during the preceding days or even over the past months.

Although most athletes with diabetes use subcutaneous injections to control their disorder, a few obtain much better control through use of an insulin pump, a pocket-sized device that is easily attached to clothing, which delivers continuous subcutaneous short-acting regular insulin with variable dosage rate depending on meal time and exercise. Athletes can safely use an insulin pump, but its use does not inevitably improve blood sugar control; and although the pump potentially provides greater flexibility regarding the timing of meals and exercise, it is somewhat cumbersome in some sports in that it requires tubing and a needle implanted in the skin of the abdomen. The pump has to be detached for some activities, especially water sports and some contact sports. It is not practical to pad the pump for contact sports.

Type 2 diabetes is sometimes treated with insulin, but more often it is initially treated with diet and exercise. If these are unsuccessful, health providers usually try one of the oral hypoglycemic agents as listed in table 4.2 on page 45. Each of these medications works in a different way. None of them can be used for type 1 diabetes.

DIABETES AND EXERCISE

Exercise can reduce morbidity and improve the quality of life for most people with diabetes mellitus and is reviewed in Colberg and Swain (2000). Because exercise increases sensitivity to insulin, people with type 1 diabetes who exercise regularly need less insulin to maintain normal blood sugar. Exercise contributes to better weight control, improvement in self-image, and decreases in hypertension and lipid-related cardiovascular risk factors. Regular exercise to control blood lipids is important in that both type 1 and type 2 diabetes significantly increase the incidence of both **hypercholesterolemia** and **hypertriglyceridemia.** Hypertension also occurs more frequently in diabetic than in nondiabetic people, and because exercise can help control blood pressure, it may help prevent some of the vascular complications associated with diabetes that are exacerbated by hypertension.

The psychological benefits of athletic participation are extremely important; for people with diabetes, participation in sports confers a feeling of mastery over the chronic disease that seems to affect most other aspects of their lives. Reduced insulin requirements and improvements in glycemic control through exercise help improve self-esteem at all ages.

Problems can arise, however, when people with poorly controlled type 1 diabetes exercise. In some cases aerobic exercise can lead to either hypoglycemia or hyperglycemia, depending on the direction in which the individual errs in trying to adjust insulin doses for the effects of exercise. For example, Joan is a 14-yr-old high school freshman whose friend is going out for cross-country and talks Joan into accompanying her for fun. Joan has had diabetes for 4 yr and did not participate in any sports in middle school. She did very little running in the summer and has had to decrease her daily insulin doses only slightly in the past. When she begins two practices a day in August, she discovers she is developing frequent low blood sugars, usually 4 to 6 h after her workouts. A call to her physician helps her reduce her insulin dosage further to adjust to the marked increase of intense exercise in her daily routine. Resistance training can also seriously exacerbate some of the side effects of diabetes. Before going into further detail, we first describe what is supposed to happen in healthy individuals as they exercise.

Normal Glucose Metabolism and Exercise

Glucose and **free fatty acids (FFAs)** are the body's primary energy sources in the blood. Muscles utilize fuel stored in the form of **glycogen** and triglycerides (fat). Under normal circumstances, only a small percentage of the body's total energy comes from metabolizing protein.

When people begin an exercise session, breakdown of glycogen in their muscles provides an immediate source of energy in the form of **adenosine triphosphate (ATP)**. As exercise continues, muscles begin to utilize blood glucose and FFAs. The predominant source of energy depends on the duration and intensity of the exercise. Glycogen stored in the liver—and converted to glucose for transport to the muscles—tends to be the primary energy source as the *intensity* of exercise increases and the muscles deplete their own stored glycogen, whereas FFA consumption increases with greater *duration* of exercise. During endurance training, the body increasingly utilizes FFAs; highly trained endurance athletes "burn" a higher proportion of FFAs than do untrained individuals.

In healthy people, insulin levels naturally decrease during exercise:

- Exercise diminishes the need for insulin to facilitate glucose transport into muscle cells.
- Exercise increases insulin sensitivity by enhancing the binding of insulin to receptor sites on the muscle cells.
- Insulin blocks the breakdown of both glycogen and fat in the liver; therefore, decreased insulin levels permit the liver to break down more glycogen and fat.
- The increased adrenaline (epinephrine) produced during exercise suppresses insulin secretion, facilitating mobilization of hepatic glucose and avoiding hypoglycemia.

For similar reasons, people with diabetes can use lower doses of insulin when they exercise. Physically fit athletes exhibit increased insulin binding as well as an expanded number of insulin receptor sites in their cells.

Insulin is not the only hormone that regulates availability of energy. It is opposed in its action by several other hormones, called insulin antagonists—primarily **glucagon, epinephrine, norepinephrine, cortisol,** and **growth hormone.** The intricate balance among these hormones is what permits the healthy body to fine-tune its energy expenditures and is discussed in detail in Landry and Allen (1992). Soon after exercising muscles begin utilizing glucose, an interesting interplay occurs between insulin and its antagonists. We mentioned previously that exercise leads to a decline in insulin levels. But the decline in plasma glucose during exercise stimulates production of glucagon, a pancreatic hormone that generally works in a manner opposite to that of insulin in that glucagon *increases* blood sugar levels. The combination of higher glucagon and lower insulin levels in the blood tells the body that a lot of fuel is needed as soon as possible—and in response, the liver breaks down glycogen to release more glucose into the bloodstream. And whereas insulin ordinarily inhibits production of FFAs, high glucagon/low insulin levels release this inhibition, thus increasing blood levels of FFAs. The liver then begins generating even more glucose from glycerol (from breakdown of the FFAs) as well as from lactate that is released from the muscles. This process is called **gluconeogenesis.** Increases in rates of glycolysis and gluconeogenesis are regulated by the counter-regulatory hormones. Epinephrine and norepinephrine, whose levels increase during exercise, promote the breakdown of glycogen and fat. Cortisol and growth hormone, which also increase during exercise, also stimulate the breakdown of glycogen in response to declining plasma glucose concentrations but appear to be more important in prolonged exercise.

Glucose Metabolism and Exercise in People With Diabetes

In athletes with type 1 diabetes, subcutaneous insulin administration cannot mimic the normal, gradual decline of insulin levels during exercise. Injected insulin may be absorbed into the bloodstream more rapidly during exercise, creating excessive insulin levels; yet athletes who inject too little insulin may have insufficient glucose available to their exercising muscles. Note that although there has been concern about higher risks of hypoglycemia in people who inject insulin into exercising limbs (e.g., a runner's injection site would be the legs), that risk has never been well proven. While it is usually recommended that a person with diabetes use a nonexercising body part such as the abdomen for insulin injection before exercise, the site of the injection may not be as important as once thought.

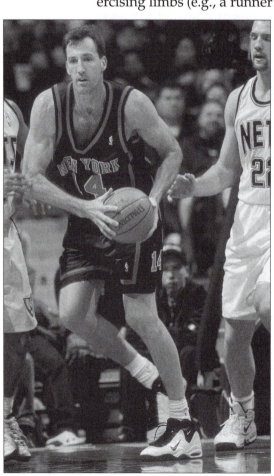

■ **Figure 4.1**   Diabetes did not prevent Chris Dudley from a career in professional basketball.
© Ezra O. Shaw/Getty Images

Exercise and Type 1 Diabetes

Exercise can be quite beneficial to people with type 1 diabetes in that it helps to keep down weight, lowers blood pressure, lowers lipid levels in the blood, and reduces the required insulin dosages. If athletes are able to maintain good control of their blood sugar levels, there is no reason they cannot participate in sports, even on the professional level (figure 4.1). Yet there is a risk of hypoglycemia or hyperglycemia when an athlete is unable to gauge *how much* to lower insulin doses before a bout of exercise. Because exercise enhances absorption of the injected insulin, overestimating the correct dosage can lead to severe hypoglycemia. Underestimating the correct dosage (i.e., overestimating the effects of exercise), on the other hand, can lead to marked and prolonged hyperglycemia and ketosis—especially when adolescents with poorly controlled diabetes exercise with the express purpose of lowering their blood sugar. People with type 1 diabetes who want to participate in sports must carefully plan their insulin injections, especially if daily workouts vary in timing, intensity, or duration.

Young people who have had type 1 diabetes for <10 yr usually can engage in resistance training with no great risk of complications. Because resis-

Table 4.2 Medications Used for Control of Type 2 Diabetes

Medication	Action
Sulfonylureas	Stimulate pancreatic production of insulin
Biguanides	Decrease liver production of glucose
Alpha-glucosidase inhibitors	Slow absorption of dietary starches
Thiazolidinediones	Increase insulin sensitivity
Meglitinides	Stimulate pancreatic production of insulin

Reprinted, by permission, from F.J. Cerny and H.W. Burton, 2001, *Exercise physiology for health care professionals* (Champaign, IL: Human Kinetics), 62.

tance training can cause transient periods of hypertension, however, people with long-standing type 1 (or even type 2) diabetes may need to avoid strength training activities. If they have already begun to experience any kind of retinopathy or musculoskeletal complications of diabetes, activities such as heavy weightlifting or training for football can severely exacerbate existing pathologies.

Exercise and Type 2 Diabetes

Most people with type 2 diabetes control their disease through diet, weight reduction, oral hypoglycemic agents, and physical exercise. As Creviston and Quinn (2001) discussed, exercise remains a very important part of therapy for type 2 diabetes, not simply for its role in weight reduction but more important because it increases insulin sensitivity. In fact, increased physical activity often can prevent the onset of type 2 diabetes in individuals who are at risk for the disease. It is not even necessary to engage in repeated bouts of exercise to see a benefit: Insulin sensitivity declines 12 to 16 h after any single bout of exercise that is sufficiently vigorous to deplete glycogen.

Hypoglycemia is infrequent in people with type 2 diabetes who treat their disease with diet and exercise alone. Because people who take oral hypoglycemic agents may increase their insulin sensitivity by exercising, they may need to reduce the dose of such agents. Table 4.2 lists the medications that are available for people with type 2 diabetes who cannot otherwise control their blood sugar levels.

WORKING WITH ATHLETES WHO HAVE DIABETES

Your most important roles are

- to identify athletes who have diabetes and to obtain as much information as possible on their condition and its history and treatment;
- to be certain that athletes choose a sport that will not exacerbate existing problems;
- to meet periodically with athletes and review their records to monitor their blood sugar—principally by performing frequent blood sugar tests and by intelligently matching insulin doses to their exercise patterns; and
- to discuss with athletes (and, when appropriate, with their parents) their diets, to satisfy yourself that they are eating appropriately for a person with diabetes.

Even the most careful monitoring can't prevent all problems, however, and the following discussion should help you know how to deal with those that arise.

Preparticipation and Periodic Evaluations

Your first defense against complications in athletes with diabetes is prevention. *Preparticipation evaluations of athletes with diabetes should establish that the athletes have a good program of self-monitoring and have achieved good metabolic control* before *participating in organized athletics.* The cornerstone of good metabolic control is the modern portable glucose meter that can determine accurate blood glucose in 1 min. Insist that athletes with diabetes demonstrate a willingness to check blood sugar on a regular basis, preferably four times a day. Be sure that the athlete is using the meter properly—which means that you must know how to do so yourself. (See *Checking Blood Sugar With a Blood-Glucose Meter.*) Obtain and keep on file the results of a recent glycosylated hemoglobin assay; it will permit you to determine if the athlete has been able to maintain good metabolic control over the past several months. The athlete must be willing to keep written records of blood sugar as well as insulin doses. This is especially important if the exercise requirements of the sport vary from day to day.

Because hypoglycemia is a common complication of exercise for people with diabetes, ask athletes about their past experiences with that problem. Ask also about their ability to detect hypoglycemia at its earliest stages. The longer people have had diabetes, the more important this matter becomes, since they can lose some of the symptoms—such as increased sweating, weakness, and hunger—that younger individuals experience. As these early warning signs become less intense, more severe hypoglycemic reactions may develop because of a delay in treatment.

If there is a family history of early coronary artery disease, stroke, or hypertension, obtain a thorough evaluation of the athlete's lipoprotein profile. Such a history should not disqualify a person with diabetes from participating in sports, but it should heighten the athlete's awareness of the importance of controlling blood lipids. People with diabetes are more susceptible than others to problems with high cholesterol, high levels of triglycerides, and hypertension—and well-planned and monitored exercise is a good way to help alleviate these risk factors for cardiovascular disease. When appropriate, insist that the athlete obtain periodic tests that will demonstrate continuing control of lipids and hypertension.

Checking Blood Sugar With a Blood-Glucose Meter

1. The glucose meter must have fresh batteries.

2. The chemical strips designed for the meter must be available.

3. A lancet (a small pointed instrument like a needle) must be available to puncture the skin.

4. The skin should be cleansed with alcohol, and a fresh puncture should be made in the tip of a finger. This is often done with a spring-loaded device.

5. Blood is squeezed from the finger onto the chemical strip to cover the appropriate area on the strip. (Newer strips can be placed on the blood drop in the finger, and the blood is drawn into the strip.)

6. The strip is inserted into the glucose meter.

7. The glucose meter will beep or flash the measurement when it is available.

8. The lancet should be disposed of in a sharps container.

Note: Glucose meters have a memory chip that stores the previous measurements, which is helpful when you're trying to determine recent glycemic control.

Children and adolescents with type 1 diabetes rarely exhibit any long-term effects of the diabetes until after they have had the disease for 10 yr or more. Young adults with type 1 diabetes and all people with type 2 diabetes should be examined carefully for any evidence of microvascular changes, neurological changes, or musculoskeletal complications that exercise may aggravate. Individuals with long-standing poor control of their diabetes are of particular concern, because sudden improvement in their hyperglycemia can exacerbate diabetic retinopathy and neuropathy. Before such athletes begin a new type of exercise or participation in sports, they should have appropriate specialists carefully assess their retinas and evaluate the health of their kidneys. These evaluations should be done on an annual basis.

Following are other items to watch carefully:

- Diabetic neuropathy often results in loss of light touch sensation and proprioception. Because even mild loss of pain sensation may predispose athletes to problems with foot lesions, their feet should be inspected carefully by the athletes themselves or their caregivers on a continuing basis. Wearing good athletic shoes with a wide, nonpointed toe box will reduce stress to the feet. In the presence of neuropathy, aerobic sports that are easy on the legs and feet, such as swimming, biking, and golf, would be the best activities.

- Poor control of diabetes can produce restricted joint flexibility (the current thinking is that glycosylation of connective tissues makes the collagen less flexible). Watch out for reduced flexibility in diabetic athletes.

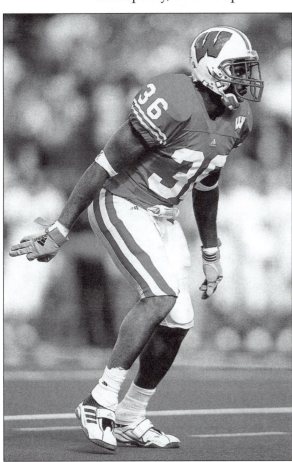

■ **Figure 4.2** Properly controlled diabetes will not keep a person from success in athletics. Michael Echols earned a college football scholarship after being diagnosed with diabetes in high school. He excelled at the University of Wisconsin and was drafted by the Tennessee Titans professional football team.

Courtesy of University of Wisconsin.

Selection of Athletic Activities

Sports activities of greatest benefit to people with diabetes are those that promote aerobic conditioning and, ideally, that they can continue for a lifetime. Athletes with type 1 diabetes who are in good metabolic control can participate in virtually any activity. Many highly successful athletes at the collegiate and even on the professional level have type 1 diabetes (see figure 4.2). Discourage people with type 1 diabetes from participating in high-risk sports, however, where unexpected hypoglycemia could produce a life-threatening situation—sports such as scuba diving, rock climbing, and parachuting. Regardless of the sport chosen, the athlete with diabetes must be committed to frequent monitoring of blood glucose and close attention to diet. Coaches or athletic trainers should ensure that athletes with diabetes test their blood glucose frequently and ingest appropriate amounts of calories sometime during the activity. Appropriate caloric levels vary from person to person and depend on the activities they are involved in. It is important for the inactive athlete with diabetes to start with a modest intensity and quantity of exercise and gradually increase the routine over weeks or months.

Dealing With Hypoglycemia

The greatest risk of hypoglycemia in exercising diabetics typically occurs 6 to 14 h after exercise—or sometimes even the next day. Because exercise depletes muscle glycogen, these stores must be replenished from glucose in the bloodstream during rest. Glycogen resynthesis can reduce blood glucose to dangerous levels. To counteract this effect, athletes must reduce insulin doses and increase caloric intake following strenuous exercise; failure to follow this routine can result in severe hypoglycemia.

Despite excellent metabolic control and frequent blood glucose monitoring, some athletes with diabetes will still experience hypoglycemia. Every athlete needs to be aware of the warning signs of hypoglycemia, which may vary from person to person. Symptoms of mild hypoglycemia include dizziness, fatigue, hunger, mental confusion, and headache; these symptoms tend to occur when the blood glucose is declining. Most individuals begin to develop symptoms when their blood sugar is in the range of 45 to 60 mg/dl. When this occurs, the athlete should ingest the most readily available source of sugar, such as fruit juices, oral glucose tablets, or sometimes candy if that is the only source of sugar available. It is best to supplement these items with foods containing complex carbohydrate and protein to provide a more sustained glycemic response.

For example, Larry has had diabetes for 6 yr and is a junior on the high school football team. He has excellent control but occasionally develops hypoglycemia. His athletic trainer and coaches have learned to recognize a personality change that usually accompanies his low blood sugars. Larry is usually an even-tempered boy, so when he gets ornery or easily frustrated, they know to have him stop and check his blood sugar. There is a cooler on the field that contains oranges, apples, and sports drinks so that Larry has a source of sugar readily available if the result of the blood sugar test confirms that he is low.

If an athlete with diabetes becomes semiconscious or unconscious and protection of the airway is in doubt (usually when blood glucose has dropped below 40 mg/dl), do not give her anything by mouth. Ideally, you should be able to obtain a glucose level rapidly—*which means you and other responsible authorities should become familiar with how to use each individual's blood sugar monitoring devices.* It is helpful if you can confirm that hypoglycemia is the problem—but when in doubt, assume that the athlete is hypoglycemic and *do not delay* trying to increase the blood sugar. The treatment of choice for unconscious athletes with diabetes is a subcutaneous or intramuscular injection of 1 ml of glucagon. This will cause a rapid release of glycogen from the liver and will rapidly increase blood sugar. *All athletic trainers—as well as any other health providers responsible for field coverage of athletes with diabetes—should have such injectable glucagon readily available and should know when and how to use it.* Like epinephrine, glucagon has a relatively short shelf life and must be repurchased approximately yearly.

You should also presume that hypoglycemia is the cause if a person with diabetes develops a seizure. In this case you can't administer glucose by mouth. If no intravenous fluids are available, intramuscular or subcutaneous injection of glucagon is again the treatment of choice. As soon as the athlete becomes conscious, give her supplemental oral carbohydrate and protein. Occasionally athletes are vomiting, or at least quite nauseated, which will delay their ability to ingest oral carbohydrate. Table 4.3 provides a quick reference to what an athlete's signs and symptoms are telling you about her blood sugar level.

Consuming Calories During Exercise

Most athletes with diabetes mellitus find it necessary to ingest some calories immediately before and during exercise to help counter the effects of insulin. Different people's caloric needs vary significantly; most people figure out what works

Table 4.3 Comparisons of Hypoglycemia and Hyperglycemia Signs and Symptoms

Onset	Hypoglycemia Rapid onset, occurring within minutes	Hyperglycemia Slow onset, occurring over a span of hours and even days
Neurological changes	Irritability, mental confusion, dizziness, bizarre behavior, slurred speech, memory loss, headache, dilated pupils; in severe cases, seizures and coma	Lethargy
Skin	Cold, clammy; profuse sweating*	Warm and dry
Muscular changes	Weakness, fatigue, muscle tremors, incoordination, ataxic gate	Weakness and fatigue
Cardiorespiratory changes	Weak, rapid pulse	Rapid pulse (tachycardia)
	No odor on breath	Deep, rapid breathing (Kussmaul respirations) and characteristic odor of acetones on breath
Genito-urinary/ gastrointestinal changes	None	Nausea and vomiting, excessive urination, excessive thirst, excessive eating

* = Some people with long-standing diabetes may lose the ability to sweat.

Reprinted, by permission, from S.J. Shultz, P.A. Houglum, and D.H. Perrin, 2000, *Assessment of athletic injuries* (Champaign, IL: Human Kinetics), 432.

for them individually. Athletes can estimate the amount of carbohydrate they will need during exercise based on duration and intensity of the activity. The key figure to remember is that 1 g of glucose provides about 4 kcal of energy. Assume, for example, that a person will be engaging in vigorous endurance activity that will burn about 600 kcal/h (10 kcal/min). If the exercise intensity is 50% of the athlete's maximum oxygen consumption, then—according to exercise physiology studies of the sources of calories consumed during exercise—approximately 50% of the energy needed (5 kcal/min, or 1.25 g/min of glucose) will be derived from glucose oxidation (a more intense bout of exercise consumes a higher percentage of glucose; a lower-intensity bout, less). The athlete planning 30 min of such exercise should therefore take a supplemental feeding of 30 min × 1.25 g/min glucose = 37.5 g glucose, which we round to about 30 to 40 g of carbohydrate (which is, after all, just long chains of glucose) to help prevent hypoglycemia. Examples of snacks with 30 to 40 g carbohydrate appear in table 4.4.

Adequate food replacement is important for the athlete with type 1 diabetes. Increased fluid loss due to **glycosuria** may add to the risk of dehydration.

If an athlete with type 1 diabetes is taking insufficient insulin, hyperglycemia will follow exercise and can be prolonged—leading in some cases to production of ketones and other metabolic acids. Should this athlete try to exercise again without having replenished his glycogen stores, he will feel quite ill during exercise and develop DKA.

Exercise and Complications of Diabetes

People with type 1 diabetes not only need to prevent DKA, but they also want to prevent or delay the long-term complications of diabetes. Although the exact

Table 4.4   Examples of Snacks Containing 30-40 g Carbohydrate (CHO)

Food	Amount	g CHO
Apple juice	8 oz	30
Cola	12 oz	39
Pop-Tarts® (blueberry)	1 serving	30
Granola	1/2 c	45
Raisins	1/3 c	40
Oranges	2 medium	30
Banana	1 1/2 medium	30
Saltine crackers	15 crackers	30
Honey	2 Tbsp	30

Adapted from Clark, 1997, *Sports nutrition guidebook*, 2nd ed. (Champaign, IL: Human Kinetics), 122-123.

mechanisms of the complications are not totally understood, it is thought that the glycosylation of molecules throughout the body plays a role in many of them. Most people with type 1 diabetes develop complications only after they have had the disease at least 10 yr, and often much longer. The most significant complications of type 1 diabetes affect the body's small blood vessels. The changes in the blood vessels in the retina of the eye (leaking vessels at first, and eventually abnormal proliferation of vessels) can lead to blindness. Changes in vessels in the kidneys can lead to kidney failure. The elevated cholesterol and blood lipids may cause hardening of the arteries (arteriosclerosis), predisposing the affected individual to premature stroke or myocardial infarct (heart attack). Diabetes may adversely affect the function of peripheral nerves, leading to decreased sensation in the feet and lower legs, and can also affect the function of the autonomic nervous system, causing gastrointestinal dysfunction. Diabetic neuropathy can also produce pain in the feet and legs and make the skin extremely sensitive.

If a person has long-standing diabetes of either type, *exercise may increase the risk of some of these complications.* Any changes in the eyes' retinal blood vessels can worsen with fluctuations in blood sugar. Rapid changes in blood pressure that occur with exercise may also produce hemorrhages in the eyes in individuals with retinal disease. A person with diabetic neuropathy has an increased risk of musculoskeletal injuries to soft tissues and joints. Always be on the watch for indications of these complications.

Drug Interactions

A large number of drugs can alter the body's response to insulin. When working with an athlete with diabetes, you are usually forced to assume (rightly or wrongly) that the athlete's physician carefully monitors all drug interactions. There are three specific substances, however, that some adolescent athletes may be hesitant to discuss with their doctors. These athletes are just as likely to be hesitant to talk with you, of course, but by knowing about potential interactions, and by doing your best to establish a rapport with and gain the respect of athletes, you may be able to head off some potentially dangerous drug interactions.

- *Ethanol* enhances the glucose-lowering effect of insulin. Do your best to convince athletes with diabetes *never* to drink alcohol. Any use of alcohol increases the risk of hypoglycemia.

- *Anabolic steroids* also enhance the effects of insulin. It is dangerous for any athlete to use these illegal drugs, but it is especially dangerous for those with diabetes.

- *Birth-control pills* (and estrogens in general) can reduce the effects of insulin. In many states, sexually active adolescent girls are able to obtain birth control pills without their parents' knowledge and without seeing their regular doctor. If nothing else, make it generally known in group discussions with female athletes how such drugs can affect the body's response to insulin and that blood glucose monitoring is even more important for anyone starting these medications.

General Recommendations

With a knowledge of the effects of exercise on diabetes, you can help prevent many problems rather than having to deal with them after they occur. Here are basic principles you can both teach your athletes with diabetes and help them to implement:

- An athlete with diabetes going from a relatively sedentary lifestyle to a significant increase in exercise should *gradually* increase her fitness activity over several weeks to allow her to adjust her insulin doses as well as her diet.

- An athlete with diabetes should diligently monitor his blood glucose levels not only during this transition but also during the entire season to help prevent hypoglycemia with its complications. Suggest monitoring glucose *at least* two times a day, and preferably four times a day, during changes in his routine.

- Whenever possible, an athlete with diabetes should exercise on a daily basis (or at least four or five times a week)—preferably at the same time every day—to avoid big changes in day-to-day insulin doses and diet.

- An athlete with diabetes should try to avoid rising insulin levels during exercise, timing her insulin administration so that peak insulin activity does not occur during the exercise session or immediately following it.

- An athlete with diabetes must be sensitive to any symptoms of hypoglycemia, especially after a particularly exhausting or prolonged activity; any increase in appetite or feelings of weakness or fatigue in the hours following exercise should alert him to monitor his blood glucose more frequently, and probably to further reduce his evening insulin dose and increase his caloric intake.

- When starting an exercise routine or with changes in intensity or duration, the athlete should check blood sugar at one or two o'clock in the morning to check for postexercise late-onset hypoglycemia.

- Instruct athletes with long-standing diabetes to be particularly faithful in performing thorough warm-up, stretching, and cool-down exercises to counteract the progressive stiffening of connective tissues that often accompanies poorly controlled diabetes.

- If the athlete's preexercise blood glucose levels are elevated, she may need to defer exercise and administer insulin to improve control.

- An athlete with diabetes should never drink alcohol or use anabolic steroids.

- Young women taking birth control pills should find a physician with whom they can comfortably discuss the interaction between these drugs and insulin; they also should monitor blood sugar closely when starting or stopping oral contraceptives.

- Athletes with diabetes should understand that if their blood glucose levels are poorly controlled, severe hyperglycemia and ketosis can contribute to dehydration during exercise, and that these problems may occur even in relatively well controlled individuals during a viral illness.

SUMMARY

1. *Identify the signs and symptoms of type 1 (insulin-dependent) and type 2 (non-insulin-dependent) diabetes.*

Diabetes mellitus is characterized by a deficiency of the hormone insulin or by the inability of the body to use insulin. Without insulin or the ability to utilize it, cells cannot metabolize glucose to produce energy. Type 1 diabetes, also called insulin-dependent diabetes mellitus or juvenile-onset diabetes, is an autoimmune disorder that destroys the islet cells in the pancreas, where insulin is made. Without insulin, blood sugar rises to dangerous levels and the body begins to produce ketones and a variety of organic acids.

Type 2 diabetes—also known as non-insulin-dependent diabetes mellitus or adult-onset diabetes—usually develops in adults over age 40 and is most common in people over age 55. It is increasing in prevalence worldwide. Recent data suggest that it can begin developing early in overweight adolescents. Type 2 diabetes is characterized not by a lack of insulin but rather by resistance to the action of insulin—which leads the body to produce higher insulin levels than would normally be the case.

2. *Discuss the diagnosis and treatment of type 1 and type 2 diabetes.*

Symptoms of type 1 diabetes include excessive hunger, excessive thirst, abnormally frequent urination, and weight loss. A random blood glucose level greater than 200 mg/dl usually confirms the diagnosis, which rarely needs to be verified with a glucose tolerance test (GTT). If the person is asymptomatic, such as usually occurs with type 2 diabetes, diabetes is diagnosed when the fasting blood sugar is more than 126 mg/dl or the 2-h blood glucose in an oral glucose tolerance test is greater than 200 mg/dl.

Exercise is an important component of treatment for people with type 2 diabetes, because it increases insulin sensitivity. Though exercise can also be an important adjunct therapy for type 1 diabetes, it is not nearly as important as optimal management of insulin. Most people with type 1 diabetes require at least two injections a day, each consisting of a dose of short-acting and a dose of long-acting insulin. Injections are usually given before breakfast and dinner. For the first year or more, when islet cells are still producing insulin, the individual might be able to get by with only one injection a day. Blood sugar is usually much easier to control during this period.

3. *Explain the importance of monitoring glucose levels when designing a treatment plan.*

Frequent glucose monitoring is important to help people adjust insulin dosing for changes in diet and exercise. Glucose monitors are now small, portable, and very accurate. All people with diabetes should keep careful records of blood glucose and insulin doses. Review of the written records can reveal the degree of metabolic control and stabilization of blood sugar during the preceding days or even over the past months.

4. *Describe the role exercise plays in improving the quality of life and reducing the morbidity associated with diabetes.*

Physical exercise is beneficial for most people with type 2 diabetes and many people with type 1 diabetes. Exercise helps with weight control and glycemic control and tends to enhance self-image for young people with diabetes. Exercise also helps control hypertension and lipid-related cardiovascular risk factors. You need to be knowledgeable about the metabolic responses to exercise in athletes with diabetes. With proper metabolic control, individuals with either type 1 or type 2 diabetes can participate in most athletic activities.

5. *Explain the need for adequate caloric intake for the active patient with diabetes and recognize the symptoms and treatment for hypoglycemia and hyperglycemia.*

Athletes who are able to maintain good control of their blood sugar levels can participate in sports, even on a professional level. Yet a risk of hypoglycemia or hyperglycemia exists when an athlete is unable to gauge *how much* to lower insulin doses before a bout of exercise. Because exercise enhances absorption of the injected insulin, overestimating the correct dosage can lead to severe hypoglycemia.

For Further Information

Print Resources

American Diabetes Association. 1996. *The American Diabetes Association complete guide to diabetes: The ultimate home diabetes reference.* Alexandria, VA: American Diabetes Association.

American Diabetes Association. 2002. Standards of medical care for patients with diabetes mellitus. *Diabetes Care* 25(1): 213-29.

Colberg, S.R. 2001. *The diabetic athlete.* Champaign, IL: Human Kinetics.

DeFronzo, R.A., ed. 1998. *Current therapy of diabetes mellitus.* St. Louis: Mosby.

Jimenez, C.C. 1997. Diabetes and exercise: The role of the athletic trainer. *Journal of Athletic Training* 32(4): 339-43.

Web Resources

American Diabetes Association
www.diabetes.org
The American Diabetes Association is the nation's leading nonprofit health organization, providing diabetes research, information, and advocacy. The mission of the organization is to prevent and cure diabetes and to improve the lives of all people affected by diabetes.

Centers for Disease Control and Prevention—Diabetes Public Health Resource
www.cdc.gov/diabetes/
A public health Web site sponsored by the CDC's National Center for Chronic Disease Prevention and Health Promotion.

This condition is characterized by dizziness, fatigue, hunger, mental confusion, and headache; these symptoms tend to occur when the blood glucose is declining and has a rapid onset. Most individuals begin to develop symptoms when their blood sugar is in the range of 45 to 60 mg/dl. When symptoms occur, the athlete should ingest the most readily available source of sugar, such as fruit juices, oral glucose tablets, or sometimes candy if that is the only source of glucose available. It is best to supplement these items with foods containing complex carbohydrate and protein to provide a more sustained glycemic response. If an athlete with diabetes becomes semiconscious or unconscious and protection of the airway is in doubt, do not give her anything by mouth.

Underestimating the correct dosage (i.e., overestimating the effects of exercise), on the other hand, can lead to marked and prolonged hyperglycemia and ketosis. This can occur in adolescents with poorly controlled diabetes who exercise with the express purpose of lowering their blood sugar. Hyperglycemia has a slow onset and is characterized by a patient who is lethargic, warm and dry, and weak or fatigued; has a rapid pulse, deep, rapid breathing, and a characteristic acetone odor on his breath; and may present with nausea, vomiting, excessive urination, excessive thirst, and excessive eating. People with type 1 diabetes who want to participate in sports must carefully plan their insulin injections, especially if daily workouts vary in timing, intensity, or duration.

CHAPTER 5

Eye, Ear, and Maxillofacial Pathologies

OBJECTIVES

Upon completion of this chapter the reader will be able to do the following:

1. Identify the signs and symptoms, injury mechanisms, and common injuries and infections of the eye and recognize the need for appropriate medical referral

2. Recognize injuries and conditions of the ear and determine the appropriate management

3. Describe maxillofacial pathologies that frequently occur in sports and identify potential complications associated with these injuries

4. Recognize the potential association among concussions, cervical injuries, and other injuries to the head and face

5. Identify the importance of protective devices for the teeth and eyes in competition

Athletes must keep their eyes on the ball or, at the very least, watch the action closely during practice and competition; unfortunately, the face frequently ends up *in the way* of the action. Facial injuries are common in some sports such as basketball, baseball, racket sports, and wrestling. Sports that offer face protection, such as football, see fewer facial injuries. Injuries to the face can run the gamut from nosebleeds to disfiguring fractures. Eye injuries are common and sometimes critical in nature. You need to know when to apply palliative measures and merely wait a few minutes before letting an athlete back into the game, when to have an athlete sit out the game while receiving first aid, and when to head straight for the emergency room. The information in this chapter will help you assess eye, ear, and facial injuries appropriately.

Case Study

A 17-yr-old wrestler awakes in the morning with a red, painful right eye. It continually tears and itches, and it hurts when he blinks. He does not recall getting anything into his eye. Because he has pain, the athletic trainer refers him on an urgent basis to a primary care physician, who discovers that the young man's **visual acuity (VA)** is 20/20 in the left eye and 20/60 in the right eye and that the **conjunctiva** are very swollen and red. Ophthalmoscopic examination under a black light after application of **fluorescein** reveals a dendritic (branching) pattern on the cornea. After the eye exam, the physician notices a vesicular rash on the forehead of the athlete, who reports that he previously had herpes in the same spot. Because the physician suspects herpes keratoconjunctivitis, she arranges immediate referral to an ophthalmologist. The ophthalmologist confirms the diagnosis and prescribes antiviral eyedrops to combat the herpes and cortisone eyedrops to minimize inflammation. With close follow-up and use of the drops, the athlete's infection resolves and he has normal vision. If left untreated, the herpes could have caused permanent scarring that would require a corneal transplant.

EYE TRAUMAS, INFECTIONS, AND DISORDERS

You probably will see more traumas than infections in athletes' eyes, but you should be prepared to suspect either condition, depending on an athlete's symptoms. Some traumas to the eye look frightening but are more or less benign. Others are quite dangerous and if left untreated can lead to blindness. By becoming familiar with the material in this chapter, you will have a good idea of what to do when an athlete experiences problems with eyes or other parts of the face—and, more important, you'll understand under what circumstances you should transport an athlete immediately to the nearest emergency room.

Eye Trauma

Trauma to the eye can occur in a variety of ways. A common mechanism of injury is a poke in the eye. Other common injury mechanisms include blunt trauma from a racket, ball, fist, or elbow. Determining the mechanism of injury is an essential component to a thorough evaluation and is essential information to pass along when the athlete is referred to a physician. As discussed in Garcia (1996), initial assessment of an eye injury includes the following:

- Assessing eye movements in all four directions to make sure that the eyes work together—this is called **conjugate gaze.** If the eyes do not move together, this is called **disconjugate gaze.**

Terms and Definitions

anisocoria—Inequality in pupil size that sometimes occurs naturally.

cellulitis—A spreading bacterial infection of the dermis and subcutaneous tissue; it typically begins as a small area of tenderness, redness, and swelling, and may progress to fever, chills, and swollen lymph nodes close to the infected area.

ciliary muscles—Tiny muscles within the eye that cause the lens to change shape to focus light on the retina and thus change the opening of the iris to accommodate different intensities of light.

conjugate gaze—Normal vision, when both eyes work together to point at the same place.

conjunctiva—The mucous membrane lining the inner surface of the eyelids and the outer surface of the eyeball.

cornea—The transparent, tough outer coating of the eye that covers the pupil and iris.

crepitus—A grating sound or sensation in joints, lungs, or skin.

diplopia—Double vision.

disconjugate gaze—A condition wherein the eyes do not move together.

external hordeolum—The common **sty,** which is a mild infection of the glands of Moll or Zeis in the eyelid.

fluorescein—A dye that fluoresces under black light; when applied to the eye, it can allow the examiner to see very small abrasions of the cornea.

glands of Moll/glands of Zeis—Microscopic glands in the eyelid that produce an oil that coats tears to keep them from evaporating too quickly. Infection of one of these glands produces a **sty.**

glaucoma—A condition of elevated intraocular pressure. If left untreated, glaucoma can cause permanent visual loss or blindness.

globe—The eyeball.

internal hordeolum—Infection of the **meibomian glands**.

mandible—The lower jaw.

meibomian glands—Microscopic glands in the eyelid, similar to the glands of Moll and Zeis. Infection of one of these glands produces a **sty.**

rectus muscles—The four muscles that control eye movement. Each of the four is attached to the back of the globe (eyeball). The *medial* and *lateral* rectus muscles move the eye side to side; the *superior* and *inferior* recti move the eye up and down.

sclera—The tough, fibrous coating of the exterior of the white part of the eyeball.

sty—Infection of one or more of the glands in the eyelid.

subconjunctival hemorrhage—Bleeding in the white of the eye. More specifically, a relatively harmless rupturing of tiny veins in the sclera as a result of a **Valsalva maneuver.** Typically results in a bright red triangle next to the iris.

temporomandibular joint (TMJ)—The joint at which the lower jaw attaches to the side of the skull.

Valsalva maneuver—An effort to forcibly expel air while intentionally blocking the exit of air from mouth and nostrils (as is often done when trying to clear the eustachian tubes during air travel).

visual acuity (VA)—A measure of the eye's ability to resolve two adjoining lines. The most common expression of VA is as a measurement of the smallest letters you can read on a standardized chart at 20 ft. This is usually expressed as a ratio of the distance you are from the chart to the distance at which a person with normal eyesight could read the same line. If a person's VA is 20/40, then at a distance of 20 feet from a chart that person can see what a normal person would see at 40 feet. Normal vision is 20/20.

vitreous humor (also called simply **vitreous**)—The clear, colorless gel that fills the eyeball behind the lens.

zygomatic arch (or **zygoma**)—The curved bone along the front or side of the skull beneath the eye opening (orbit); the cheekbone.

- Checking for **diplopia** (double vision), because diplopia usually accompanies disconjugate gaze.
- Noting if there is pain in the eye and the nature of any pain—whether the athlete feels like something is in her eye, if she feels generalized pain, and so forth.
- Checking for photophobia—whether light shining into the eye causes pain.
- Asking the athlete whether a flash of light appeared at the moment of impact.
- Checking whether the pupil is very constricted.
- Looking for blood in the iris.
- Checking whether any part of the white of the eye is bright red.
- Checking for asymmetry in pupil size, using a handheld light. Normal reaction of pupils to light is brisk and symmetrical—shining a light in one eye should also produce brisk pupillary constriction in the other eye. But note: *Be sure that pre-participation physical exams (chapter 19) include information about asymmetrical pupil sizes.* One to two percent of normal individuals have more than 1 mm of asymmetry in pupil size (a condition known as **anisocoria**). It is important to maintain a record of individuals who have this condition, to prevent incorrect assumptions after a head or eye injury that unequal pupil size is a result of the injury.

Corneal Abrasions

Any trauma that abrades or lacerates the **cornea** (figure 5.1) will cause pain, watering of the eye, and photophobia. For example, Jorge complains of eye pain after getting poked in the eye during a basketball practice. He states that it feels like something is in the eye and that it hurts every time he blinks. After 5 or 10 min the eye is still watering and is painful. You refer him to a physician, who diagnoses a corneal abrasion and gives him antibiotic eyedrops to prevent infection.

As with Jorge, most people with corneal abrasions will tell you that every blink causes pain as the eyelid moves over the injured surface of the cornea. Such injuries are best diagnosed by a physician using fluorescein dye and illuminating the eye with a black light in a dark room (figure 5.2). The eye must be examined with a magnifying lens. Any irregularity of the cornea will take up the dye. It is important to examine the entire eye—including under the eyelids—with a bright light to ascertain whether a foreign body is present. Although deep lacerations need atten-

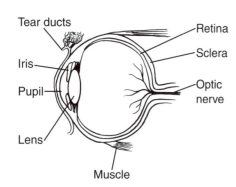

■ Figure 5.1   The anatomy of the eye in cross-section. The cornea is the clear covering over the pupil and iris of the eye.

Reprinted, by permission, from L.A. Cartwright and W.A. Pitney, 1999, *Athletic training for student assistants* (Champaign, IL: Human Kinetics), 62.

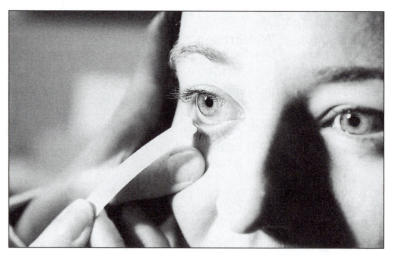

■ Figure 5.2   Instilling fluorescein dye using a dye strip, which needs to just touch the lower lid. This dye makes it much easier for a physician or properly trained athletic trainer to identify abrasions with a black light.

tion from an eye specialist, primary care providers can care for small abrasions and lacerations by treating with antibiotic eyedrops and checking on the individual's progress by phone or in an office visit in 12 to 24 h. Corneal lesions that do not heal in 24 to 36 h usually need to be seen by an eye specialist. Patients who wear contact lenses must be particularly cautious. If there is any concern that an abrasion exists, the patient should not wear contacts until she is evaluated. Poorly cleansed, torn, or old contact lenses may be the source of a nontraumatic abrasion. In addition, following trauma to the eye, it is imperative that the patient remove the contact lens to avoid further aggravation (see *Eyewear and Contact Lenses*).

Although standard treatment primarily included having the patient wear an eye patch to prevent painful blinking, today most eye specialists prefer to leave the eye unpatched because a patch itself can cause trauma. Instruct the athlete not to rub the eye, since this will cause more trauma to the cornea. It is good practice to have the athlete wear a pair of sunglasses. This will reduce photophobia and will help discourage rubbing of the eye.

Eyewear and Contact Lenses

Eyewear that is used in sports and recreation may include both corrective lenses to improve visual acuity and protective lenses to reduce the risk of injury. It is estimated that one-third of all people participating in sports require corrective lenses to improve vision.

Contact Lenses

Contact lenses are a common form of corrective eyewear used by athletes. They allow for greater peripheral vision as well as correction of visual irregularities, and athletes find them desirable for cosmetic reasons as well. They do not provide the protection of sports goggles. Contact lenses may be dislodged or lost, thus requiring that wearers keep a duplicate set of lenses available. Those who wear contact lenses must adhere faithfully to the guidelines for their use and care. Infected solutions, torn lenses, and improper wear are all common causes for eye infections and abrasions.

Protective Lenses

Eye protection is recommended for people who play racket sports such as squash, handball, racquetball, and paddleball. Protective lenses should also be worn for those sports that involve a projectile (such as a ball or stick) that can potentially cause ocular damage. Athletes must keep in mind, however, that although eye-protection devices are designed to reduce the risk of injury, they cannot guarantee the prevention of injury.

Guidelines

- Eye protection is recommended for participants in collision and contact sports who use corrective lenses (including contacts).
- All participants in racket sports such as squash, handball, racquetball, and paddleball should have eye protection that conforms to standards of the American Society for Testing and Materials (ASTM). This protection should include closed lenses, because open-lens (no-lens) protection has been shown to be ineffective.
- Athletes should consider eye protection in sports that use a projectile of a size, consistency, or speed capable of causing ocular injuries. This protection should meet ASTM standards.
- If external lenses are used for protection (sport spectacles), they should be made of polycarbonate plastic or CR-39 (a type of hard plastic).
- All one-eyed participants (those whose best correction in their weaker eye is 20/80 or worse) in collision and contact sports should wear eye protection.

Adapted from NCAA Committee on Competitive Safeguards and Medical Aspects of Sports 2001.

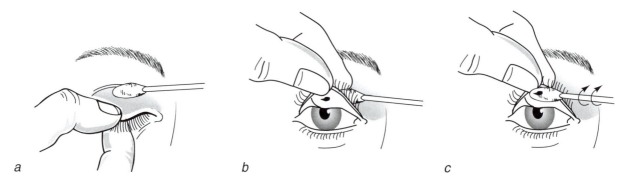

a   *b*   *c*

■ **Figure 5.3**   Everting the eyelid to find a foreign body.

The tiniest foreign body in the eye can produce a great deal of discomfort. If the increased tearing does not wash the particle out, irrigation with saline may help. If the particle is caught on the **sclera** or cornea, sometimes you can remove it by simply touching it gently with a moist, sterile cotton swab. If the foreign body is caught on the inside of the upper eyelid, you'll need to evert the lid before the object becomes visible. Figure 5.3 illustrates this technique: Gently apply pressure on the top of the upper lid with a cotton swab and gently pull the eyelashes out (*a*). Then pull them up over the swab (*b*) (or, for the lower lid, apply the swab to the bottom of the lid, gently pulling the lashes out and down). Finally, remove the object by touching it with another moist, sterile cotton swab (*c*). This procedure is usually not particularly uncomfortable to the patient. If the foreign body is removed from the lid, the symptoms will usually resolve with no further treatment unless the cornea has also been abraded.

Trauma to the Globe or Surrounding Tissues

The eyeball, or **globe,** is housed in the bony orbit, protected above by the orbital rim, below by the cheekbone (zygoma), and on the sides by the nose and the cheekbone. Large objects, such as large balls, strike the face and orbit before causing any trauma to the eye. Small objects, however, such as tennis balls and baseballs, can strike the eyeball itself and cause significant trauma. When an object strikes the eyeball, an increase in pressure within the eyeball can be transmitted to the bony orbit, the lower portion of which (the inferior orbit) is very thin, leading to an orbital blowout fracture (figure 5.4). This fracture tends to trap the inferior **rectus muscle,** preventing the person from being able to look up with that eye, and therefore resulting in double vision (diplopia) during an upward gaze (figure 5.5). This injury requires immediate care from an ophthalmologist.

If a blow to the eye fractures the iris, bleeding in the anterior chamber can occur, producing a hyphema (figure 5.6). The blood in the anterior chamber of the eye can rapidly cause an inflammatory reaction and pain. Spasm of the **ciliary muscles** (those that control the opening of the iris and the shape of the lens) produces pain, and the pupil becomes very constricted. The blood sometimes layers out in the lower portion of the iris—and if the person has a blue or light-colored iris, close inspection of the iris may permit you actually to see the meniscus of fluid. Immediately refer a patient with this injury to an ophthalmologist or an emergency facility. If possible, the patient should be transported in a seated or upright position.

When the globe is depressed, the retina can peel off the inside of the eyeball and float into the **vitreous humor** (the gel that fills most of the globe). This condition can be difficult to diagnose; although detachment is associated with a deficit in the field of vision, an athlete may not immediately notice a small deficit, and detached retinas do not always produce significant pain. The most common symptom is a

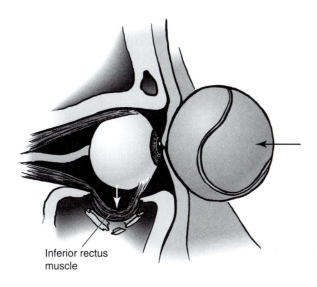

Inferior rectus
muscle

■ **Figure 5.4** A blowout fracture occurs from blows to the eyeball. The force can fracture the inferior orbital rim, which can trap the inferior rectus muscle.

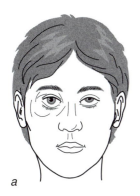

a

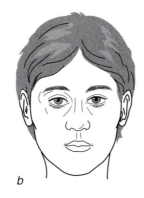

b

■ **Figure 5.5** When the athlete is asked to gaze upward, *(a)* the normal left eye moves up while the injured right eye still appears to look straight ahead. If the athlete is not asked to do this, *(b)* the eyes appear normal, as they do on the right.

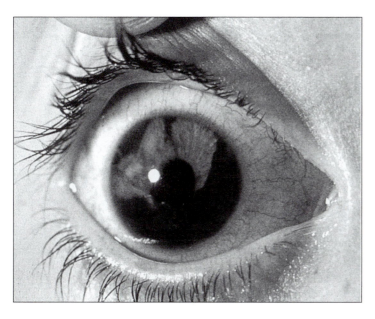

■ **Figure 5.6** Bleeding from a fractured iris, resulting in a hyphema.

Reprinted, with permission, from Trobe, J.D. *The Physician's Guide to Health Care,* 2nd edition. San Francisco: American Academy of Ophthalmology; 2001.

flash of light contemporaneous with the blow to the eye. Any flash of light occurring with trauma warrants an immediate phone call to an ophthalmologist and an office visit within a few hours.

Some mild trauma causes only temporary blurring of vision, ciliary spasm, and watering—and within 10 to 15 min the athlete feels fine and has normal visual acuity. Occasionally a **subconjunctival hemorrhage** appears as a bright red triangle adjacent to the iris (figure 5.7). It looks frightful but is often painless. The hemorrhage typically results from a **Valsalva maneuver**—a process (often done unconsciously) whereby the athlete stops his mouth and nose to keep from expelling air but pushes with his diaphragm and chest muscles as if to expel air forcefully (air travelers may also perform this maneuver during flight to clear the eustachian tubes). The action increases venous pressure to the extent that small scleral vessels rupture. Valsalva maneuvers occur frequently in weightlifting, forceful coughing, and vomiting, and in women during labor.

As an example, Stephanie, a 17-yr-old shot putter, consults you because of bright red blood on the white part of her eye. She reports no pain and no history of an injury. She states that her vision is normal, but everyone keeps asking her what happened. You send her to a physician, and with further questioning, she remembers an intense weightlifting session using heavy weights the day before her visit with you. The physician examines her eye and reports that the exam is normal except for the hemorrhage and that it will take several days to resolve. He does not restrict her activity. Subconjunctival hemorrhages are not dangerous, and they heal with no treatment. If you see an athlete with a subconjuctival hemorrhage as a result of possible trauma to the eye, check carefully for signs of a more severe injury to the rest of the eye.

Eye Infections

Infections can occur in and around the eyeball itself, or in the skin surrounding the eye. **External hordeolum** is the medical term for the common **sty,** which is a mild infection of the **glands of Moll or Zeis** in the eyelid (figure 5.8). These sebaceous glands produce a thin layer of oil that covers tears to slow their evaporation. A deeper infection on the inside of the eyelid is called an **internal hordeolum**—an infection of the **meibomian glands,** whose function is similar to that of the glands of Moll or Zeis. Both kinds of infections are treated in the same way: Sties rarely

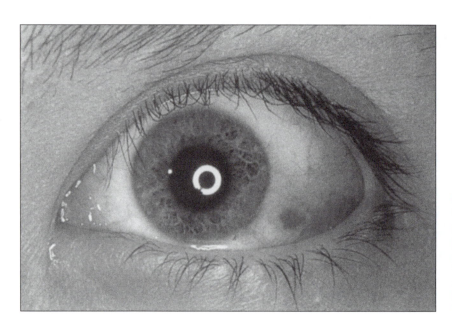

■ **Figure 5.7** Subconjunctival hemorrhage. This condition usually looks more serious than it really is.

Reprinted, with permission, from Trobe, J.D. *The Physician's Guide to Health Care,* 2nd edition. San Francisco: American Academy of Ophthalmology; 2001.

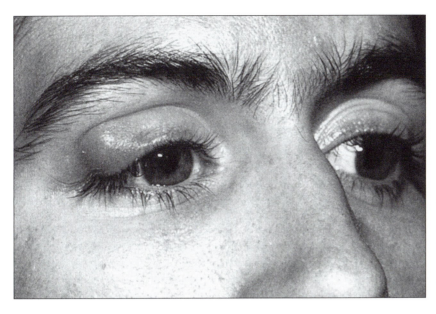

■ **Figure 5.8** A common sty—in this case, an external hordeolum.

Reprinted, with permission, from Trobe, J.D. *The Physician's Guide to Health Care,* 2nd edition. San Francisco: American Academy of Ophthalmology; 2001.

require surgical attention and often drain and resolve within 3 to 5 days. Treatment usually consists of frequent application of warm compresses, at least four times a day for 5 to 10 min at a time. Note: If the entire eyelid and surrounding tissue are swollen and warm, the infection is more serious and probably indicates **cellulitis,** which can occur without a sty or predisposing lesion. Cellulitis requires an urgent visit to a physician for antibiotic therapy.

The most common eye infection is conjunctivitis, which involves the conjunctival vessels that include the vessels on the sclera (figure 5.9). Numerous cold viruses, as well as a number of bacteria, cause conjunctivitis (commonly called pinkeye). Unfortunately, it is virtually impossible to distinguish viral conjunctivitis from its bacterial counterpart. Conjunctivitis can start in only one eye but within 1 to 2 d usually involves the other eye. There may be increased tearing and mattering of the eye, especially upon awakening in the morning. Conjunctivitis does not significantly affect visual acuity; although rarely painful, it may cause

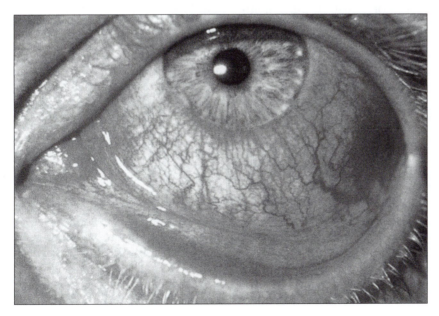

■ **Figure 5.9** Conjunctivitis (pinkeye).

Reprinted, with permission, from Trobe, J.D. *The Physician's Guide to Health Care,* 2nd edition. San Francisco: American Academy of Ophthalmology; 2001.

mild itching. Although doctors cannot know whether the cause is bacterial or viral (antibiotics have no effect against the viral form), they often prescribe antibiotic eyedrops just in case the cause is bacterial. Sometimes the best remedy is time and warm compresses. Warn people with conjunctivitis that the infection is quite contagious—no one else should use the same towel or pillow as an infected person; and those with conjunctivitis should wash their hands every time they touch their faces. Most cases of conjunctivitis last 7 to 10 d. Tell infected individuals to consult a physician if they experience significant pain and photophobia, which suggest corneal involvement and perhaps infection by a herpes virus—a potentially much more serious infection than one that is caused by cold viruses as discussed in the case at the beginning of this chapter.

Misuse of contact lenses can lead to eye infections. Most contact lenses, whether or not they are disposable, are made of soft plastic and can be worn for extended periods—and leaving lenses in the eye for periods longer than prescribed can lead to eye infections. Wearing infected lenses for a long time can permanently scar the cornea. Any redness or irritation associated with contact lenses warrants investigation and may require a consultation with the eye doctor who prescribed the lenses. Athletes should always have glasses as a backup to their contact lenses in case infection or other circumstances prevent them from wearing the contacts (see *Eyewear and Contact Lenses*, page 59).

Eye Allergies

Conjunctivitis caused by environmental allergens can be difficult to distinguish from that caused by infection. It usually can be diagnosed by a history of allergies, a history of similar problems at the same time each year (e.g., certain pollens are more common in the spring, others in the fall), and the prominence of itching as a symptom. It often accompanies symptoms of allergic rhinitis. Allergic conjunctivitis can be treated with oral antihistamines, antihistamine eyedrops, or a combination of the two. Some anti-inflammatory eyedrops are available only by prescription.

Glaucoma

Glaucoma is a condition of elevated intraocular pressure resulting from blockage of the flow of fluid in the anterior chamber of the eye. When left untreated, glaucoma is a common cause of permanent visual loss. Treatment has traditionally consisted of eyedrops that relieve the blockage; a more recent treatment uses a laser to painlessly punch a hole in the iris, thus relieving the pressure. In its acute form, symptoms develop suddenly and consist of red, painful eye and a marked decrease in visual acuity. People with these symptoms must see an eye specialist immediately. More often than not, however, glaucoma has no subjective symptoms. As the disease advances, a person may notice peripheral vision disappearing—but by this point, it may be too late to prevent blindness. High-risk groups are people with a family history of glaucoma, African Americans over the age of 40, and anyone over the age of 60. People in these populations should have a dilated-pupil eye exam (not just an air-puff pressure exam) every 2 yr.

EAR TRAUMA, INFECTIONS, AND DISORDERS

Direct trauma to the external ear (auricle) can cause hemorrhage and a hematoma. A hematoma involving muscle or skin usually leads to the body's inflammatory process healing the injury with no sequelae. When a hematoma occurs adjacent to cartilage, the cartilage can be destroyed during the inflammatory process as the hematoma is absorbed. An auricular hematoma may result in a deformity

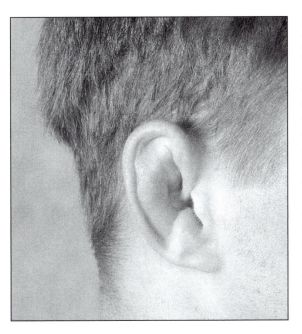

■ **Figure 5.10**   A cauliflower ear resulting from an auricular hematoma.

Reprinted, by permission, from S.J. Shultz, P.A. Houglum, and D.H. Perrin, 2000, *Assessment of athletic injuries* (Champaign, IL: Human Kinetics), 355.

known as cauliflower ear (figure 5.10). Damage to the ear may be reduced by evacuating the blood. Numerous methods exist for removal of blood in the auricle. Most practitioners drain the blood using sterile technique with a needle and syringe and pack the ear with a compression dressing. If one of your athletes sustains a hematoma of the ear, a physician should be consulted in the first 48 to 72 h after the injury. Once the hematoma begins to form scar tissue, it can no longer be drained.

A direct blow over the opening of the ear canal can cause high pressure in the canal and rupture the tympanic membrane. This may occur in divers due to water pressure and also can occur when a fist or open hand strikes the ear. The rupture produces immediate intense pain and usually a decrement in hearing. Most ruptures heal quickly (72 h), but the athlete must not get water in the ear canal until a physician documents that the hole in the tympanic membrane has healed. Nonsterile water entering the middle ear can cause an infection and prevent the perforation from healing. An athlete with a suspected perforation should be evaluated by a physician within 24 to 48 h of the injury.

Ear pain without trauma may be due to excessive cerumen (earwax) buildup, an infection of the ear canal (otitis externa), an infection of the middle ear (otitis media), or pain in the temporomandibular joint. The only way to diagnose excessive wax buildup is to look in the ear canal with an otoscope. If the eardrum is not visible and cerumen seems to be blocking the entire canal, the wax needs to irrigated with tepid water or hydrogen peroxide by a knowledgeable practitioner. If cerumen is the culprit, removal of the wax relieves the pain immediately.

Otitis externa is commonly known as swimmer's ear because the canal gets infected from water that sits in the ear canal after swimming. One of the signs is pain with movement of the auricle. Otitis externa typically occurs after swimming in a lake or river that has a higher bacteria level than a chlorinated pool. Occasionally people get the ear canal wet while bathing or taking a shower. Some people are prone to this condition; it may be familial, related to the shape of the ear canal. If the ear canal is shaped in a way that allows water to pool at the bottom, an infection is more likely. The bacterium that causes otitis externa is almost always *Pseudomonas aeriginosa*. A mild infection can be treated with rubbing alcohol or a mixture of alcohol and vinegar. Anything that dries the canal or makes it more acidic prevents the growth of bacteria. If the canal is red and swollen, alcohol will burn, and a physician needs to prescribe antibiotic drops. Occasionally the canal becomes so swollen that the debris and wax must be removed with special equipment in the office of an ear, nose, and throat specialist (otolaryngologist). People who are prone to swimmer's ear learn to dry the canal carefully after swimming or instill alcohol or an eardrop to prevent an infection.

Otitis media is an infection behind the eardrum. It is highly associated with the common cold and allergic rhinitis because of the associated dysfunction of the eustachian tubes, the mucosa-lined connections between the throat and the middle ear (figure 5.11). Any process that irritates the mucosa of the nose and makes the eustachian tubes function abnormally is associated with otitis media. Typically

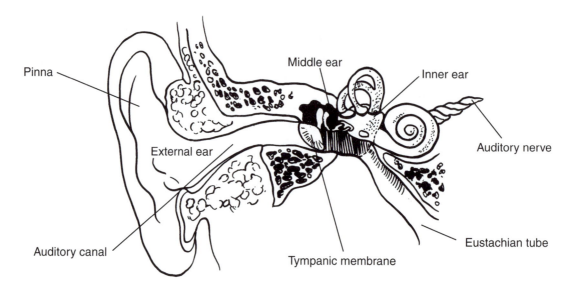

■ **Figure 5.11**   The anatomy of the middle ear.

Adapted, by permission, from L.A. Cartwright and W.A. Pitney, 1999, *Athletic training for student assistants* (Champaign, IL: Human Kinetics), 130.

otitis media occurs after a person has had a cold for a week or more. If the eusta-chian tube will not open to ventilate the middle ear, air is absorbed and a vacuum develops. More mucus is therefore secreted, which fills the middle ear. Without an infection, this state is called a middle ear effusion; it frequently accompanies the common cold, producing what is often referred to as a *plugged ear* because it can cause a mild hearing deficit. If any bacteria make their way from the throat up the eustachian tube and into the middle ear, an abscess develops. This abscess causes swelling and bulging of the eardrum, which is often very painful. The bacteria that cause ear infections are the same as those that inhabit the nose and can cause sinus infections. Most ear infections will resolve with no treatment. Complications occur if the infection spreads into the bone around the ear (mastoiditis) or gets into the bloodstream to cause pneumonia or meningitis. Because of these complications, it is common practice for physicians to treat otitis media with an antibiotic, usually for 7 to 10 d.

Temporomandibular joint (TMJ) dysfunction may cause ear pain because the joint lies just anterior to the external ear canal. The TMJ is easily palpated just anterior to the tragus or by inserting a finger into the ear canal and palpating the anterior wall of the canal. Typically the person with TMJ pain has been vigorously chewing something like a bagel, meat, or too much chewing gum. Any dental or orthodontic work that changes a person's bite may result in TMJ pain.

MAXILLOFACIAL INJURIES

Trauma to the head and face tends to cause profuse bleeding, making field ex-amination emotionally stressful. As with any injury, it is important to help the athlete stay calm. And remember the ABC rule: Check *a*irway, *b*reathing, and *c*ir-culation. Consider any blow to the head that alters consciousness as a potential cervical spine injury until the athlete can respond to questions about the neck. Checking the ABCs and ruling out a cervical spine injury are critical factors in on-field decisions. Remember, however, that even seemingly minor maxillo-facial injuries can be associated with an underlying concussion. When dealing with these injuries it is important not to be "misled by the obvious." If an athlete sustains an injury mechanism that is sufficient to cause a hematoma, nosebleed, or facial laceration, she may have sustained a blow that could cause a concussion. The nosebleed is the obvious injury; the possible underlying concussion is less obvious. The careful practitioner will care for the obvious and evaluate for the less obvious.

Larynx

Trauma to the larynx can cause swelling or bleeding (or both) that compromises the airway. Although the initial spasm may frighten the athlete, it usually subsides in seconds. If there is significant injury to the larynx, the thyroid cartilage (Adam's apple) may lose its prominence. Hoarseness or persistent loss of voice implies an injury to the larynx. **Crepitus** in the neck may be caused by a fracture of the cartilage with leakage of air into the subcutaneous tissue (subcutaneous emphysema). Because of the potential for airway compromise, an athlete with a significant injury to the larynx should be taken immediately to the nearest emergency facility.

Oral Trauma

Increased use of protective mouth guards has diminished the incidence of injuries to the teeth. Yet such injuries still occur in sports that do not require mouth guards and when athletes fail to use them. Most athletes find custom-made mouth guards more comfortable than off-the-shelf devices and therefore are more likely to use them. Custom-made guards also seem to provide more protection from injury. Because custom-made guards are significantly more expensive than the other type, you must decide whether your budget can justify their use.

If a tooth is completely knocked out (extruded), it must be handled properly to optimize chances that it can be reimplanted:

- Handle the tooth only by the crown.
- Do not rub the tooth to remove dirt.
- Rinse the tooth with saline solution to remove dirt; use tap water if you have no saline.
- If the tooth is clean and it is obvious where it goes, try to replace it as soon as possible into the socket. Have the athlete bite down gently on gauze to keep the tooth in place. If a mouth guard is available and is not distorted, it can make an excellent splint.
- If the tooth is too soiled or if it is not clear how it should fit into the socket, store it in a proper environment. Conscious adults can store the tooth under the tongue or in the cheek until a dentist is available. Otherwise, store the tooth in a small cup containing the athlete's saliva. Milk is a good alternative storage medium; and commercial solutions for tooth storage are available that can be kept in powder form in the medical bag.
- Ensure that the athlete sees a dentist immediately (within 2 h). A tooth that is not reimplanted within 2 h is much less likely to survive. As discussed by Roberts (2000), an avulsed tooth should be reimplanted within 30 min for best results.

Fractures to the teeth are classified based on the specific tissue affected. Some fractures may involve only the surface or enamel of the tooth (i.e., a chip) (figure 5.12, fracture *a)*, whereas more severe fractures may involve the root or expose the inner pulp of the tooth (figure 5.12, fractures *b-d)*.

Chipped teeth can be very uncomfortable. Covering the sharp edge with beeswax or a similar material will temporarily relieve the discomfort. If the chip is

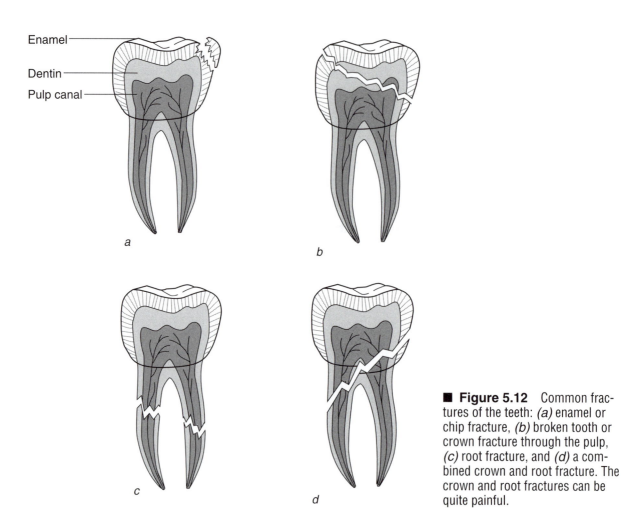

Enamel
Dentin
Pulp canal

a   *b*

c   *d*

■ **Figure 5.12**   Common fractures of the teeth: *(a)* enamel or chip fracture, *(b)* broken tooth or crown fracture through the pulp, *(c)* root fracture, and *(d)* a combined crown and root fracture. The crown and root fractures can be quite painful.

available, save it. A dentist may be able to bond it back to the tooth. If that cannot be done, the sharp edges of the chipped tooth should be filed smooth by a dentist. Dentists should evaluate loose teeth to look for fractures of the roots. Sometimes the dentist can stabilize loose teeth with specially constructed splints.

Nose

Because of its prominence on the face, the nose is traumatized frequently. It is very vascular and bleeds with little trauma. Most episodes of nosebleed occur from injury to the anterior plexus, which is the complex of tiny, fragile blood vessels in the front of the nose on both sides of the septum. The first step in treating nasal trauma is to stop the bleeding. Have the athlete remain upright (usually sitting), with direct pressure over the nose; compression of the nose is more effective if the nares (the nostrils) are held together to apply pressure on the septum. The pressure should be held constantly for at least 10 min (the most common error is removing the pressure too soon). If the bleeding does not subside after 30 min of compression, take the individual to the nearest emergency facility.

Once the bleeding has stopped, a knowledgeable professional should assess the nose for evidence of fracture. Asymmetry or crepitus with palpation indicates a fracture. As discussed by Stackhouse (1998) one should also look for septal deformity or any evidence of a septal hematoma—a mass of (usually) clotted blood within the septum (figure 5.13). A septal hematoma should be drained by a physician because the inflammatory reaction can destroy cartilage and result in an in-

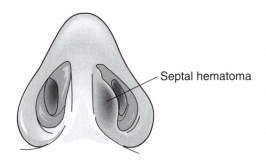

■ **Figure 5.13**   Septal hematoma. The hematoma appears as a bulge into the patient's left nostril. The patient's right nostril (on the left of the picture) is normal. The bulge can be seen as a blue mass on the nasal septum when examined with speculum and light. (The otoscope with an ear speculum can be used to examine the nostril and septum.)

dentation in the slope of the nose (commonly called a saddle nose deformity). Most nasal fractures do need to be seen eventually, but not necessarily as an emergency. Athletes with a gross deformity or depression of the nasal bridge clearly should be evaluated the same day as the injury. Otherwise, most ear, nose, and throat specialists prefer to reduce nasal fractures several days after the injury, after the swelling has subsided.

Maxillary Fractures

Fractures to the midface usually are caused by a high-energy injury such as a blow from a stick, fist, or hard ball. They are classified as Le Fort I, II, or III, depending on whether nasal bones and cheekbones are involved (figure 5.14). Other than bruising, signs of a fracture are lengthening of the face, mobility of the midface, malocclusion of the teeth, nasal deformity, or flattening and splaying of the naso-orbital region. Some of these injuries can impede the airway; often the athlete will not be able to talk or will be able to talk only poorly. Because of the risk of bleeding and of blockage to the airway, take the athlete immediately to an emergency facility.

Mandibular Fractures

Blows to the jaw (**mandible**) are common in collision sports. If an athlete can open her jaw and close it comfortably without much pain, she probably does not have a fracture—especially if she can bite down comfortably without malocclusion. The

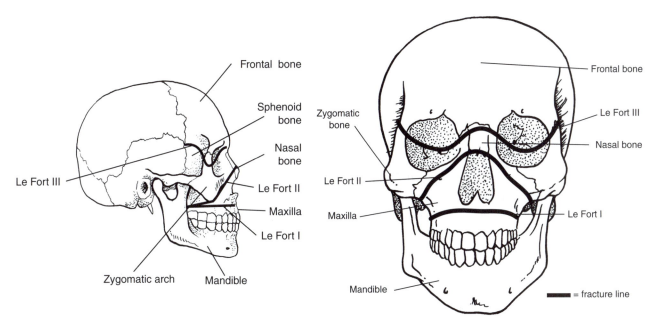

■ **Figure 5.14**   Bones of the face and the location fractures classified as Le Fort I, II, and III. Though it is by no means up to you to diagnose such fractures, it is important for you to understand this terminology for two reasons: (1) so that you will be able to interpret correctly physicians' notes regarding these types of fractures and (2) so that you will be aware of how complex such injuries can be.

Adapted, by permission, from L.A. Cartwright and W.A. Pitney, 1999, *Athletic training for student assistants* (Champaign, IL: Human Kinetics), 131.

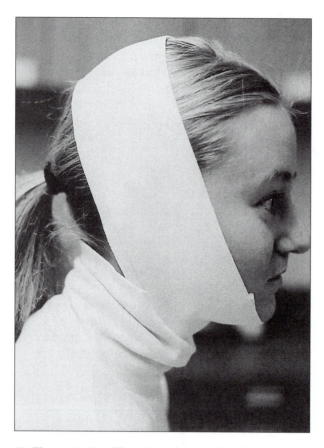

■ Figure 5.15 Wrapping a fractured jaw for transporting the patient to an emergency facility.

common signs of a jaw fracture are change in bite, mobility of the mandible in segments, pain while opening the mouth, inability to bite or chew, deviation of the jaw on opening, numbness of the lower lip, or bruising of the gums and floor of the mouth. Fractures usually occur at the angle of the jaw (the condyle). Condyle fractures may produce pain and tenderness in the area just in front of the ear, in addition to some of the signs mentioned previously. You may need to wrap the athlete's jaw to support it during the trip to the hospital. Simply wrapping a bandage under the chin and over the head will keep a fractured jaw stable (figure 5.15).

Fractures of the Cheekbone

Fractures of the cheekbone **(zygoma)** typically result from a high-velocity blow from a stick, fist, or hard ball. Because the cheekbone is so close to the eye, always suspect secondary eye injuries. A zygoma fracture may produce flatness of the cheek, limited mandibular opening, change in sensation of the cheek, swelling and bruising of the tissue, air in the soft tissue (emphysema), subconjunctival hemorrhage, sinking of the eye into the socket, double vision, limitation of eye movement, discontinuity in the bone of the orbital rims, or bruising inside the mouth. Any of these symptoms calls for an immediate trip to the nearest emergency facility.

Temporomandibular Joint Injuries

The **temporomandibular joint (TMJ)** is a hinge joint that can be injured by any blow to the mandible. As in the knee joint, a crescent-shaped cartilage (meniscus) in this joint is quite susceptible to injury. Injury to the joint may limit opening of the jaw (normal opening is more than 4.0 cm, or 1.5 in.) or cause deviation to the side of the injury on opening the jaw, severe pain with opening or biting, malocclusion, crepitus of the joint, or inability to close the mouth. If the disability does not improve or resolve within an hour or so, the athlete needs a dental evaluation for a possible fracture.

Acute dislocations of the TMJ can occur from yawning or from trauma. The athlete will be unable to close the mouth, and the skin will have a dimple in front of the joint. If the dislocation is unilateral, the mandible will be deviated to one side. When the TMJ is dislocated, the mandible is sitting in front of the articular eminence and cannot return to the normal position because of muscle spasm (figure 5.16a). To reposition the mandible, the practitioner should sit in front of the athlete and place the thumbs over the molars with the other fingers under the chin. Pressing down and slightly back on the posterior part of the mandible while raising the chin will relocate the TMJ (figure 5.16b). Do not attempt this if a condylar fracture is suspected. A fracture can mimic a dislocation, and you do not want to displace a fracture. (If the relocation attempt is unsuccessful, immediately transport the athlete to an emergency facility for X rays.) After completing the reduction, apply

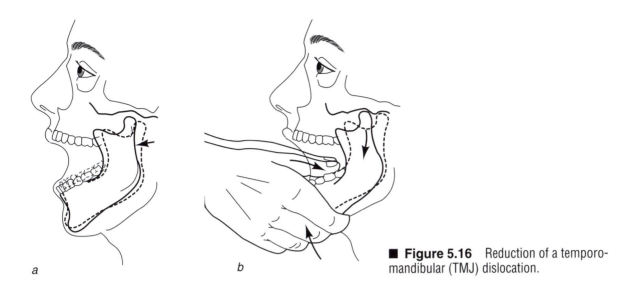

a   b

■ **Figure 5.16** Reduction of a temporo-mandibular (TMJ) dislocation.

For Further Information

Print Resources

Handler, S.D. 1991. Diagnosis and management of maxillofacial injuries. In *Athletic injuries to the head, neck and face,* ed. Torg, J., chapter 40. St. Louis: Mosby Yearbook.

Kaufman, B.R., and F.R. Heckler. 1997. Sports-related facial injuries. *Clinics in Sport Medicine* 16(3): 543-61.

Krasner, P. 2000. Management of sports-related tooth displacements and avulsions. *Dental Clinics of North America* 44(1): 111-35.

NCAA Committee on Competitive Safeguards and Medical Aspects of Sports. 2001. Eye safety in sports. Revised 1999. *2000-2001 NCAA Sports Medicine Handbook,* 68-69. Indianapolis: NCAA.

Trobe, J.D. 2001. *The physician's guide to eye care,* 2d ed. San Francisco: Foundation of the American Academy of Ophthalmology.

Web Resources

National Library of Medicine and National Institutes of Health
www.nlm.nih.gov/medlineplus/eyeinjuries.html
A Web site maintained by the National Library of Medicine and National Institutes of Health (NIH) with public information on eye injuries, eye disease, and vision correction.

National Eye Institute
www.nei.nih.gov
The National Eye Institute (NEI) is the primary NIH organization for research on eye injuries. The NEI conducts and supports research that helps prevent and treat eye diseases and other vision disorders. This research leads to sight-saving treatments, reduces visual impairment and blindness, and improves the quality of life for people of all ages.

ice to the jaw and tell the athlete not to open the mouth completely; otherwise the dislocation can recur. Chewing will be difficult for several weeks. A dentist should be consulted to help manage the TMJ injury, because it can produce pain for weeks after an injury and occasionally produce chronic symptoms. Some athletes with TMJ pain benefit from use of a dental splint (worn primarily during sleep).

Most people with TMJ pain need to avoid chewing until they are more comfortable. They often need to use analgesic or anti-inflammatory medication (such as ibuprofen) for several weeks after the injury.

SUMMARY

1. *Identify the signs and symptoms, injury mechanisms, and common injuries and infections of the eye and recognize the need for appropriate medical referral.*

Trauma to the eye can occur in a variety of ways. A common mechanism of injury to the eye is the poke in the eye. Other common injury mechanisms include blunt trauma from a racket, ball, fist, or elbow. Determining the mechanism of injury is an essential component to a thorough evaluation and is essential information to pass along when the athlete is referred to a physician.

Signs and symptoms of eye injuries include inability to move the eye in all four directions, diplopia (double vision), pain, a sensation associated with a foreign object, photophobia (light sensitivity), redness or bleeding into the sclera or white of the eye, changes to the pupil or iris, a flash of light with contact, and partial or complete loss of vision. Infections often are associated with redness, photophobia, a "weepy" or tearing eye, pain, and a sensation of irritation. Allied health professionals must make appropriate medical referral for any patient with changes in vision, photophobia, a known mechanism associated with fracture, diplopia, or pain.

2. *Recognize injuries and conditions of the ear and determine the appropriate management.*

Auricular hematomas and injuries that can rupture the tympanic membrane are the most common injuries to the ear. Auricular hematomas must be managed by a physician within the first 48 to 72 h of the injury. Draining the hematoma and providing compression will allow for the best result and the least cosmetic deformity to the ear; once the hematoma begins to form scar tissue, it can no longer be drained. Ruptures to the tympanic membrane usually result from a blow to the ear. They are painful and usually present with a decrement in hearing. Most ruptures heal quickly (72 h), but the athlete must not get water in the ear canal until a physician documents that the hole in the tympanic membrane has healed. An athlete with a suspected perforation should be evaluated by a physician within 24 to 48 h of the injury.

3. *Describe maxillofacial pathologies that frequently occur in sports and identify potential complications associated with these injuries.*

While most maxillofacial injuries take the form of lacerations and hematomas, fractures can occur to the maxilla, mandible, zygomatic arch, nose, and supporting bones of the eye. Injuries to this region can result from direct or indirect trauma. Although the majority of these injuries are not life threatening, it is imperative to treat any injury resulting in neurological or sensory deficits as a potential catastrophic injury.

4. *Recognize the potential association among concussions, cervical injuries, and other injuries to the head and face.*

Allied health personnel responding to a head or face injury should consider any blow to the head that alters consciousness as a potential cervical spine injury until the athlete can respond to questions about the neck. Checking the ABCs (*a*irway, *b*reathing, and *c*irculation) and ruling out a cervical spine injury are critical factors in on-field decisions. Remember, however, that even seemingly minor maxillofacial injuries can mask an underlying concussion. When dealing with these injuries, it is important not to be "misled by the obvious." If an athlete sustains an injury mechanism that is sufficient to cause a hematoma, nosebleed, or facial laceration, she may have sustained a blow that could cause a concussion and should therefore be evaluated and referred appropriately.

5. *Identify the importance of protective devices for the teeth and eyes in competition.*

Using protective devices can significantly reduce injuries to the teeth and eyes. Mouth guards have been shown to decrease the likelihood of tooth-related injury. Most athletes find custom-made mouth guards more comfortable than off-the-shelf devices and therefore are more likely to use them. Because custom-made guards are significantly more expensive than the other type, you must decide whether your budget can justify their use. Eye protection is recommended for participants in collision and contact sports who use corrective lenses (including contacts). All participants in racket sports such as squash, handball, racquetball, and paddleball should have eye protection that conforms to standards of the American Society for Testing and Materials (ASTM). All one-eyed participants (those whose best correction in their weaker eye is 20/80 or worse) in collision and contact sports should have eye protection.

CHAPTER 6

Gender-Based Pathologies

OBJECTIVES

Upon completion of this chapter the reader will be able to do the following:

1. Define the components of the female athlete triad

2. Recognize the signs, symptoms, and treatment strategies for disordered eating

3. Explain the difference between primary and secondary amenorrhea

4. Discuss the determinants of bone mineral density

5. Discuss various irregularities in the menstrual cycle and reproductive system

It was not until 1967 that a woman first completed the Boston Marathon (after illegally entering the race) and not until 1972 that women were officially allowed to enter the race. Title IX of the Educational Amendments Act was passed that same year, prohibiting sex discrimination in any educational program or activity at educational institutions that receive federal funding. The number of female athletes participating in sports has increased dramatically over the last quarter century, with one of every three high school girls participating in varsity sports. With more participation at the high school and college levels, more opportunities exist for women to receive elite coaching, strength training, medical expertise, and media attention.

During the 1990s, the media focused increasing attention on the success of women involved in sports. In the last years of the 20th century and at the beginning of the 21st, three new magazines in the United States were devoted to women's sports—fueled in large part by public interest in women who won Olympic gold medals in softball, ice hockey, and soccer. The national exposure will no doubt inspire increasing numbers of adolescent and preadolescent girls to participate in all types of sports. Women's participation in sports results in countless short- and long-term benefits—including more positive body image, lowered rates of teen pregnancy, and reduced risk of breast cancer and osteoporosis (Freedson et al. 2000).

Unfortunately, overzealous or obsessed female athletes risk adverse health consequences and are more likely to encounter these consequences than their male counterparts. You probably will have many opportunities to recognize these pathological conditions and intervene in an appropriate manner. Moreover, there are a number of health problems of the reproductive system that athletes have in common with the rest of the population. Some of these disorders require prompt professional attention. Others are at best annoying, but sometimes temporarily debilitating, and require your patience and understanding when a female athlete may be unable to participate in a workout or even a competition.

Case Study

A 17-yr-old cross-country runner has just completed cross-training to recover from a second stress fracture, and you are part of her rehabilitation team. As she weighs herself, you overhear her tell a classmate that she "can never gain weight." As she is 5 ft 4 in. (163 cm) and weighs 108 lb (49 kg), you suspect her public claims about inability to gain weight might be a red herring to hide an underlying determination to *lose* weight—that is, you are concerned about a possible eating disorder. After gaining her confidence, over several discussion sessions you tactfully begin to explore various reasons why she in fact wants to lose weight, how she is losing the weight, her competitive status at this weight when she is fully recovered from her current injury, her menstrual status, and the reasons for the recurring stress fractures.

FEMALE ATHLETE TRIAD

One interrelated group of pathologic disorders has been termed the female athlete triad, and the Task Force on Women's Issues of the American College of Sports Medicine has developed a position stand on this issue (ACSM 1997). The **female athlete triad** is an interrelated group of disorders consisting of disordered eating, amenorrhea, and osteoporosis. This chapter covers each disorder separately, as well as other reproductive and gender-based issues you may encounter in dealing with female athletes of any age.

Terms and Definitions

amenorrhea—The absence of menstrual bleeding for at least 90 d.

anorexia athletica—A term coined by Sundgot-Borgen that refers to eating disorders in female athletes that do not strictly fit the definition of anorexia nervosa but that are clearly pathological and related to sport.

anovulation—The occurrence of a menstrual cycle that is not related to release of an egg (ovum).

dysmenorrhea—Painful menses.

endometriosis—Possible cause of dysmenorrhea related to abnormally placed uterine cells in pelvic cavity. The cells may be attached to the ovaries, fallopian tubes, uterus, or anywhere in the pelvic cavity.

female athlete triad—An interrelated group of disorders consisting of disordered eating, amenorrhea, and osteoporosis.

hirsutism—Excessive hairiness; in women, it usually manifests as an adult male pattern of hair distribution.

hysterectomy—Surgical removal of the uterus.

menarche—The beginning of menstrual functioning.

nonsteroidal anti-inflammatory drug (NSAID)—Any medication that blocks inflammation and is not chemically related to a corticosteroid (e.g., ibuprofen).

oligomenorrhea—Infrequent menstrual bleeding, typically at intervals of more than 40 d.

osteoporosis—The loss of bone mineral density and the inadequate formation of bone, leading to bone fragility and possible risk of fracture.

ovariectomy—Surgical removal of an ovary.

polycystic ovary syndrome (PCOS)—Includes the following signs and symptoms: irregular or absent menses, numerous cysts on the ovaries in many but not all cases, high blood pressure, acne, elevated insulin levels associated with insulin resistance, infertility, excess hair on the face and body, thinning of the scalp hair, and obesity.

premenstrual syndrome (PMS)—Usually occurring during the 10 d prior to menstruation, marked by emotional instability, irritability, insomnia, and headache.

Eating Disorders

Disordered eating describes a wide array of possibly harmful behaviors—including unhealthy caloric or fat restriction, and bingeing and purging—usually intended to maintain a thin physique. It is important to remember that not all athletes who have problems maintaining weight meet the strict criteria for anorexia nervosa or bulimia nervosa (see table 6.1). Although women in certain activities (dance, gymnastics, distance running, lightweight crew) are particularly at risk for disordered eating patterns, athletes in any sport can develop these disorders.

Significant controversy exists over whether eating disorders are more prevalent among athletes as compared to nonathletes, in part because research studies vary widely in how they define the seriousness of disorders. Some researchers have reported rates of anorexia nervosa as high as 6.5% in a group of ballet dancers (Garner and Garfinkel 1980). A study of female collegiate athletes in many different sports found that 14% used self-induced vomiting and 16% used laxatives to control their weight (Rosen et al. 1986). Using an inventory scale of eating disorders, Sundgot-Borgen (1994) found that 22.4% of elite Norwegian athletes were at risk for an eating disorder. Approximately 10% of the women in this study were classified as having anorexia nervosa or bulimia, with another 8% classified as having an eating disorder "not otherwise specified," or what they termed **anorexia**

Table 6.1   Diagnostic Criteria for Eating Disorders

Anorexia nervosa	Bulimia nervosa
1. Failure to maintain body weight at or above a minimally normal weight for age and height (i.e., body weight less than 85% of expected weight, either from weight loss or because the individual failed to gain weight during a period of growth)	1. Recurrent episodes of binge eating
2. Intense fear of gaining weight or becoming fat, even though underweight	2. Recurrent inappropriate compensatory behavior to prevent weight gain, such as self-induced vomiting; misuse of laxatives, diuretics, enemas, or other medications; fasting; or excessive exercise
3. Disturbance in the way in which one's body weight or shape is experienced, undue influence of body weight or shape on self-evaluation, or denial of the seriousness of the current body weight	3. Bingeing and purging at least twice a week for 3 months
4. In postmenarchal females, amenorrhea	4. Self-evaluation is unduly influenced by body shape and weight

Reprinted with permission from the *Diagnostic and Statistical Manual of Mental Disorders,* Fourth Edition. Copyright 1994 American Psychiatric Association.

athletica. Stein et al. (1997), however, comparing female athletes to nonathlete college women, found the prevalence of disordered eating to be fairly similar (as high as 20%) in both groups.

It is not easy to recognize athletes who are suffering from a disordered eating pattern or pathological weight loss. People with mild disorders often lack physical evidence, and those with longer-term disorders are sometimes surprisingly adept at hiding their symptoms until the condition becomes quite serious. Advanced symptoms include bloating, edema, swollen salivary glands, lanugo (dense, downy hair growth, especially on the arms, face, and torso), callus formation around the nails from recurrent purging, and discolored tooth enamel. Anorexia nervosa is diagnosed by using diagnostic criteria published by psychiatrists in the *Diagnostic and Statistical Manual* (4th ed.) (DSM-IV). A woman has anorexia nervosa if she

- has lost 15% of her body weight,
- has demonstrated unhealthy attitudes toward eating,
- has a severe body image disturbance, and
- has amenorrhea.

Before such advanced symptoms appear, however, look for the following red flags that should alert you to possible problems:

- Worsening athletic performance
- Preoccupation with food, calories, and weight
- Noticeable weight loss or gain
- Frequent weighing
- Avoidance of food-related social activities

- Wearing baggy clothes or layered clothing
- Excessive exercise
- Bathroom visits after meals
- Increasing criticism of one's body
- Depression
- Fatigue
- Social isolation (especially at mealtimes)
- Teammates' concerns

Additional clues relate to other parts of the female athlete triad, including amenorrhea and stress fractures. Although amenorrhea usually appears before there is dramatic weight loss, athletes often don't share such problems with athletic trainers or coaches. If you conscientiously educate all your athletes about the symptoms and dangers of anorexia nervosa, however, you may be fortunate in learning about an individual's menstrual problem from a teammate who is concerned about her—or, in some cases, from a physician to whom the athlete goes because of her menstrual problems. Most athletes do not fit the diagnostic criteria for anorexia nervosa, even though they may exhibit some of the symptoms.

When you suspect a problem, you need to feel comfortable about addressing it, and you should know to whom you can refer an athlete. Schedule a confidential meeting with the athlete to discuss concerns in a caring but direct manner. Be prepared for the athlete to deny that anything is wrong. Many people with eating disorders have become adept at hiding their problem, denying its existence and rationalizing their thoughts and behaviors. For the anorexic who has usually been quite rigid in her restrictive eating behavior, it may be effective to suggest she use her strength and discipline to overcome the problem. *Reassure the athlete that her spot on the team will not be in jeopardy unless her disorder becomes so severe that it compromises her performance or her general health.* Be prepared in advance to assemble a multidisciplinary team consisting of a medical physician, a psychologist or psychiatrist familiar with eating disorders, and a nutritionist to both evaluate and treat individuals in need of help:

- The physician should have experience caring for athletes with eating disorders. In severe cases, chronic malnutrition resulting from eating disorders can affect almost every organ system in the body. The most severe consequences are cardiac dysrhythmias; electrolyte abnormalities; and psychiatric depression, including risk of suicide.
- Psychological counseling is needed to evaluate and treat both the primary psychological problems that may have led to the disordered eating pattern and any secondary psychological problems associated with the disease itself. Athletes may suffer from the usual causes of eating disorders such as societal pressure, low self-esteem, prior or ongoing sexual abuse, and family dysfunction; but other factors may also relate directly to their sport—such as an extenuating injury, a coach's comments, peer pressure, or the stress of competition (Sundgot-Borgen 1994).
- A nutritionist can help the affected athlete learn to monitor caloric intake so that she can endure the physical stress of practice and competition. The nutritionist also can help the athlete set realistic weight goals and find alternative weight-control methods if they are ever appropriate in the future.

Because an eating disorder is a chronic illness, any athlete suffering from such a disorder requires long-term support of family members and consistent follow-up with members of the multidisciplinary team. The family must be educated about the seriousness of the problem so that they can understand the probable long-term

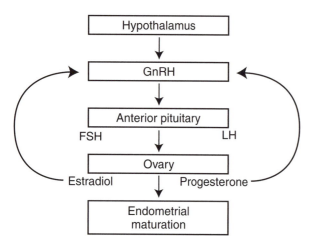

■ Figure 6.1 Hormonal influences on menstrual cycle.

struggle that dealing with the problem will require—and have realistic expectations of the treatment process. The prognosis depends on early intervention, the severity of the disorder, the individual's willingness to seek help, and the family's ability to cooperate with the treatment program. In a study of anorexia by Lowe et al. (2001), follow-up after 21 yr found that 51% of the patients had recovered, 21% had partially recovered, and 10% still met full diagnostic criteria for anorexia nervosa. Even more sobering was that 16% had died due to causes related to anorexia nervosa.

Amenorrhea

The menstrual period results from a complex set of hormonal interactions involving the hypothalamus and pituitary gland in the brain along with the ovaries and uterus. Any interruption or reduction in the hypothalamic or pituitary hormones can cause ovarian dysfunction (figure 6.1). **Amenorrhea** is classified as primary or secondary depending on the patient's pubertal development. Primary amenorrhea denotes no history of menstrual bleeding by age 14 *without* development of secondary sexual characteristics or by age 16 *with* otherwise normal development. Secondary amenorrhea is defined as the 3-month absence of menstrual bleeding in a woman with previously regular menses.

The prevalence of amenorrhea in the general population is believed to be 2% to 5%. Although athletes are variously reported to have a higher incidence of amenorrhea than nonathletes, the statistics are suspect because they are so astoundingly variable—published reports range from 3.4% to 66%!

In many young women, it is difficult to cleanly separate extreme exercise from eating disorders as a cause of amenorrhea. By definition, all women with anorexia suffer from amenorrhea; however, amenorrhea can result from excessive exercise even in women who eat normally. Note, moreover, that although disordered eating or the stress of training, or a combination of these two factors, is the usual cause of amenorrhea in athletes, this diagnosis is appropriate *only after other potential causes are excluded*—including (among many possible factors) pregnancy, pituitary tumors, thyroid disease, and side effects of many different medications or hormonal agents (figure 6.2).

The mechanism of exercise-induced amenorrhea is not well understood. The most popular theory is that a chronic imbalance of calories consumed versus calories expended creates an "energy drain" that decreases basal metabolic rate and causes hypothalamic dysfunction—which, in turn, leads to diminished estrogen production by the ovaries, and amenorrhea. The other major theory is that, because exercise can raise cortisol levels, these levels inhibit production of hypothalamic hormones—which in turn leads to lack of stimulation of the ovaries to produce estrogen and progesterone. In either theory, the hypothalamus is the mediator of the hormone dysfunction, leading to the term hypothalamic amenorrhea—of which amenorrhea stemming from exercise and that caused by anorexia are examples, as well as amenorrhea resulting from the actions of certain drugs (Sundgot-Borgen 1994).

Ovarian dysfunction and lack of estrogen put athletes at risk for premature bone loss. In theory, an athlete could restore her menstrual function through proper nutrition, modification of training regimens, and maintenance of body weight. In reality, because most athletes (whether they have anorexia or not) often are not

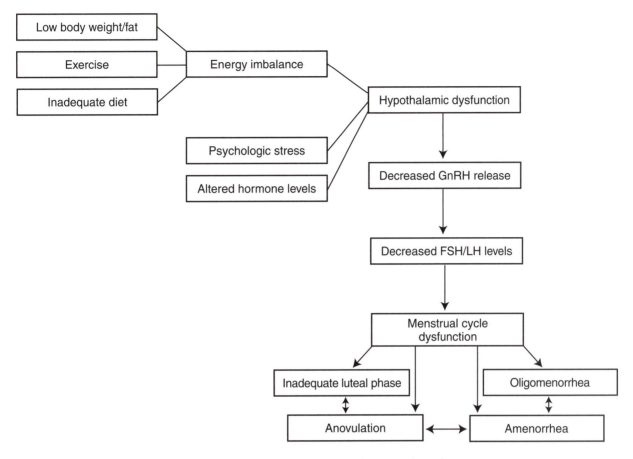

■ **Figure 6.2**   Amenorrhea and menstrual irregularity can result from a variety of causes.

willing to make the necessary changes in their training schedules to alter their menstrual status, they require hormonal supplementation to regulate their menses and, it is hoped, to protect against premature bone loss.

Osteoporosis

A woman who suffers from disordered eating, poor calcium intake, and menstrual dysfunction is at increased risk of premature bone loss and not achieving peak bone mass—and women who fail to attain their optimal peak bone mass by age 20 enter menopause with a suboptimal bone mineral density, which theoretically increases their risk of osteoporosis. For this reason, early intervention is warranted when menstrual regularity has been disrupted for at least 3 months, especially in teenagers.

Osteoporosis is defined as the loss of bone mineral density and the inadequate formation of bone, leading to bone fragility and possible risk of fracture. Besides hormone levels, weight-bearing exercise is one of the main determinants of bone mineral density. Therefore, although athletes with disordered eating patterns are at risk for osteoporosis, constant weight-bearing exercise often provides enough stimulation so that bone mineral content remains normal for an athlete's age and weight. In a study of athletes with a history of stress fractures, Bennell and colleagues (1996) found that bone mineral density in athletes with stress fractures was lower than in other athletes but higher than in nonathletes. The implication is that, at least for short-term health, athletes (who place extra stress on their bones) may require greater bone mineral density than the general population.

Table 6.2   Calcium Sources: Dietary

Source of calcium	Serving size	Amount of calcium (mg)
Milk and dairy products		
Yogurt, low fat	1 c	415
Milk, low fat (2%)	1 c	315
Cottage cheese, low fat	1/2 c	75
Cheddar cheese	1 oz	205
Green vegetables		
Turnip greens	1 c	250
Broccoli	1 c	180
Spinach	1 c	145
Legumes and soy products		
Soymilk	1 c	300
Tofu	1/2 c	260
Kidney beans	1 c	60

Although the data are controversial and require further research for confirmation, Hergenroeder and colleagues (1997) found that a 12-month regimen of oral contraceptives led to improved bone mineral density in young women (ages 14-28 yr) with hypothalamic amenorrhea. In addition to hormonal treatment of amenorrhea to prevent premature bone loss, many women should strongly consider calcium supplementation if they find it difficult to consume the recommended dietary allowance of calcium (1,200-1,500 mg/d) (see table 6.2). Supplements should include calcium, such as calcium carbonate tablets (sold under various brand names for relief of acid indigestion) along with a multivitamin containing 400 IU of vitamin D to aid absorption.

Case Study

A 16-yr-old girl comes to you worried about her menstrual cramps. The cramps seem to precede her actual period by about 48 h. She has tried using nonsteroidal anti-inflammatory drugs (NSAIDs) without relief. She denies any chance of having a sexually transmitted disease since she has never had intercourse or oral sex. She has seen her family physician, who has recommended starting oral contraceptives to treat this problem. The cramps have interfered with competition at least three times in the last 12 months. Based on your knowledge of dysmenorrhea, you offer advice in terms of standard treatments for this disorder, predictable timing of the menstrual cycle with hormonal therapy, and a good chance of decreased severity of the cramps. Finally, you tell her that the oral contraceptives do not provide an excuse to change her sexual practices in terms of becoming sexually active or using barrier contraception.

DISORDERS OF THE REPRODUCTIVE SYSTEM

There are a multitude of disorders of the reproductive system and a multitude of causes. You need to be aware of the potential causes of such disorders, and you also need to know when you should refer an athlete to a medical specialist to rule out a more serious disease. Because menstrual disorders can lead female athletes to miss practices or even competitions, you may be the first person to learn of certain symptoms that warrant closer scrutiny.

A common belief about young female athletes is that those who push themselves the hardest appear more likely to experience delayed **menarche.** Yet a neat cause-and-effect relationship related to performance does not seem to exist, in that delayed menarche in itself—even in young women who do not begin their athletic experience until after menarche—is still somewhat associated with good athletic performance. It is possible that delayed menarche (or slowed physical maturity) confers some athletic advantage, perhaps because of the physical characteristics that tend to go with late menarche—such as lower weight for a given height, longer legs, narrower hips, and less relative body fat. Regardless of an athlete's prowess, you should refer to a physician any young woman who has shown no signs of pubertal development by age 14 or who has not had her first menses by her 16th year.

In addition to delayed menarche, which is not inherently problematic as long as it is not delayed *too* long, several disorders show up fairly often in young women—especially oligomenorrhea, anovulation, dysmenorrhea, and pre-menstrual syndrome. Endometriosis is rare in school-age females, but if you work with women in late adolescence or older, you no doubt will encounter this disorder.

Oligomenorrhea

Oligomenorrhea is defined as menstrual cycles that are more than 40 d in length—or, more qualitatively, simply as irregular menstrual bleeding. In some ways, you can think of oligomenorrhea as a step on a continuum toward amenorrhea. One important question is whether oligomenorrhea has been present since menarche or if it developed later (especially if it developed after the young woman began intense athletic training).

Irregular bleeding from the onset of menarche may point to a serious problem that a gynecologist should evaluate, such as adrenal enzyme deficiency or, more commonly, **polycystic ovary syndrome (PCOS),** which occurs in about 3% of adolescent and adult women. About 40% of young women with PCOS are obese; many exhibit **hirsutism,** masculinization, or persistent acne that is unresponsive to traditional treatments. PCOS represents a spectrum of disorders associated with increased androgen production from the ovaries or adrenal glands. The ovaries of affected patients may appear normal to large, with associated cystic structures inside. The consequences of this disorder include irregular menses and metabolic abnormalities, including insulin resistance, high levels of triglycerides, and low levels of high-density lipoprotein (HDL) cholesterol. Treatment of this disorder will require consultation with a physician who is comfortable in its management. Medications may include oral contraceptives that may regulate menses and suppress further hair growth in some patients. Other patients may require treatment with other medications or cosmetic procedures. Long-term patients may have problems with ovulation induction and fertility, which are beyond the scope of this book.

Oligomenorrhea can be caused by a variety of other disorders besides PCOS, such as complications from a progesterone intrauterine device, chronic illness or traumatic injuries, or food poisoning. Endometrial cancer, ovarian cysts, and Graves' disease are other possible causes of oligomenorrhea. It is important to rule out more serious causes before concluding that irregular menses are related to an athlete's lifestyle or environment, or both.

Excessive exercise can lead to missed periods, as can poor nutrition, low body fat, emotional stress, and use of anabolic steroids. There is little need to treat oligo-menorrhea in most adolescents, whose menses often are somewhat irregular until the various parts of the complex ovulatory system begin functioning together effectively. If a young athlete's menses become irregular after previously being regular, however, you should explore with her the possible causes and take appropriate steps to correct the problem, which usually means changing diet or backing off a bit on training (which may not be practical for many athletes). Women with a history of oligomenorrhea or amenorrhea tend to exhibit lowered bone mineral density even after their menses return to normal. Evidence exists, in fact, that oli-gomenorrhea can be just as deleterious to a woman's bone health as amenorrhea. Therefore it is important to deal with this problem as soon as it is discovered and to help an athlete learn the cause and take appropriate action to return menses to normal as quickly as possible.

Anovulatory Cycles

Anovulation means simply the occurrence of a menstrual cycle that is not related to release of an egg (ovum). Because of the immaturity of young women's ovulatory systems (and some inconsistency in the hormones produced by the hypothalamus and pituitary), many of their menses (from 50% to 80% of cycles) may be anovulatory during the first couple of years after menarche. Although such cycles sometimes differ little from ovulatory cycles, they may be characterized by excessive and prolonged bleeding. Most women with oligomenorrhea experience some anovulatory cycles.

There are two primary concerns about anovulatory cycles:

- For women who are trying to become pregnant, anovulatory cycles obviously are problematic.
- Prolonged lack of ovulation can lead, via several successive physiological steps, to excessive estrogen levels that overstimulate the endometrium—which, over a long time, can lead to a precancerous condition.

Although laboratory assays for various hormones can unambiguously identify anovulatory cycles, you generally will refer an athlete for such tests only when you suspect a serious underlying medical problem. Common symptoms of anovulatory cycles are excessive bleeding, a cycle that lasts more than 41 d, and absence of usual premenstrual symptoms (e.g., cramping, bloating, breast tenderness).

Chronic anovulation may point to PCOS or another disorder involving androgen production or metabolism. Sporadic anovulation can be caused by endocrine disorders (e.g., overproduction of adrenal hormone, or thyroid pathologies) or by use of certain prescription drugs such as spironolactone (brand name Aldactone®), which is sometimes used to treat premenstrual syndrome. Often, however, sporadic anovulation is a result of lifestyle or environmental factors that are to varying extents under the control of the athlete.

Once you have ruled out more serious problems, consider lifestyle and environmental factors. The hypothalamic control that leads eventually to ovulation can be suppressed by excessive exercise, other forms of stress, anorexia, or an inappropriate ratio of lean body mass to fat. Women for whom these factors cause anovulation should modify their behavior or environment accordingly—as with oligomenorrhea, this usually means changing their diets to include more calories (and often more fat) and cutting back on their training levels. In many cases, they also should be prescribed calcium supplements (with vitamin D) and hormone-replacement therapy (HRT) to stem any loss of bone mineral density, especially in a woman less than 30 years of age. HRT is more controversial in the peri- and postmenopausal woman and probably needs to be based on other symptoms.

For many athletes who find that changes in diet or training are not practical, hormonal treatment with estrogen and progesterone is often useful in regulating the cycle and providing the hormonal stimulation necessary for normal bone metabolism.

Dysmenorrhea

Of the two types of **dysmenorrhea,** primary dysmenorrhea affects up to 90% of menstruating women, whereas secondary dysmenorrhea is rare. It is important to distinguish dysmenorrhea from premenstrual syndrome (PMS), both of which cause pain or discomfort and both of which are associated with menses.

Primary Dysmenorrhea

It is generally believed that primary dysmenorrhea is related to elevated production of endometrial prostaglandins, which increase both the strength and the frequency of uterine contractions. Primary dysmenorrhea usually begins during adolescence, usually no earlier than 6 months after the first period. It is most common in teenagers and in women in their 30s and typically presents as painful cramps in the lower central abdomen at the beginning of and during menstruation—usually starting on the first and ending on the second or third day. Pain may be intermittent and spasmodic, radiating in some cases to the lower back or to the backs of the legs. Other common symptoms are fatigue, headache, light-headedness, nausea, diarrhea, fever, and depression. Symptoms in about 10% of women are severe enough to restrict normal activity. Although the symptoms can clearly compromise an athlete's performance, the good news is that exercise (at least in moderation) appears to ameliorate the symptoms; athletic women generally have fewer problems than nonathletes.

Many women obtain adequate symptomatic relief by taking **nonsteroidal anti-inflammatory drugs (NSAIDs)**—such as ibuprofen, naproxen, or mefenamic acid (brand name Ponstan®)—the day before they expect symptoms to begin. Applying a heating pad to the abdomen can also help alleviate symptoms.

Women often can ameliorate symptoms by reducing their levels of emotional and physical stress, by engaging in moderate aerobic exercise if they are not already exercising, and by getting plenty of rest. Oral contraceptives, when appropriate for a woman's health and lifestyle, generally completely eliminate symptoms as long as the pills are taken. Although the treatments have not yet been confirmed by multiple laboratories, limited data have suggested that low levels of omega-3 fatty acids, thiamine, and/or magnesium may contribute significantly to dysmenorrheic symptoms. Empiric supplementation with these substances may reduce the severity of these symptoms.

About 10% of affected women do not respond even to oral contraceptives. In these cases it is especially important to determine whether secondary pathologies are present.

Secondary Dysmenorrhea

Secondary dysmenorrhea is caused not by poorly functioning components of the normal reproductive cycle but rather by secondary pathologies such as pelvic inflammatory disease; endometriosis; uterine fibroids; benign tumors or cysts; or inflammation or infection of other abdominal tissues such as the fallopian tubes, uterus, or intestines. Intrauterine devices (IUDs) can also cause the disorder. Symptoms—most often a strong aching sensation in the lower abdomen—generally begin several days before the menstrual period and continue throughout the period. The disorder is relatively rare in younger athletes but becomes more common in later adolescence.

Because there is no single cause of secondary dysmenorrhea, few generalizations can be made about treatment. The basic approach is to treat the underlying pathology, providing symptomatic relief as appropriate.

Premenstrual Syndrome

Whereas the pain of primary dysmenorrhea usually coincides with the beginning of a menstrual period, the pain and discomfort of **premenstrual syndrome (PMS)** begin a week to 10 d before the period. PMS may be associated with symptoms such as lower abdominal cramps, abdominal bloating, back pain, breast tenderness, headache, water retention, cravings for certain foods, diarrhea, constipation, or dizziness. Emotional or mental symptoms can include depression, anxiety,

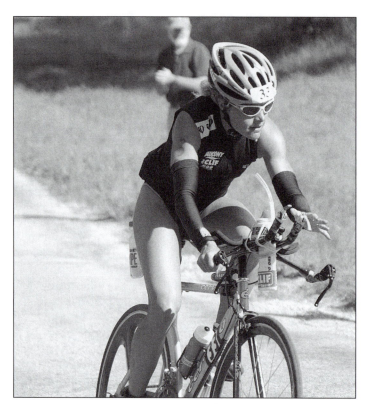

■ Figure 6.3   Premenstrual disorder and other menstrual irregularities can affect performance.

mood swings, anger, aggression, irritability, sleepiness, insomnia, or inability to concentrate. Symptoms often peak at the beginning of the menstrual period and may be accompanied by dysmenorrheic cramping; symptoms usually end a few days after menstrual bleeding begins. The disorder can be quite debilitating.

Treatment involves addressing individual symptoms: Headaches are generally treated with NSAIDs, bloating with diuretics, and anxiety and depression with a variety of anxiolytic or antidepressant medications. Physicians generally advise women with insomnia to avoid caffeine and to follow standard guidelines for maximizing sleep. Several researchers have reported that daily calcium supplements can reduce PMS symptoms, including cramping (Thys-Jacobs et al. 1998). The most effective medication studied for the treatment of PMS is fluoxetine (Prozac®). In women with severe PMS, treatment with fluoxetine or a similar antidepressant should be considered.

Endometriosis

Depending on the statistics one reads, **endometriosis** affects from 3% up to 15% of women in the United States and is one of the main reasons that women undergo hysterectomies. Although it most often occurs in women who are in their late 20s, endometriosis occasionally is observed in teenage girls. You probably will see it only rarely unless you work regularly with older athletes—but since it *can* occur at almost any age, you should be aware of the symptoms and treatments.

The endometrium is the membrane that lines the uterus. Each month that a woman does not become pregnant, this tissue is sloughed off during the menstrual period; it then begins to regrow and thicken until the next period. In endometriosis, endometrial cells develop outside of the uterus, attaching themselves as *implants* to various tissues—most often on the ovaries, the outer surfaces of the uterus, the fallopian tubes, the intestines, or the lining of the abdominal cavity. Implants also may occur on the vagina; on the liver; on old surgical scars; and, rarely, even in tissues outside the abdomen such as the brain or the lungs. The cause is unknown. Though implants are rarely cancerous, they can cause a great deal of pain.

Endometrial implants respond to menstrual cycle hormones in the same way that normal endometrial tissue responds—they grow during the month, then break down and bleed during menstruation. But because there is no way for the sloughed tissue and blood to exit the body, this process leads to pain, inflammation, and eventually scarring, and often to infertility.

Although most women with endometriosis are asymptomatic, the most prevalent symptoms are abdominal pain and infertility. Less-common symptoms are low back pain, irregular menstrual bleeding, diarrhea, constipation, or blood in the urine. The abdominal pain typically occurs 24 to 48 h before the onset of menses and declines after the end of the period. In some women, sexual intercourse, urination, or bowel movements cause pain. Both intensity and course of the pain are highly variable, changing from month to month and sometimes disappearing without treatment. In many women, however, the pain and cramping become worse with time.

The only way to diagnose endometriosis unambiguously is to directly view the implants and by biopsy of suspected tissue—usually accomplished by laparoscopy under general (or sometimes local) anesthesia on an outpatient basis.

Symptomatic treatment of endometriosis involves use of analgesics—NSAIDs, such as ibuprofen, or sometimes narcotics for more intractable pain—or hormones such as birth-control pills that, by reducing estrogen levels, reduce the cyclical growth of the implants. Other hormones used for symptomatic relief are medroxyprogesterone (brand name Depo-Provera®) and danazol (brand name Danocrine®), which provide effective relief but have considerable negative side effects and cannot be used on a long-term basis.

More aggressive treatments seek to eliminate or at least shrink the implants themselves, typically using either hormones or hormone analogs. Common treatments are analogs to gonadotropin-releasing hormone—such as leuprolide (brand name Lupron®), which is injected subcutaneously, and nafarelin (brand name Synarel®) which, administered as a nasal spray, induces temporary menopause. Unfortunately, because the accompanying decline in estrogen levels can lead to osteoporosis, such treatments usually are limited in duration. The standard 6-month regimen of nafarelin generally leaves about 60% of women free of symptoms: Half of these remain asymptomatic 6 months after the end of treatment (Minjarez and Schlaff 2000).

More severe cases of endometriosis are treated with surgery. Most cases are amenable to laparoscopic surgery, in which implants are destroyed by lasers or by cauterization, or sometimes are mechanically excised. The worst cases require open surgery, sometimes including **hysterectomy** and **ovariectomy.**

Even with the most drastic treatment, endometriosis and its accompanying symptoms can sometimes return. The symptoms finally disappear after menopause.

SUMMARY

1. *Define the components of the female athlete triad.*

The female athlete triad—disordered eating, amenorrhea, and osteoporosis—is common, and you should be familiar with the red flags listed in this chapter that may point to deeper problems. It is important to intervene as quickly as possible when you suspect such problems in a young woman, because eating disorders can develop into critical short-term problems and sometimes even be fatal.

2. *Recognize the signs, symptoms, and treatment strategies for disordered eating.*

Disordered eating describes a wide array of possibly harmful behaviors—including unhealthy caloric or fat restriction, and bingeing and purging—usually intended to maintain a thin physique. Not all athletes who have problems maintaining weight meet the strict criteria for anorexia nervosa or bulimia nervosa. It can be difficult to recognize athletes who are suffering from a disordered eating pattern or pathological weight loss. People with mild disorders often lack physical evidence, and those with longer-term disorders are sometimes surprisingly adept at hiding their symptoms until the condition becomes quite serious. Advanced symptoms include bloating, edema, swollen salivary glands, lanugo (dense, downy hair growth, especially on the arms, face, and torso), callus formation around the nails from recurrent purging, and discolored tooth enamel.

For Further Information

Print Resources

Agostini, R., ed. 1994. *Medical and orthopedic issues of active athletic women.* Philadelphia: Hanley and Belfus.

Minjarez, D.A., and W.D. Schlaff. 2000. Current reproductive endocrinology: Update on medical treatment of endometriosis. *Obstetrics and Gynecology Clinics* 27(3): 641-51.

Thompson, R.A., and R.T. Sherman. 1993. *Helping athletes with eating disorders.* Champaign, IL: Human Kinetics.

Web Resources

The Women's Sports Foundation

www.womenssportsfoundation.org/cgi-bin/iowa/sports/index.html
Founded in 1974 by Billie Jean King, the Women's Sports Foundation is a charitable educational organization dedicated to ensuring equal access to participation and leadership opportunities for all girls and women in sports and fitness. The Web site includes information about many issues related to women's sports, including pertinent health-related topics.

Red flags that should alert you to possible problems include poor athletic performance; preoccupation with food, calories, and weight; noticeable weight loss or gain; frequent weighing; avoidance of food-related social activities; wearing baggy clothes or layered clothing; excessive exercise; bathroom visits after meals; poor body image; depression; fatigue; social isolation (especially at mealtimes); and concern expressed by teammates and coaches.

During treatment, ensure the athlete that her spot on the team will not be in jeopardy unless her disorder becomes so severe that it compromises her performance or her general health. Treatment should include a multidisciplinary team consisting of a medical physician, a psychologist or psychiatrist familiar with eating disorders, and a nutritionist. Access to such a team will also assist with proper diagnosis and referral. An eating disorder is a chronic illness; any athlete suffering such a disorder requires long-term support of family members and consistent follow-up with members of the multidisciplinary team. The athlete's family must be educated about the seriousness of the problem so that they can understand the probable long-term struggle that dealing with the problem will require—and have realistic expectations of the treatment process. The prognosis depends on early intervention, the severity of the disorder, the individual's willingness to seek help, and the family's ability to cooperate with the treatment program.

3. *Explain the difference between primary and secondary amenorrhea.*

Interruption or reduction in hypothalamic or pituitary hormones that influence the menstrual cycle can cause ovarian dysfunction. Amenorrhea is classified as primary or secondary depending on the patient's pubertal development. Primary amenorrhea denotes no history of menstrual bleeding by age 14 *without* development of secondary sexual characteristics or by age 16 *with* otherwise normal development. Secondary amenorrhea is defined as the 3-month absence of menstrual bleeding in a woman with previously regular menses.

The prevalence of amenorrhea in the general population is believed to be 2% to 5%. Athletes are reported to have a higher incidence of amenorrhea than nonathletes; however, the statistics in these reports vary greatly.

In many young women, it is difficult to separate extreme exercise from eating disorders as a cause of amenorrhea. By definition, all women with anorexia suffer from amenorrhea; however, amenorrhea can result from excesses of exercise even in women who eat normally. Note, moreover, that although disordered eating or the stress of training, or a combination of these two factors, is the usual cause of amenorrhea in athletes, this diagnosis is appropriate only after other potential causes are excluded. The mechanism of exercise-induced amenorrhea is not well understood. Most theories involve the impact of energy balance on the hypothalamus. The hypothalamus mediates hormone function.

Ovarian dysfunction and lack of estrogen put athletes at risk for premature bone loss. An athlete could restore her menstrual function through proper nutrition, modification of training regimens, and maintenance of body weight. However, most athletes (whether they have anorexia or not) often are not willing to make the necessary changes in their training schedules to alter their menstrual status; they require hormonal supplementation to regulate their menses and, it is hoped, to protect against premature bone loss.

4. *Discuss the determinants of bone mineral density.*

Women who suffer from disordered eating, poor calcium intake, and menstrual dysfunction are at increased risk of premature bone loss and not achieving peak bone mass—and women who fail to attain their optimal peak bone mass by age 20 enter menopause with a suboptimal bone mineral density, which theoretically increases their risk of osteoporosis. Early intervention is warranted when menstrual regularity has been disrupted for at least 3 months.

Osteoporosis is defined as the loss of bone mineral density and the inadequate formation of bone, leading to bone fragility and possible risk of fracture. Besides hormone levels, weight-bearing exercise is one of the main determinants of bone mineral density. Therefore, although athletes with disordered eating patterns are at risk for osteoporosis, constant weight-bearing exercise often provides enough stimulation so that bone mineral content remains normal for an athlete's age and weight.

5. *Discuss various irregularities in the menstrual cycle and reproductive system.*

Various reproductive system disorders are extremely common. Symptoms of premenstrual syndrome and of primary dysmenorrhea can range from mildly annoying to debilitating. Do your best to encourage women athletes to seek medical help for such problems, even if the treatments are only palliative. You should also be aware of the symptomatic differences between primary and secondary dysmenorrhea, since the latter results from underlying pathologies that a gynecologist should address.

Anovulatory menstrual cycles are common in young women; but a gynecologist should assess chronic anovulation, because it can lead eventually to serious endometrial pathology. Endometriosis is rarely seen among young adolescents, but if you work with women in their late teens and early 20s or later years, you probably will encounter this common disorder. It is variously treated, depending on the severity of symptoms, with analgesics, hormones, or surgery.

PART II

INFECTIOUS CONDITIONS AND ALLERGIES

CHAPTER 7

Dermatological Pathologies

OBJECTIVES

Upon completion of this chapter the reader will be able to do the following:

1. Describe the signs and symptoms of a variety of skin lesions common in active populations

2. Explain the common course of treatment for various skin conditions

3. Determine which skin conditions require immediate medical referral

4. Discuss the guidelines for sports participation for athletes with specific skin conditions

Skin problems receive a lot of attention, in part because they tend to be so visible. One challenge for health care professionals and those they serve is the difficulty of describing skin symptoms using words when visual aids would be so much easier. The necessity of using words to describe essentially visual phenomena makes it important that anyone encountering skin problems be able to use and understand a common vocabulary.

Here is a brief introduction to dermatological terminology: Any bump on the skin (i.e., a raised area) may be called a **papule.** A spot of any size is described as a **macule.** (Therefore a fine macular, papular rash is one with tiny spots that are raised on the skin.) A papule with pus in the center is called a **pustule.** Some rashes are so fine that the skin feels like sandpaper; hence the rashes associated with streptococcal infections are sometimes described as sandpapery. Some rashes are **pruritic** (i.e., itchy). A large blister on the skin is a **bulla** (plural, bullae). A very tiny blister is a **vesicle.** A scaly rash feels and appears like the scales on a fish. **Erythema,** or redness, is usually due to increased blood flow to inflamed skin. It is always important to describe accurately the size and location of the affected area.

To understand skin disorders, you need to know the basic anatomy of the skin. The skin has three basic layers. The outermost layer, or epidermis, is composed of keratin—tough, proteinaceous material that provides an excellent barrier to infectious agents and other noxious substances. The next layer is the dermis, which contains tiny blood vessels and sensory nerves. Within the dermis also lie the sweat glands, hair follicles (where the hair grows), and oil glands (which lie at the base of the follicles). The subcutaneous layer is made up of fat and connective tissue as well as larger blood vessels and nerves.

Case Study

Treesha, a 15-yr-old basketball player, has developed a rash on her leg in an area that has been in contact with a rubber knee sleeve. She has been wearing the sleeve for many months without a problem but recently washed the sleeve in soap and water. She reports that the rash is very itchy and is spreading. It itches at night and interferes with her sleep. She has tried hydrocortisone on the rash, without much relief.

You refer Treesha to a physician, who finds the rash to be quite red, with well-demarcated borders corresponding to the edges of the sleeve. A few vesicles are scattered throughout. There are a few pustules within the rash (bumps with yellow centers) and a few outside the large area of the rash. Her scratching has also caused linear abrasions in various places.

The distribution of the rash demonstrates that Treesha has developed sensitivity to the knee sleeve (contact dermatitis); the pustules suggest a secondary infection. To treat the infection, the doctor gives her dicloxacillin, an oral antibiotic, to kill the bacteria that are causing the infection. For the itch, he prescribes 0.1% triamcinolone, a medium-strength corticosteroid ointment that will be more effective than the over-the-counter hydrocortisone she has used. He suggests that oral diphenhydramine (popular brand name Benadryl®) might help the itch at night. The physician also instructs Treesha to discard the knee sleeve, since its age apparently has combined with the effects of washing to produce a chemical to which she is sensitive. He said it is possible that her skin might tolerate a new sleeve but advises her to use a cotton liner under the sleeve. A few days later, her skin and her symptoms have markedly improved.

TRAUMA

Because the skin is the first line of defense against trauma to the body, there are myriad ways in which the skin is damaged.

Terms and Definitions

bulla—A large blister, usually larger than 2 cm in diameter.

cellulitis—A spreading bacterial infection of the dermis and subcutaneous tissue; it typically begins as a small area of tenderness, redness, and swelling and may progress to fever, chills, and swollen lymph nodes close to the infected area.

erythema—Abnormal skin redness, usually resulting from congestion of capillaries.

macule—A spot of any size on the skin.

papule—Any bump on the skin.

pruritic—Itchy.

pustule—A papule with pus in the center.

vesicle—A very small blister, usually less than 1 cm in diameter.

Traumatic Blisters

The most common form of trauma to the skin is caused by friction against another object such as a shoe or racket. Moisture on the skin increases the friction, the first response to which is redness and tenderness. Athletes sometimes refer to such areas as *hot spots,* since they feel warm to the touch. Continued friction causes the epidermis to separate from the dermis, whereupon fluid accumulates to cushion the underlying dermis to cause a bulla, or blister. The fluid eventually can cause pressure that painfully stimulates the nerves in the dermis. A blood blister may form if the friction causes a break in a small blood vessel in the dermis.

Most blisters resolve with little treatment, provided the athlete avoids further friction in that area. Ice massage can be helpful in providing pain relief to a hot spot; icing alone, however, will not reduce the friction. A variety of dressings (e.g., petroleum jelly, petroleum-based ointment) can reduce friction, but avoid bulky dressings, which can increase the friction. Sometimes the pressure from a blister is so painful that the fluid needs to be drained. Note, however, that the epidermis over the blister is protective and should remain in place, because its removal would expose the tender dermis, causing more pain and increasing the risk of infection. Draining a blister under sterile conditions with a sterile needle and syringe will relieve the pressure, yet leave the epidermis intact. The needle hole is a potential portal for bacteria, so cover it with an antibacterial ointment to reduce the chance of infection. This simple procedure can be performed by a health professional other than a physician if that practitioner is knowledgeable about sterile technique. Infected blisters are very painful and can cause a deeper infection, such as a **cellulitis,** that may require hospitalization and intravenous antibiotics.

Preventing blisters involves mainly reducing friction and preventing clothing (especially socks) from becoming wet from perspiration. To reduce friction, many athletes apply petroleum jelly or other oil-based moisturizers to the skin. Powder or cornstarch also can serve to reduce friction and absorb moisture. Applying antiperspirant to the bottom of the feet also appears to help prevent blisters, as does wearing acrylic rather than cotton socks (or acrylic sock liners), because the acrylic material both reduces friction against the skin and wicks moisture away from the skin. Blister formation may also indicate a poor shoe fit; shoes may be either too large or too small.

Burns

Burns are categorized in three grades of severity. A first-degree burn involves only the epidermis and superficial dermis, producing redness and tenderness.

The common sunburn is a first-degree burn. A second-degree burn causes blistering, with separation of the epidermis and dermis much like what occurs with a traumatic blister. Second-degree burns are quite painful and are more prone to infection than first-degree burns. Treat the blistering like any traumatic blister, being careful to prevent infection once a blister opens. A third-degree burn involves the deep dermis and damages the blood vessel and nerves deep in the skin. Many third-degree burns require skin grafts to prevent excessive scarring. Any burn that has areas of anesthesia (decreased feeling) must be seen by a physician and evaluated for the need for surgical consultation and skin grafting.

Consider questions of playability on an individual basis; clearly, you must weigh the extent and severity of the burn. Note that trauma to a second-degree or third-degree burn can lead to infection of more tissue than was originally involved in the burn. It is generally a good idea to keep athletes on the sidelines if they have any blistering that could open as a result of trauma incurred during the workout or competition.

The vast majority of the burns athletes experience are from the sun—a potential problem in any outdoor sport that involves skin exposure during the daytime. Most sunburns are essentially first-degree burns, but more prolonged exposure can lead to blisters and a second-degree burn. Sunburn is more likely to occur during the hottest part of the day. People with fair complexions (e.g., those of northern European heritage) are more prone to burns, yet even a very dark-skinned person (e.g., of black African descent) can burn during long exposure to the sun's ultraviolet rays.

Proper use of clothing, sunscreen, or both can prevent sunburn. Remember that cloud cover may not protect against sunburn, because ultraviolet rays can penetrate clouds. Remind athletes to use water-insoluble sunscreens, since sweating can wash off water-soluble products, and to reapply sunscreen every few hours. The sun protection factor (SPF) represents how much longer the sunscreen wearer can stay in the sun before experiencing a burn than would occur without the sunscreen. For example, if the skin burns in 5 min, applying an SPF 15 sunscreen would allow 15 times 5, or 75 min, in the sun before the skin would burn. The SPF reflects the approximate protection under ideal conditions with reapplication of screen every 2 h. People rarely apply sunscreen as often as is recommended, and sunlight is often more intense than in the experimental conditions. Therefore, make sure athletes use a sunscreen with a minimum SPF of 15; those with fair skin must use stronger sunscreen to prevent burns. This is especially true for athletes with a family history of skin cancer. The SPF is only used to measure the UVB ultraviolet light ray protection because those rays are responsible for causing sunburn. The UVA light rays penetrate the skin more deeply, and this spectrum of light is not blocked by most sunscreens. UVA causes skin damage without the burn. There is no standard for UVA protection in the United States. An excellent review on sunscreens appears in *Consumer Reports* ("Sunscreens," 2001).

Calluses

Areas of friction on the hands and feet eventually cause a callus—a thickening of the epidermis to protect the underlying dermis. Calluses can be distinguished from other skin lesions because the dermal lines responsible for fingerprints (or footprints) are preserved in a callus. Other lesions, such as viral warts, distort the dermal lines.

When calluses become too thick, and especially if they are tender, it is prudent of athletes to trim them with a callus shaver, emery board, or callus file (use of razor blades should be reserved for the physician's office). As discussed in Burkhardt

(1999), care must be taken not to remove too much of a callus, seeing that it developed in the first place to protect underlying layers from friction—removing too much callus may lead to a hot spot and eventually a blister. Occasionally, friction causes a small amount of bleeding under a callus, which then turns dark. This process is common in the heel, where it is called *black heel*. Basketball players often get black heel, and weightlifters can get *black palm* from the friction between the weights and their hands.

Preventing unwanted calluses is largely a question of determining the cause of the friction. Unacceptably large calluses on the feet often arise from shoes that fit poorly; in this instance, athletes can prevent calluses by wearing properly fitting shoes that also offer sufficient padding to absorb the shock of running. Court-sport athletes are prone to calluses on the ball of the foot as well as along the great toe. Runners often get calluses on the ends of the toes if shoes do not fit properly. Athletic trainers should routinely check for excessive callus formation during prepractice taping. Educate your athletes in proper preventive foot care. Callus pads, for use in any shoes, are available in most pharmacies. Some athletes find that wearing two pairs of socks helps eliminate friction.

Chafing

Athletic clothing can chafe and produce abrasions. Because long-distance runners are prone to this problem on their upper legs, they generally wear shorts with longer legs and lower-friction fabric. Chafing by a polyester or synthetic shirt can give male runners *jogger's nipples*, causing pain and even bleeding. Cool compresses are soothing to chafed skin; antibiotic ointment or even simple petrolatum can help relieve the discomfort.

Proper clothing that is soft and nonabrasive can help prevent chafing, as can use of a lubricating ointment to prevent friction. Tape can also help—preferably a kind with minimal adhesiveness (circular adhesive bandages work for nipples).

DERMATITIS/ECZEMA

Athletes work out so frequently, and therefore bathe and shower frequently, that they often develop dry skin—especially in colder climates where indoor heat dries the air. *Eczema* is a general term that covers many kinds of skin inflammation, or dermatitis. Some irritants are highly specific, as in contact dermatitis; others remain unknown to the sufferer. No matter the specific nature or stage of eczema, a universal symptom is itching.

Contact Dermatitis

Contact dermatitis is a rash caused by a localized allergic reaction to a specific substance. As in our case study at the beginning of the chapter, the reaction causes redness and may cause blistering. It almost always itches. The classic example of contact dermatitis is poison ivy, caused by an oily substance (urushiol) in the sap of the leaves (figure 7.1).

Treatment of contact dermatitis first involves eliminating exposure to the offending substance or object. Ice or cool compresses can soothe the itch, whereas exercise or a warm shower may make it worse. Topical corticosteroid cream or ointment usually reduces the inflammatory response and the itch. Oral antihistamines also may relieve the itching; the most effective over-the-counter antihistamine for contact dermatitis is diphenhydramine (Benadryl); the most effective prescription antihistamine is hydroxyzine. If the reaction is widespread (which can occur with poison ivy), oral corticosteroids can dramatically reduce symptoms.

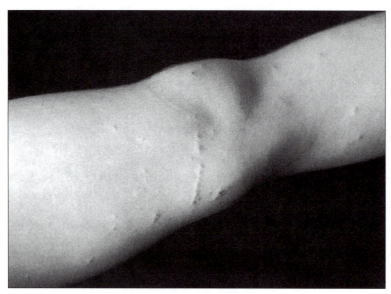

■ **Figure 7.1** Contact dermatitis. The line of papules and vesicles is typical for contact dermatitis caused by poison ivy.

Courtesy of Dr. Gary Willliams

Atopic Dermatitis

The most common kind of eczema is atopic dermatitis, in which a person's skin is genetically predisposed toward extreme sensitivity to a variety of irritants. It is a chronic disease whose appearance depends on whether the eruptions are in an acute stage. Acute exacerbations produce papules and 1- to 2-mm vesicles on a background of erythema (figure 7.2). Eventually these lesions become scaly. Extreme, relentless itching often leads to uncontrolled scratching, which in turn can lead to secondary infections and abnormally thickened skin. Treatment is aimed largely at relieving the itching to break the vicious cycle that involves scratching and (when appropriate) at treating secondary infections with antibiotics.

Chronic Eczema

Chronic eczema thickens the skin and exhibits larger papules. Chronic eczema can cause hypopigmentation (lighter skin) or hyperpigmentation (darker skin). Children tend to be affected on extensor surfaces such as the fronts of the knees and the backs of elbows, whereas adults tend to get it on the flexural surfaces of the knees (back of the knees) and front of the elbows.

Both allergies and psychogenic stress can exacerbate eczema. The skin of people with eczema dries very easily and may react to any irritant with increased lesions and itching. Both harsh soaps and frequent bathing can dry sensitive skin. In susceptible individuals, certain strains of bacteria, particularly *Staphylococcus aureus* and *Streptococcus pyogenes*, may trigger dryness and inflammation.

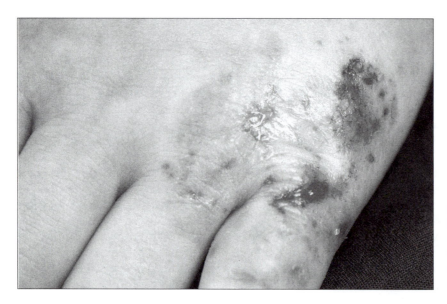

■ **Figure 7.2** Infected eczema. Note the weepy appearance and darkness (indicating redness) of the scaly area. These are signs of infection.

Courtesy of Dr. Gary Williams

Treatment and Prevention of Dermatitis

Most varieties of dermatitis require the same general treatments: relieving the symptoms and avoiding the irritant (when possible). Secondary infections in all cases are treated with antibiotics.

A good non-alcohol-based moisturizer lotion or cream can help treat mildly dry skin (alcohols can irritate the skin and dry it out even further). Some people use the rule of thumb that perfumed moisturizers tend to contain alcohol, but the best way to determine which products are alcohol free is to read labels. Note that on cosmetic labels the term *alcohol* used by itself refers to ethyl alcohol. Moisturizers may be labeled alcohol free and yet contain other so-called *fatty alcohols*—such as cetyl, stearyl, cetearyl, or lanolin alcohol—that do not dry the skin as does ethyl alcohol or isopropyl alcohol (the ingredient in rubbing alcohol). Eucerin®, Aquaphor®, and Lubriderm® are common moisturizers that contain no alcohol.

Treat inflamed skin with topical corticosteroid ointment. Ointments are generally better than creams for treating itchiness associated with dry skin. It is common to begin with a medium-strength prescription ointment, increasing the strength only if lower doses do not satisfactorily control the itching. Table 7.1 lists popular prescription topical medications in order of decreasing strength. People should use the mildest corticosteroid that works—overuse of more potent corticosteroids can break down the skin and invite infection. When itching persists and is especially problematic at night, over-the-counter antihistamines such as diphenhydramine (Benadryl) or prescription antihistamines such as hydroxyzine often provide relief. Unfortunately, the better antihistamines for itching tend to be quite sedating and are appropriate for most people only at night. For some individuals, however, these medications do not cause drowsiness and can therefore be used during the day. Widespread flares of dry skin, especially with a lot of redness and itching, may indicate a low-grade bacterial infection that will require prescribed oral antibiotics.

It is not possible to completely prevent eczema in people who are unusually sensitive to various irritants. The obvious first step is to avoid contact with anything that historically has caused difficulties. It is often wise to avoid wool clothing and to dress as much as possible so that the body does not become too warm. Many people with eczema find it helpful to use skin cleansers designed for sensitive skin (they do not contain alcohols or perfumes), and to bathe or shower in lukewarm (not hot) water.

Table 7.1 Topical Corticosteroid Medications

Group	Generic name	Brand name
I	Clobetasol propionate	Temovate®
	Betamethasone dipropionate	Diprolene®
	Halobetasol propionate	Ultravate®
II	Mometasone furoate	Elocon®
	Halcinonide	Halog®
	Fluocinonide	Lidex®
	Desoximetasone	Topicort®
III	Amcinonide	Cyclocort®
	Betamethasone valerate	Valisone®
	Diflorasone diacetate	Florone®
IV	Triamcinolone	Aristocort®
	Flurandrenolide	Cordran®
V	Hydrocortisone butyrate	Locoid®
	Hydrocortisone valerate	Westcort®
VI	Alclometasone dipropionate	Aclovate®
	Fluocinolone acetonide	Synalar®
VII	Hydrocortisone	Hytone®
	Hydrocortisone + pramoxine	Pramosone®

Medications are grouped from most potent (I) to least potent (VII). Note that for the same compound, ointments are more potent than creams, which are more potent than lotions. Most of these medications come in more than one concentration. All are prescription except for 1% hydrocortisone.

INFECTIONS

Although standard skin infections afflict athletes as often as anyone else, athletic activity actually fosters some other infections. Whatever the cause of an infection, you should be familiar with common symptoms so that you can help athletes seek treatment as soon as possible and so that you can help prevent the spread of infections.

Bacterial Infections

Bacterial infections of the skin tend to occur when there has a been a break in the integrity of the epidermis, such as occurs with an abrasion or a blister. Some are relatively benign, whereas others occasionally have serious side effects.

Staph, Strep, and Pseudomonas Infections

The two most common skin pathogens are *Staphylococcus aureus* and *Streptococcus pyogenes.* Staph infections are more likely to exhibit drainage and pus. Strep tends to cause redness and a clear exudate. Either staph or strep can cause impetigo, a highly contagious superficial infection with yellow crusts (figure 7.3). Classically occurring on the face and nose of children, impetigo can affect athletes of any age—especially those who had this infection as a child. It is difficult to distinguish between staph and strep simply from the appearance of the infected skin. Impetigo is quite contagious but more so in children than in adults. It tends to be spread by skin-to-skin contact more than on surfaces such as towels and clothing. A prescription-strength topical antibiotic (e.g., mupirocin, brand name Bactroban®) is often the first choice for treatment. If the topical antibiotic is not effective, impetigo can be treated with oral antibiotics (usually derivatives of penicillin, erythromycin, or cephalexin). Over-the-counter topical antibiotics such as bacitracin may not be as effective but are worth a try for a localized patch of impetigo. If there is any spreading of the rash during use of a topical antibiotic, a physician should be consulted. Usually the rash will improve in 24 to 48 h if the topical antibiotic is going to work.

When staph invades deeper tissues, it has a tendency to wall itself off and form an abscess. A firm mass usually suggests a deep abscess. Commonly called a *boil,*

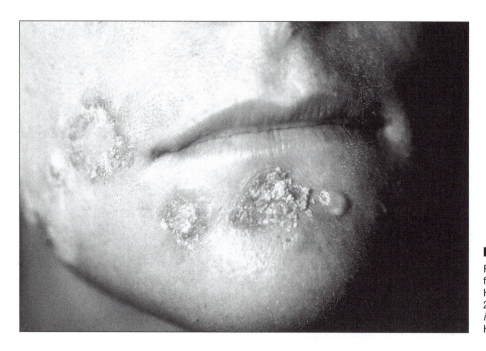

■ **Figure 7.3**   Impetigo.

Reprinted, by permission, from S.J. Shultz, P.A. Houglum, and D.H. Perrin, 2000, *Assessment of athletic injuries* (Champaign, IL: Human Kinetics), 411.

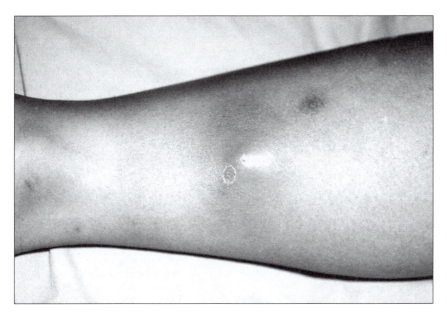

■ **Figure 7.4** Furuncle (boil).

Reprinted, by permission, from S.J. Shultz, P.A. Houglum, and D.H. Perrin, 2000, *Assessment of athletic injuries* (Champaign, IL: Human Kinetics), 411.

this lesion is also known as a *furuncle* (figure 7.4). Multiple furuncles that merge into a single large lesion are sometimes called a *carbuncle.* They are all characterized by pain, inflamed skin around a pus-filled lesion, and often fever. Boils frequently require incision and drainage, especially when the center is fluctuant (i.e., feels somewhat like a balloon filled with water) or develops a yellow center or head. Initially a physician will prescribe warm soaks and may prescribe systemic antibiotics such as dicloxacillin or cephalexin. Erythromycin may be ineffective in that many strains of staph throughout the world are resistant to it. Because boils can be contagious, athletes should not share towels or washcloths.

Strep that spreads and invades the deeper tissue causes an infection called *erysipelas,* which causes redness and warmth but is less likely to form an abscess than staph. For example, Kari is a soccer player with a 3-d-old abrasion on her lower leg. She states that over the past 24 h the skin around the abrasion has been getting red and the skin is getting tender. The abrasion itself is dry and has drainage. Because of concern about infection, you refer Kari to a physician who concurs and puts her on an antibiotic. The physician states that with only redness, the cause is probably strep and that the condition is erysipelas. It is usually treated with warm soaks and the same antibiotics as for a staph infection. If Kari has a fever or the infection does not respond to oral antibiotic, intravenous antibiotic therapy may be required. Athletes in sports requiring skin-to-skin contact cannot participate until they have been on oral antibiotics for 48 to 72 h, and any lesion must be dry with no oozing or potential for drainage. Wrestling is the sport where questions arise most often about skin lesions. Refer to *Skin Infections and Wrestling,* page 109.

Folliculitis, which literally means inflammation of the hair follicles, is usually associated with a low-grade infection. The presence of papules, especially with white or yellow centers, indicates that the infection is probably contagious—in which case you should treat the athlete as for impetigo (figure 7.5). If it is a localized patch, a topical over-the-counter antibiotic can be used. If it is widespread or getting worse despite good topical treatment, a physician should be consulted.

A superficial infection of *Pseudomonas aeruginosa* is a form of folliculitis associated with inadequately disinfected whirlpools or hot tubs. It appears 1 to 2 d after exposure, on the areas of the skin that were in contact with the swimsuit and that experienced prolonged contact with the water. It causes numerous red papules

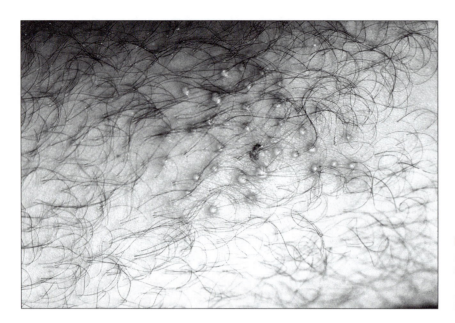

■ **Figure 7.5** Folliculitis.

Reprinted, by permission, from S.J. Shultz, P.A. Houglum, and D.H. Perrin, 2000, *Assessment of athletic injuries* (Champaign, IL: Human Kinetics), 410.

that itch. The rash disappears on its own, requiring only palliative treatment for the itching.

Acne Mechanica

The exact cause of acne is not fully understood, but it appears that plugging of the sebaceous (oil) glands in the skin invites a low-grade infection of the area with propionibacteria that inhabit the skin. Athletes are particularly susceptible to acne mechanica—a kind of acne that results from pressure, heat, and irritation from such things as shoulder pads, helmets, or tight clothing. As with any other form of acne, treatments for acne mechanica aim to prevent plugging of the pores and to kill the associated bacteria.

Topical agents such as 5% or 10% benzoyl peroxide are generally helpful. Use of topical tretinoin (retinoic acid; common brand name is Retin-A®) at bedtime is also helpful for athletes who tend to develop plugged pores (blackheads and whiteheads), as this product is specifically designed to prevent plugging. Topical antibiotics such as erythromycin and clindamycin are also helpful for those who cannot tolerate benzoyl peroxide (it is too drying for some people).

Physicians generally prescribe oral antibiotics only when the topical medicines are not effective or for acne on the back where topicals are difficult to apply. Although tetracycline or its relatives doxycycline and minocycline are usually the treatment of choice, many other antibiotics are effective for acne if the tetracyclines fail. The tetracyclines have the disadvantage of making the skin more sensitive to sun, so athletes who are receiving this medication and spend much time practicing outdoors need to be watched more carefully than others for signs of sunburn. Athletes who develop scarring, especially with deep cysts (cystic acne), should be referred to a physician as soon as possible to discuss treatment with oral isotretinoin (Accutane®). (Note that both tretinoin and isotretinoin can cause birth defects, and doctors should use caution when prescribing these substances for young women of childbearing age.) Isotretinoin has been associated with severe depression and, in a small number of patients, even suicide. Because severe acne is associated with depression, it is not clear if the medication or the acne is causing the depression in those individuals.

To help treat and prevent acne mechanica, athletes should take measures to keep moisture away from the skin—for example, wearing a clean polypropylene

T-shirt underneath uniforms and bathing immediately after exercise. If athletes are *not* using tretinoin, isotretinoin, or any other peeling agents, they may benefit from a topical salicylic acid agent (literally dozens are on the market, in both nonprescription and prescription strengths).

Pitted Keratolysis

Excessive sweating can lead to pitted keratolysis on the bottoms of the feet. The most obvious symptom is a distinctive strong, bad odor, which is the reason most athletes with this condition first seek treatment; the skin may be only slightly red, with some areas of tiny pits in the epidermis. Both the pits and the odor are caused by a species of corynebacterium. Treatment is with over-the-counter 5% or 10% benzoyl peroxide. Prescription erythromycin lotion is also effective. Athletes can prevent recurrence by frequent, thorough washing with soap and water, followed by complete drying of the feet (some athletes use a hair dryer). Foot or body powder may help keep the skin dry, as can going barefoot when possible, wearing socks made of cotton or absorbent synthetic material, changing socks often (athletes can take several pairs to school with them), wearing well-ventilated shoes, and permitting shoes to dry at least 24 h before wearing them again (necessitating regular alternating use of two or three pairs of shoes). Some athletes use standard antiperspirants on their feet. Even more potent antiperspirants are available by prescription—such as 20% aluminum chloride hexahydrate (Drysol® is a common brand).

Fungal and Yeast Infections

Fungi thrive in moist, warm, dark environments. It's not surprising that athletes, who produce so much perspiration, experience more than their share of fungal infections. Tinea is a superficial fungal infection that is named for the infected area: tinea pedis (athlete's foot) for infection of the toes or feet, tinea cruris (jock itch) for the groin area, tinea capitis for the scalp, and tinea corporis for the trunk (figure 7.6).

Fungal infections typically cause itching as well as redness, cracking, and scaling of the skin. Scratching infected skin may cause a burning sensation. There is often a raised border, sometimes with satellite lesions (small macules surrounding a larger macule). Well-circumscribed lesions with raised borders represent

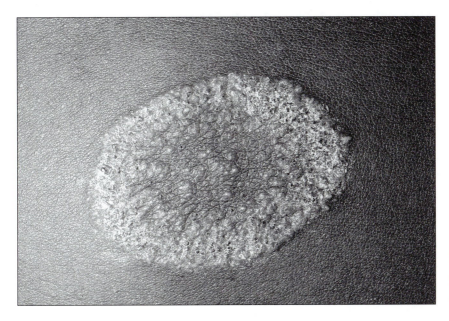

■ **Figure 7.6** Tinea corporis. This slightly pruritic lesion had been present for 2 weeks.
Courtesy of Dr. Gary Williams

the classic tinea corporis lesion—hence the common name ringworm. Of course, the causative agent is a fungus, not a worm. Although all tinea infections (even athlete's foot) were traditionally referred to as ringworm, the term is losing favor and is best avoided because of the confusion and alarm it causes among the lay public.

Treatment of infected areas includes effective drying, sometimes even with a hair dryer. Bright light can help but is not practical for the groin. Over-the-counter topical medications (such as miconazole and clotrimazole) and prescription medications (such as ketoconazole and econazole) all work equally well for these infections, which rarely require systemic antifungal agents. Over-the-counter tolnaftate will work for mild infections. Creams are usually better than powders and aerosols because they penetrate the skin better. If no improvement in the condition occurs after 2 to 3 weeks of topical antifungal therapy or if the condition worsens, a physician should be consulted.

Case Study

Joe is a 14-yr-old wrestler who appears with two dime-shaped spots, one on each forearm. The spots have raised borders. Joe states that he had ringworm the previous year, and he thinks he has it again. He was wrestling an opponent last week who had a suspicious rash. You refer him to a physician, who recommends use of topical miconazole cream twice a day for 4 weeks and allows him to wrestle as long as he promises to use the topical medication and keep the spots covered for the next week when he is on the mat.

Occasionally fungi can invade the fingernails or toenails, resulting in thickening and cracking of the nails. The infection often distorts the nail and makes it darker in color. Although the infection rarely causes pain, people often seek treatment because the infected nail is so unattractive. Treatment for fungal nail infections requires an oral antifungal agent that is taken for many months—about 6 months for fingernails and about 12 months for toenails. Griseofulvin is an older antifungal agent to which fungi are occasionally resistant; moreover, it sometimes causes stomach upset and headaches, is occasionally toxic to the liver, and is strongly contraindicated in women who take certain kinds of oral birth control hormones. The newer antifungals such as ketoconazole, fluconazole, and itraconazole are probably more effective, but they also exhibit various side effects. Rare serious side effects may include liver toxicity. These medications are also very expensive.

Pityriasis versicolor is a very mild yeast infection of the trunk. Previously (and incorrectly) believed to be a tinea fungus, it used to be called tinea versicolor. The most visible symptom of pityriasis versicolor in light-skinned people is pale areas that do not tan along with surrounding uninfected skin; darker-skinned athletes may exhibit areas with less pigmentation any time of year. This mild infection will sometimes clear with application of an over-the-counter selenium shampoo or such prescription topical treatments as econazole foaming solution or ketoconazole cream. A one-time ingestion of a prescription oral antifungal agent like ketoconazole or fluconazole 1 h before a workout is often curative.

Parasites

Biologically, parasites are microscopic animals. They present a particular challenge for treatment, because biochemically they are little different from people. Fortunately, infections with such organisms are relatively rare in the developed world.

Swimmer's Itch

Swimmer's itch is associated with freshwater swimming in the hot summer months when waterfowl may deposit trematode (fluke or schistosome) parasites into lake water. In coastal areas, it is sometimes called clam digger's itch. Although these benign parasites quickly die after invading a swimmer's superficial skin, the presence of the foreign antigens causes a hypersensitivity dermatitis (i.e., a superficial allergic reaction). A macular, papular rash typically appears on areas in contact with wet swimwear. Treatment aims only at alleviating the itching, through use of a topical corticosteroid for the itch, a systemic antihistamine, or both. Only about one-third of the population is susceptible to this allergy. Prevention involves avoiding swimming in freshwater lakes when the water is warm; alternatively, swimmers should remove wet swimwear as soon as the water activity is finished and dry the skin with a towel (if infested water is not allowed to evaporate from wet skin, the parasites usually are unable to penetrate the skin).

Scabies

Scabies is a very contagious infection by a mite *(Sarcoptes scabiei)*. Mites are not insects but arachnids (with eight legs—related to spiders). Mites can infect the skin anywhere in the body but most often infect the hands and arms of adults. An intense hypersensitivity reaction to mites leads to unrelenting itchiness. The skin has the appearance of eczema, except that there may be evidence of nearly invisible burrows, just 2 to 3 mm long, where the mite has tunneled into the skin (figure 7.7). If a person with no history of eczema has a new eczematous rash that causes intense itching, scabies is a good candidate for the diagnosis. If an acquaintance or family member is also itching, this increases the likelihood that it is a scabies infection. To provide proof of the infection, a physician may scrape the rash and look for mites in the scrapings under the microscope.

Scabies is treated with presciption medications, 5% permethrin cream (Elimite®) or 1% lindane lotion (Kwell®). It is important that all infected individuals in the household be treated simultaneously.

Scabies mites live for no more than about 1 h when not on a warm body. The disease is spread by relatively prolonged skin-to-skin contact. The contact can be from sexual intimacy or merely from a parent hugging a child. Though athletes should generally avoid physical contact with people who have scabies, they needn't be afraid of simple gestures such as a handshake.

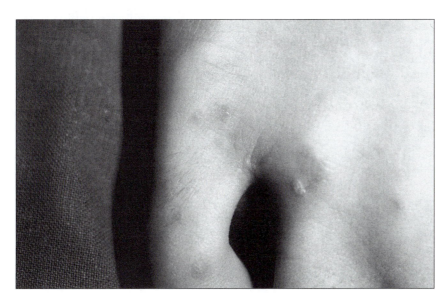

■ **Figure 7.7** Example of scabies, which is caused by mites.

Reprinted, by permission, from S.J. Shultz, P.A. Houglum, and D.H. Perrin, 2000, *Assessment of athletic injuries* (Champaign, IL: Human Kinetics), 416.

Lice

Lice are tiny insects that infect (and bite) humans anywhere there is hair, with different species specializing in different parts of the body: There are head lice *(Pediculosis capitis)*, body lice *(Pediculosis corporis)*, and pubic lice *(Pediculosis pubis)*, which are often known as *crabs*.

Lice are rarely transmitted in the athletic setting, except when athletes share combs or brushes. Body lice can be transmitted through sexual contact. All kinds of lice are treated with over-the-counter permethrin preparations such as Nix® shampoo or Rid® and other pyrethrin rinses. Prescription medications such as lindane are no more effective than the over-the-counter medications. Treatment often requires extensive effort to rid one's living quarters of nits, or louse eggs. It is usually wise to wash all clothing, bedding, and towels that have contacted the infested person, using hot water, and to dry them in a drier. Dry-cleaning is also effective, when appropriate. Many physicians also recommend vacuuming floors, rugs, and furniture.

Disagreement exists about whether all individuals in a household should be treated at the same time to prevent further spread. If the family in question is able to unambiguously identify who does and who does not have the lice, it is necessary to treat only infected individuals. In many cases, however, people are unsure whether they have identified everyone who is infected—in which case it may be safer simply to treat everyone.

Although even the most fastidious families can experience quite aggravating lice infestations, prevention measures are still useful. People should frequently inspect the hair of family members, especially schoolchildren, for lice or nits; clean their clothing and linens frequently; avoid sharing used clothing; and avoid sharing combs, hairbrushes, hair ribbons, and the like.

Viral Infections

Viruses sometimes have a long latency period before they produce symptoms, and they are not generally susceptible to chemical agents (by most definitions they are not even alive). As a result they present formidable challenges to infected individuals as well as to physicians.

Herpes Simplex

The most common *Herpes simplex* infection is the common cold sore or fever blister that occurs on the lips—and that infection is only slightly different from genital herpes (in fact, either virus can appear at either location). Lesions generally are preceded by tingling or itching in the infected area, and sometimes by fever and enlargement of the lymph nodes. Initially a lesion consists of a group of tiny (1-2 mm) vesicles filled with (usually clear) fluid. These painful vesicles eventually break open to form a raw, red area that eventually forms a scab. This process takes several days, and the entire outbreak takes 7 to 10 d to totally resolve. During the preliminary stage of an outbreak, and while vesicles are present, viruses can spread to other people through skin-to-skin contact. Because the virus lives within nerves and is never totally destroyed by the immune system, herpes tends to be a recurrent problem—it can flare up occasionally throughout an individual's life, especially during any period when the immune system is compromised. New outbreaks may be triggered by a variety of emotional or physical stressors.

In wrestlers and rugby players, and athletes in other sports where skin-to-skin contact is common, herpes infections—called *herpes gladiatorum*—are readily spread from competitor to competitor. The lesions can occur virtually anywhere on the body and in multiple patches of vesicles (figure 7.8). Because of the frequent trauma they experience during competitions, these lesions may not have vesicles.

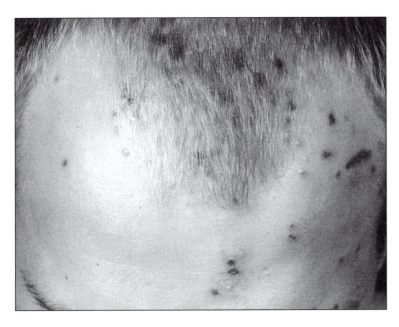

Moreover, the inoculum of virus may be so high that the vesicles may appear larger (5-10 mm) with cloudy fluid instead of clear. The key in these cases is to determine the history of previous infection or to note changes in the athlete's sensory perceptions: Bacterial infections are rarely painful, whereas herpes infections almost always cause some sensory abnormalities.

If the affected athlete is examined in a doctor's office, the lesions can be cultured for virus, since herpes viruses grow readily in vitro. Alternatively, a smear of cells from the lesion can be stained to reveal so-called *giant cells* under the microscope, which indicate a herpes infection. These procedures are done for the first appearance of the lesions or when the diagnosis is unclear.

If the lesions are diagnosed within the first 48 to 72 h of the illness, antiviral medication can be prescribed that will prevent the virus from replicating and shorten the illness. The most common antiviral is acyclovir. Table 7.2 lists the various antiviral medications used for herpes infections. Any athletic competitor with active (wet) lesions must be disqualified to prevent spread of the infection. It is unknown how long an individual sheds virus particles after the initiation of antiviral therapy. As recommended by the National Federation of High School Associations' *Sports Medicine Handbook* (NFHSA 2002), athletes in skin-to-skin sports such as wrestling must not compete until all lesions are dry and crusted over and no new lesions have appeared in the previous 48 h. Physicians may want to utilize the examination form provided by NFHSA for wrestlers with contagious skin infections (see figure 7.9).

As with herpes genital infections, herpes gladiatorum can be prevented by prophylactic use of antiviral medications (usually acyclovir).

Table 7.2 Antiviral Medications and Doses for Herpes Infections

Stage/Purpose	Drug	Strength and duration
Initial	Acyclovir	400 mg TID × 7 d
Recurrences	Acyclovir	400 mg TID × 5 d
Prophylaxis	Acyclovir	400 mg BID
Initial	Valacyclovir	500 mg BID × 7 d
Recurrences	Valacyclovir	500 mg BID × 5 d
Prophylaxis	Valacyclovir	500 mg QD
Initial	Famciclovir	250 mg TID × 5 d
Recurrences	Famciclovir	125 mg TID × 5 d
Prophylaxis	Famciclovir	250 mg BID

TID = three times daily; BID = two times daily; QD = one time daily.

Sports Medicine Advisory Committee
NATIONAL FEDERATION OF HIGH SCHOOL ASSOCIATIONS
PHYSICIAN RELEASE FOR WRESTLER TO
PARTICIPATE WITH SKIN LESION

Name: _____ Date of Exam: _____ / _____ / _____

Mark Location of Lesion(s): _____

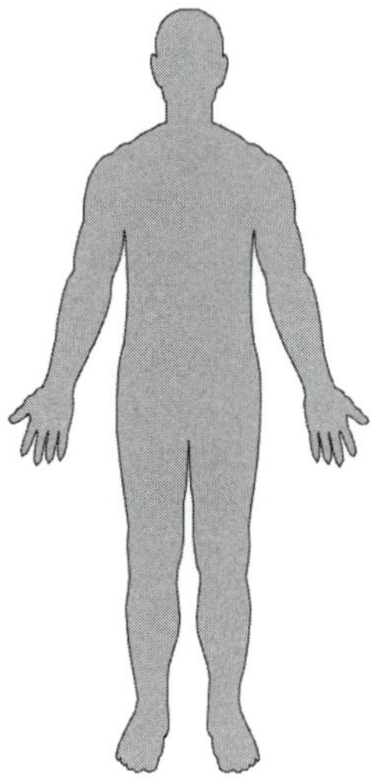

Diagnosis _____

_____

Communicable _____ Noncontagious _____

Location of Lesion(s) _____

_____

Date Treatment Started: _____ / _____ / _____

Medication(s) Used to Treat Lesion(s): _____

_____

Earliest Date May Return to Participation: _____ / _____ / _____

Physician Name (Printed or Typed) _____

Provider Signature _____ Office Phone #: _____

Office Address _____

Note to Providers: *Noncontagious lesions do not require treatment prior to return to participation (e.g., eczema, psoriasis, etc.). Please familiarize yourself with NFHS rule below. NFHS Rule 4-2-3 states:*

If a participant is suspected by the referee of having a communicable skin disease or any other condition that makes participation appear inadvisable, his coach shall provide current written documentation from a physician stating that the suspected disease or condition is not communicable and that the athlete's participation would not be harmful to his opponent. Covering a communicable condition shall not be considered acceptable and does not make the wrestler eligible to participate. This document shall be furnished at the weigh-in or upon arrival at the site of the dual meet or tournament. *Note:* If an on-site tournament physician is present, he/she may overrule the diagnosis of the physician signing this form.

Below are some treatment guidelines that suggest minimum treatment before return to wrestling.

Bacterial diseases (impetigo, boils): Oral antibiotic for 2 days and no drainage, oozing, or moist lesions.

Herpetic lesions (Simplex fever blisters, Zoster, Gladiatorum): No new lesions in 48 hours and all lesions scabbed over. No oral treatment is required.

Tinea lesions (ringworm scalp, skin): Oral or topical treatment for 7 days on skin and 14 days on scalp.

Scabies, head lice: 24 hours after appropriate topical management.

Conjunctivitis: 24 hours of topical or oral medication and no discharge.

Molluscum contagiosum: 24 hours after curretage.

■ **Figure 7.9** Physician release form from the National Federation of High School Associations.

Reprinted, by permission, from National Federation of State High School Association, 2002, *Sports Medicine Handbook* 2: 46.

From *Essentials of Primary Care Sports Medicine* by G.L. Landry and D.T. Bernhardt, 2003, Champaign, IL: Human Kinetics.

Skin Infections and Wrestling

The National Federation of High School Associations (NFHSA) Wrestling Rule Book, Section 2, Article 3 states the following:

"If a participant is suspected by the referee to have a communicable skin disease or any other condition that makes participation appear inadvisable, his coach shall provide current written documentation from a physician stating that the suspected disease or condition is not communicable and that the athlete's participation would not be harmful to his opponent" (p. 43).

Covering a communicable condition shall not be considered acceptable and does not make the wrestler eligible to participate.

Wrestlers at the high school level will have to present a form signed by a physician that outlines the diagnosis and method of treatment and present it at the time of weigh-in. Skin checks are frequently done during the weigh-in at the time of tournament competition. A tournament physician may be able to overrule the diagnosis provided on a skin lesion form. A sample form is provided.

Treatment guidelines for common skin conditions are provided in the NFHSA Handbook. These are considered the minimum criteria an athlete must meet before returning to wrestling:

- **Bacterial diseases** (impetigo, boils): Oral antibiotics for 2 d and no drainage, oozing, or moist lesions.
- **Herpetic lesions** (simplex, zoster, gladiatorum): No new lesions in 48 h and all lesions scabbed over. No oral treatment is required.
- **Tinea lesions** (ringworm, scalp, skin): Oral or topical treatment for 7 d on skin and 14 d on scalp.
- **Scabies, head lice:** 24 h after appropriate topical management.
- **Conjunctivitis:** 24 h of topical or oral medications and no discharge.

NCAA Guidelines for Skin Infections

The NCAA guidelines differ slightly. The NCAA rules stipulate the following (NCAA Committee on Competitive Safeguards and Medical Aspects of Sports 2002):

- A physician or certified athletic trainer shall examine all contestants for communicable skin diseases before all tournaments and meets.
- It is recommended that this examination be made at the time of weigh-in. The presence of a communicable skin disease (or any other condition that, in the opinion of the examining physician or certified athletic trainer, makes the participation of that individual inadvisable) shall be full and sufficient reason for disqualification.
- If a team official suspects a student-athlete of having such a condition and consults a physician (ideally a dermatologist) who determines that it is safe for that individual and his opponent to compete, that contestant's coach shall provide current written documentation from that physician to the examining physician or athletic trainer at the medical examination describing (1) the diagnosed skin disease or condition, (2) the prescribed treatment and the time necessary for it to take effect, and (3) that the skin disease or condition would not be communicable or harmful to the opponent at the time of competition. Such documentation shall be furnished at the medical examination.
- Final determination of the participant's ability to compete shall be made by the host site physician or certified athletic trainer who conducts the medical examination, after review of any such documentation and the completion of the exam.

Physicians and athletic trainers are encouraged to follow the guidelines put forth by the NCAA Committee on Sports Medicine (2002, p. 21). Guideline 2B, "Skin Infections in Wrestling," states the following:

Open wounds and infectious skin conditions that cannot be adequately protected to prevent their exposure to others should be considered cause for medical disqualification from practice or competition. These include the following:

- Bacterial skin infections
- Viral skin infections
- Parasitic skin infections
- Fungal skin infections

(continued)

(continued)

Common treatment for bacterial infections includes no participation until the athlete has been on oral antibiotics for 48 to 72 h and the lesion is dry with no oozing or potential for drainage.

An athlete with a viral infection must not compete until all lesions are dry and crusted over and no new lesions have appeared in the previous 48 h. In addition to antiviral or antibiotic treatments, covering of conditions is advisable for fungal conditions and during the later stages of treatment. Skin conditions should be covered with a securely attached bandage or nonpermeable patch.

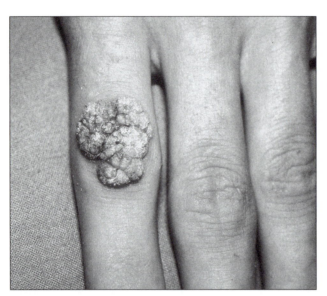

■ **Figure 7.10**   Viral wart.

Reprinted, by permission, from S.J. Shultz, P.A. Houglum, and D.H. Perrin, 2000, *Assessment of athletic injuries* (Champaign, IL: Human Kinetics), 413.

Warts

Nothing is more frustrating than the common wart (the scientific term is *verruca vulgaris*). Caused by a variety of human papilloma viruses, these lesions typically occur on the hands or the bottoms of the feet, where trauma has caused tiny breaks in the skin. Variable in diameter, warts are large papules that appear as thickened skin 1 to 4 mm above the surface of the skin (figure 7.10). Athletes often seek treatment when a wart's size causes pain during a sport activity. Although warts can be confused with calluses, careful examination shows that warts distort the normal dermal lines (the lines that create fingerprints and unique footprints), whereas calluses leaves these lines intact. Warts on the soles of the feet are called plantar warts, even though their cause is the same as that of warts elsewhere on the body. Because papilloma viruses are ubiquitous, infection seems to be related to individual differences in immune defenses. Some families seem to have more trouble than others with wart viruses.

Virtually anything that destroys the thickened epidermis may stimulate an immune reaction that destroys the viruses in the base of the wart. Warts may be frozen with liquid nitrogen or burned with a cautery tool; or they may be treated with any type of caustic acid, with care to avoid exposure to normal skin. There is no infallible cure—most warts require repeated treatments, along with a hefty dose of patience from both athlete and health practitioner. With the exception of genital warts, warts tend to clear up without treatment about half the time. Genital warts do not clear up without treatment and need to be evaluated by a physician because of the association with cervical cancer in women. Athletes must have access to the proper medical resources when dealing with conditions like genital warts. Some athletes, particularly younger ones, may be reluctant to let the athletic trainer know that they are experiencing genital warts. Thus, the trainer should make it clear to all the athletes under her care that to get a referral to appropriate resources for medical care, the athlete need say no more than "I have a personal problem that I want to see a doctor about." Chapter 9 provides an in-depth discussion of sexually transmitted diseases.

Molluscum Contagiosum

Molluscum contagiosum is a papular eruption caused by any of several different papilloma viruses. It is not very serious but can be annoying—and it's rather con-

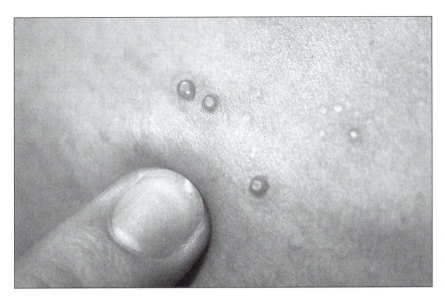

■ **Figure 7.11** Molluscum contagiosum.

Reprinted, by permission, from S.J. Shultz, P.A. Houglum, and D.H. Perrin, 2000, *Assessment of athletic injuries* (Champaign, IL: Human Kinetics), 411.

tagious. The papules contain small dots and have a clear center. Older lesions have an umbilical center that is depressed below the surface of the lesion (figure 7.11). The lesions often disappear if the tops of the papules are unroofed to stimulate an immune reaction. Physicians may freeze the lesions with liquid nitrogen, open the bumps with a sterile needle and squeeze out the fluid, or even use carbon dioxide lasers. The rash generally goes away after treatment. The lesions sometimes subside without any treatment—but if they persist and are untreated, they can remain for months or even years, during which time the disease can be transmitted through physical (including sexual) contact.

Because this infection is contagious, wrestlers, rugby players, and other athletes in sports where skin-to-skin contact is common must have their lesions treated before they compete. The latency period between exposure and symptoms is from 1 to 3 months. Prevention involves avoiding contact with an infected person.

Rashes Associated With Fever

Several common viral infections can cause faint rashes, especially after the fever subsides. Chicken pox, caused by the varicella virus (in the herpes family), deserves special mention here because, in spite of widespread vaccination programs, it still affects a small percentage of high school and college students. Spread through the air from the skin lesions, chicken pox is one of the most contagious infections known. The illness usually starts with fever, dry cough, red eyes, and headache. Rashes typically begin on the head and neck, with red macules that become papular and develop a vesicle in the center (the classic description of a lesion is a "dewdrop on a rose petal"). It is important to diagnose chicken pox promptly so that infected athletes can be quarantined from classes and social activities. People are contagious for 1 to 2 d (sometimes up to 5 d) before and about 5 d after the rash appears. By the time the lesions have crusted over, the person is generally not contagious. Symptoms appear from about 1 to 3 weeks after exposure. Treatment is palliative, with various lotions to stop the itching and sometimes prescribed oral antihistamines for the same reason.

The disease typically runs its course within 7 to 10 d in children; adults usually endure more severe symptoms and are bedridden longer than children. The primary long-term consequence is that people who have chicken pox may later develop shingles, a painful skin disease caused by viruses that remain latent within nerve cells for up to decades after the initial infection (figure 7.12).

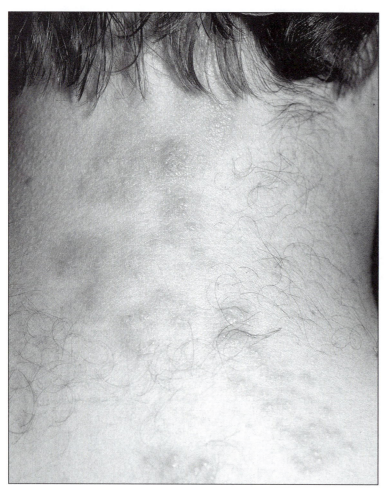

■ **Figure 7.12** Shingles (herpes zoster).

Reprinted, by permission, from S.J. Shultz, P.A. Houglum, and D.H. Perrin, 2000, *Assessment of athletic injuries* (Champaign, IL: Human Kinetics), 412.

Although prevention among susceptible individuals involves avoiding contagion from an infected person, the first line of defense against chicken pox is immunization with the varicella vaccine. Many school districts require such immunization of all students.

One rash associated with fever has grave consequences. Meningococcal infections cause meningitis, shock, and sometimes death. Such an infection is caused by the bacterium *Neisseria meningitidis*, which is present in the throats of about 1 out of 10 healthy people at any given time. Meningococcal outbreaks (defined as at least three cases within 3 months) tend to occur in college dormitories or in other locations where people—especially young adults—are confined in relatively close quarters.

The illness begins with high fever, severe headache, and sometimes vomiting. The rash usually exhibits tiny dark red macules and dark purple, superficial bruises caused by bleeding into the skin (figure 7.13). Suspicion of this infection should prompt an immediate visit to an emergency facility.

A vaccine is available that is effective against about 60% of the bacterial strains that cause this

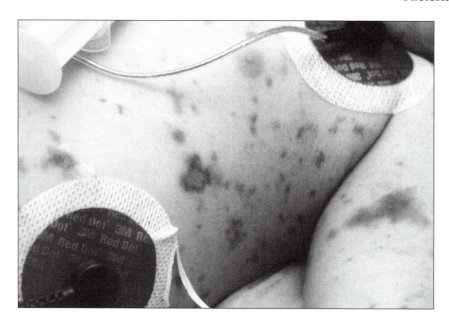

■ **Figure 7.13** Purpura associated with meningococcemia. This patient is quite ill and is in the hospital with moniters attached to his chest. The intense dark skin bruises are hemorrhages associated with meningoccocus infection.

Courtesy of Dr. Gary Williams

For Further Information

Printed Resources

Basler, R.S.W., and M.P. Seraly. 2001. Common dermatologic problems in athletes. *Patient Care* 11: 43-59.

Lillegard, W.A. 1993. Dermatologic problems in the athlete. *Sports Medicine Review*. Kansas City, MO: American Academy of Family Physicians.

NCAA Committee on Competitive Safeguards and Medical Aspects of Sports. 2002. Guideline 2b: Skin infections in wrestling. In *2002-2003 NCAA Sports Medicine Handbook*, p. 21. St. Louis: NCAA.

Sports Medicine Advisory Committee of the National Federation of High School Associations. 2002. Skin disorders. In *Sports Medicine Handbook*, pp. 43-51. Indianapolis: NFHSA.

Web Resources

American Academy of Dermatology
www.aad.org
A Web resource with links to patient information as well as information for other health care professionals.

National Library of Medicine and National Institutes of Health
www.nlm.nih.gov/medlineplus/
A searchable Web site maintained by the National Library of Medicine and National Institutes of Health. Information is available on a number of skin conditions.

Centers for Disease Control and Prevention
www.cdc.gov/ncidod/dbmd/diseaseinfo/default.htm
A helpful government site sponsored by the U.S. Department of Heath and Human Services; offers information about infectious disease, health bulletins on various topics, and current fundings and research projects.

severe infection. Health professionals often recommend vaccination for college students, especially freshmen.

SUMMARY

1. *Describe the signs and symptoms of a variety of skin lesions common in active populations.*

This chapter dealt with a wide variety of skin lesions common in active populations. A key to recognition is the ability to describe skin lesions using common terminology. In addition, understanding the origin of the skin problem will dictate referral and treatment options. Mechanical stresses; allergic response; and bacterial, viral, and fungal infections are all common origins of these problems.

2. *Explain the common course of treatment for various skin conditions.*

Treatment options are dictated by several factors, including the origin of the skin condition, the potential for spreading the infection, and the desired physical activity. The allied health professional must work with both the patient and the physician to develop treatment plans that both facilitate recovery and address the needs of the active patient.

3. *Determine which skin conditions require immediate medical referral.*

Specific skin conditions that are painful, easily spread, and nonresponsive to care must be referred to a physician. An awareness of potential complications and the ability to recognize skin conditions that are not improving can facilitate a definitive diagnosis, prevent complications, and establish an environment for an effective recovery.

4. *Discuss the guidelines for sports participation for athletes with specific skin conditions.*

Sport activities that include close contact, such as wrestling and rugby, require specific steps to prevent the spread of skin infections. Understanding the nature of the infection will dictate the course of action and limitations for participation. Specific sport-governing bodies such as the National Federation of State High School Sports Associations and the National Collegiate Athletic Association have participation guidelines for athletes with skin infections. It is the responsibility of the sports medicine team to educate coaches and participants to these guidelines and ensure that they are followed.

CHAPTER 8

Respiratory Pathologies

OBJECTIVES

Upon completion of this chapter the reader will be able to do the following:

1. Identify the characteristics of exercise-induced asthma (EIA)

2. Discuss the triggers and symptoms of EIA

3. Describe the pharmacological and non-pharmacological treatment options for EIA

4. Identify other respiratory conditions that present with symptoms similar to those of EIA

One of the most frequently encountered problems in sports medicine is the exercise-associated cough or difficulty breathing that an athlete experiences. Athletes can become alarmed, wondering how this may affect their performance; and parents may fear that their child has a serious disorder. Coaches, unfortunately, sometimes assume that the athlete is simply deconditioned—and, without investigating the problem, prescribe more vigorous exercise.

Case Study

A 17-yr-old cross-country runner has a history of exercise-associated shortness of breath and wheezing 10 min after she starts to run. The problem is especially bad on days of competition and grows worse as the season progresses. Her shortness of breath clears rapidly after practice or competition and is associated with a mild cough that lasts from a few minutes up to 1 h after completion of exercise. She has no history of asthma, lung, or cardiovascular disease; no history of atopic dermatitis or previous allergies; and no problems breathing in other situations. Family history is positive (her brother) for exercise-induced asthma. Her physical exam is completely normal, including completely clear lung fields and no murmur on examination of the heart.

You strongly suspect exercise-induced asthma, but here are some questions you might ask as you evaluate this athlete: (1) What diagnostic clues can help you decide what may be causing the symptoms? (2) What other diagnostic possibilities exist? (3) Are there simple ways in which an athletic trainer can help the athlete before her visit to a doctor? (4) What pharmacological treatments are available for the problem as it is eventually diagnosed? What are the side effects of these medications? Are the medications allowed by the sanctioned governing body for the athlete's sport, in both national and international competition?

EXERCISE-INDUCED ASTHMA

Asthma is characterized by chronic airway obstruction secondary to inflammation and hyperresponsiveness to a variety of triggers or stimuli. **Exercise-induced asthma (EIA)** is an asthma attack *triggered by exercise*—the physical exam of people with EIA is often normal, with no more than an occasional wheeze provoked with forced expiration. Most athletes with EIA have other triggers of their asthma.

In the first few minutes of exercise, bronchodilation occurs in both people with asthma and people without. In people susceptible to asthma, however, this response is transient—their lung function returns to baseline after approximately 10 min of exercise, and progressive bronchoconstriction peaks 5 to 10 min after the cessation of exercise. Lung function then gradually returns to normal over the next 20 to 40 min (figure 8.1).

Exercise provokes symptoms in 40% to 90% of people with known asthma (Kawabori et al. 1976). Among high school athletes with medical histories suggestive of possible EIA who underwent exercise challenge testing in a study by Rupp et al. (1992), approximately 30% had EIA as defined by a change in their pulmonary func-

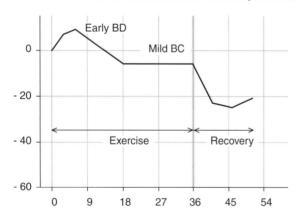

■ Figure 8.1   Exercise changes in airway function in asthmatics. BD signifies bronchodilation, and BC signifies bronchoconstriction.

Reprinted, by permission, from K. Rundell, R. Wilbur, and R. Lemanske, Jr., 2002, *Exercise-induced asthma: Pathophysiology and treatment* (Champaign, IL: Human Kinetics), 168.

Terms and Definitions

beta-2-andrenergic agonists—Medications resembling adrenaline (epinephrine) that selectively stimulate receptors in bronchial smooth muscle, causing relaxation and bronchodilation. They are selective agonists because of reduced stimulation of beta one receptors in the heart.

bronchoprovocation test—Clinical test that challenges the lungs chemically (typically with methacholine or histamine) or with another potential trigger such as exercise or temperature, and measures the effects of these potential triggers on lung function (such as forced respiratory volume or peak expiratory flow rate).

bronchospasm—Contraction of the smooth muscle that surrounds the airway, resulting in narrowing of the lumen, through which air enters and exits the lungs.

cholinergic urticaria (CU)—A condition associated with small (2-4 mm) hives in response to passive warming of the body or with exercise.

corticosteroids—Medications chemically related to cortisone and used primarily for their anti-inflammatory effect.

exercise-induced anaphylaxis—The massive release of histamine triggered by exercise, producing itchiness, hives, swelling of hands and face, and hypotension.

exercise-induced asthma (EIA)—Bronchoconstriction and mucous production associated with exercise. Asthma means hyperreactive airways. Exercise is one of many sources that produces asthmatic symptoms such as coughing, wheezing, and shortness of breath.

inflammation—A local immune response intended to protect from infection. Includes dilation of arterioles, capillaries, and the smallest veins; increased permeability and blood flow; exudation of blood plasma along with plasma proteins; and migration of white blood cells into the inflamed area. Inflammation of bronchial tissues contributes to obstruction of lumen and exacerbates asthma.

mast cell stabilizers—Medications that prevent the release of histamine from mast cells.

minute ventilation—The volume of air breathed each minute (e.g., 12 breaths/min with average tidal volume of 0.5 L/breath = minute ventilation of 6 L/min).

status asthmaticus—Emergent situation in which respiratory distress secondary to asthma is poorly responsive even to large doses of bronchodilators.

upper respiratory infection (URI)—The common cold, associated with a stuffy and runny nose, cough, and low-grade fever.

urticaria—Allergic reaction characterized by raised welts on the skin and usually accompanied by intense itching. Commonly called hives. Can be caused by internal or by external contact allergens.

vocal cord dysfunction (VCD)—Abnormal closing of the vocal cords causing difficulty breathing that mimics asthma.

tion tests. Among elite athletes, the incidence of exercise-induced asthma has been reported as 17% of long-distance runners, 30% to 35% of figure skaters, and 50% of cyclists (Helenius et al. 1997; Mannix et al. 1996; Weiler et al. 1998).

Triggers and Symptoms of Exercise-Induced Asthma

Two theories have been proposed as the main cause of EIA:

■ The water-loss theory hypothesizes that exercise results in an increased ventilation rate that bypasses upper-airway conditioning (the process of humidifying and warming the air in the upper airway). Because higher-intensity exercise involves less nasal breathing, high minute ventilation pushes the conditioning process from the upper to the lower airway. This results in a loss of water from the epithelium of the bronchial mucosa (lining of the small airways), which in turn changes the osmolarity, pH, and temperature of the periciliary fluid. Airway hyperosmolarity results in mediator release and bronchoconstriction. Bronchoactive mediators may include histamine, leukotrienes, and prostaglandins released from mast cells, epithelial cells, or both (McFadden and Gilbert 1994).

- The second theory, the heat-exchange theory, suggests that EIA symptoms can occur after exercise is terminated due to the rewarming that occurs after stopping exercise. The increased ventilation during vigorous exercise cools the airways. Stopping exercise leads to bronchial vasculature dilatation and engorgement to rewarm the epithelium. Rebound hyperemia (increased bronchial blood flow) of the bronchial vascular bed impinges and narrows the airway. Engorged vessels can also leak, leading to mediator release and bronchospasm. The main factors that influence the degree of exercise-associated airway obstruction are the **minute ventilation** (the volume of air breathed each minute), the temperature and humidity of inspired air, and the athlete's baseline airway reactivity. A higher minute ventilation due to increased intensity of exercise exacerbates EIA symptoms, as does inspiration of cool, dry air. The larger the quantity of thermal air that needs to be transferred, the cooler the airways become—the subsequent rapid rewarming results (according to this theory) in severe bronchoconstriction.

An example that is consistent with the second theory is that of a track runner who does well until, following a hard workout on a cold day, he attempts to cool down by jogging indoors where it is warmer. Under these circumstances his symptoms become very severe, with bronchoconstriction that is difficult to relieve even with several doses of bronchodilators—so-called **status asthmaticus.**

The symptoms of EIA may include wheezing, coughing, shortness of breath, or chest pain and may occur during or immediately after exercise. Generally, the symptoms are most severe for a brief time (5-10 min) and resolve between 15 and 30 min after exercise. EIA usually has a gradual onset and gradual resolution, whereas some other causes of shortness of breath seem to have an on/off switch.

Even in the absence of exercise, other triggers that aggravate the athlete's baseline asthma may exacerbate EIA. For any asthmatic athlete under your care, obtain a list of known triggers such as temperature, seasonal variability, other allergic symptoms, heartburn, and smoke exposure. Forty percent of patients with allergic rhinitis also have EIA, according to one study (Kawabori et al. 1976). A history of worsening rhinitis, sneezing, itchy eyes, or postnasal drip hints at worsening allergic symptoms that may make asthmatic symptoms worse. Though gastroesophageal reflux (manifested by heartburn) is clearly correlated with conditions such as chest pain, chronic cough, hoarseness, and bronchial asthma, reflux by itself does not appear to cause EIA—but no one has yet performed a large study to investigate this relationship. Direct as well as secondhand smoke exposure obviously exacerbates asthmatic symptoms. Many athletes avoid tobacco exposure because they are aware of this relationship. But because some athletes do not appreciate this relationship, you should ask every athlete about exposure to tobacco or other inhalants, including marijuana (you'll have to promise confidentiality to get straight answers).

Treatment of Asthma

To understand the treatment of asthma, one must understand the basic pathophysiology of the disease. Two processes are at work in most people with asthma: **Bronchospasm** is caused by contraction of the smooth muscles that surround the airway, resulting in a narrowing of the lumen through which air enters and exits the lungs; **inflammation** is mediated by many different triggers and chemicals in the body, resulting in swelling within the airway, thus further narrowing the lumen.

Treatment, both non-pharmacological and pharmacological, focuses on relieving either or both of these processes. Because most EIA can be successfully treated, you should encourage individuals with any degree of asthma to participate in athletics once their disease is optimally controlled (Cypcar and Lemanske 1994). For athletes with moderate asthma, this may mean using a single medication during certain times of the year when their symptoms are worse because of seasonal pollens, temperature, or humidity. Athletes with more severe asthma must optimize their baseline lung function before focusing on treatment of symptoms associated with exercise. Note: Any athletic trainer who cares for athletes with asthma should have a thorough knowledge of the medications that are banned by various athletic organizations (table 8.1). She should be sure that any physician treating the athlete has similar awareness.

Monitoring peak flow can help the athlete, athletic trainer, and physician assess the severity of asthma. Peak flow meters (figure 8.2) allow the athlete to detect worsening pulmonary function, sometimes even before symptoms such as wheezing or coughing occur. A physician can develop a plan to adjust medications based on the athlete's peak flow with a stepwise approach (using stronger medicine based on severity—worsening peak flows) to treatment based on the athlete's peak flow rate. A normal peak flow rate is based on the athlete's age, gender, and size. Usually when an athlete drops below 80% of his normal peak flow rate (PFR), some type of steroid (either inhaled or oral) is given in an attempt to normalize the PFR. For athletes who do not improve over a 12-h period or who drop below 50% of normal, consultation with a physician is mandatory. Asthma symptoms can worsen acutely, resulting in severe respiratory distress, wheezing, poor air exchange, and increased work of breathing with use of the accessory intercostal muscles and the abdominal muscles. When this occurs, transport to a physician for emergent evaluation and treatment if necessary. Peak flow monitoring can be performed several times a day when symptoms warrant or when a drop in peak flow occurs. Overall, this simple device allows the athlete to help in directing his own care and optimizing his lung function and, ideally, his athletic performance.

Non-Pharmacological Treatment

Non-pharmacological treatment of exercise-induced asthma includes modifying environmental triggers such as temperature or environment. The cool, dry air of an indoor ice rink, for example, may make skating difficult for hockey players. Such athletes may benefit from choosing a different sport—such as swimming, tennis, or basketball—that provides a less extreme environment for exercise.

Another standard non-pharmacological treatment is induction of a refractory period, which works in nearly

Table 8.1 Asthma Medications Permitted and Banned

Permitted	Banned

Beta-2 agonists
  Advair®*
  Salmeterol*
  Terbutaline*
  Salbutamol*
  Albuterol*
	All other beta-2 agoinists are banned

Glucocorticoids
  Flovent®*
  Nasacort®*
  Nasonex®*
  Pulmicort®*
  Rhinocort®*
  Vanceril®*
	Aerobid®
	Azmacort®
	Flonase®
	Beconase®
	Beclovent®

Mast cell stabilizers and other anti-inflammatories
  Cromolyn sodium
  Ipratropium
  Nedocromil
  Singulair®
  Theophylline	

*Restricted to inhalant or nasal forms only; medical notification form needs to be on file with United States Anti-Doping Agency.

See www.usantidoping.org/prohibited_sub/wallet_card.asp for more information.

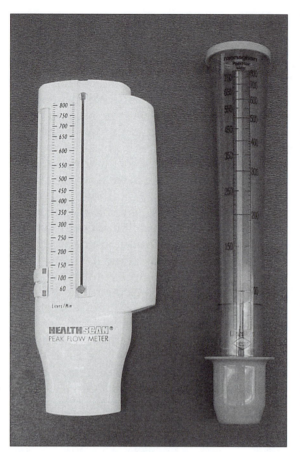

■ Figure 8.2   A peak flow meter can be useful as a tool that provides a quick, accurate record of pulmonary function.

half of people who experience EIA. Although the physiological mechanism of the refractory period remains a mystery, it works this way: For about an hour after experiencing acute EIA, many individuals experience a time during which they appear to be somewhat resistant to another EIA attack. In individuals who have a refractory period, a second bout of exercise during this period typically causes EIA symptoms less than half as severe as the first attack. *The refractory period occurs independent of any medical treatment.* If athletes commonly experience such a refractory period, have them warm up with an aerobic activity and then take 20 to 30 min to stretch. After this, they may proceed with the rest of practice or competition with reduced or even no asthmatic symptoms.

Pharmacological Treatment

Many different medications can prevent or at least ameliorate both ordinary asthma and EIA. The medications most often used to prevent EIA symptoms are **beta-2-adrenergic agonists** (stimulators), which are effective for approximately 90% of athletes with EIA. By stimulating beta-receptors on the smooth muscles surrounding the airway, these medications cause those muscles to relax, thereby enlarging the airway opening (lumen). The most popular medication in this class is albuterol, which is usually inhaled but sometimes is taken orally. Albuterol starts working within about 5 min, peaks at 15 to 60 min, and dissipates after approximately 4 to 6 h.

Typical dosage is two puffs approximately 15 to 20 min before exercise, followed by a mild exercise session in hopes of inducing a refractory period. Whereas the inhaled forms of beta-agonists are approved for use by the International Olympic Committee, oral forms are banned in international competition. For patients who are symptomatic after a bout of exercise or because of some other trigger (such as a common cold or allergy), beta-agonists are the treatment of choice due to their rapid bronchodilatory effect. Side effects include a fine tremor, jitteriness, and tachycardia.

Alternative medications used in preventing EIA are the **mast cell stabilizers.** This class of medications prevents the release of histamine from the histamine-containing mast cells that line the airway (the mechanism of how this helps prevent EIA is unclear); they also are anti-inflammatory. Because mast cell stabilizers (primarily cromolyn and nedocromil) do not result in direct bronchodilation, they are used only prophylactically—not as rescue medications once acute symptoms have appeared. Although not as effective as albuterol, this group of medications appears to have no side effects and therefore is more acceptable to some patients. As with albuterol, cromolyn has a rapid onset of action. However, the time until effects decrease is only 2 h.

Athletes must first gain optimal control of their baseline asthma (i.e., asthma independent of exercise) before they can hope to control their exercise-related symptoms. Treatment of baseline asthma often starts with the two classes of medications—beta-adrenergic agonists and mast cell stabilizers—already discussed.

Some people, however, require stronger medications. **Corticosteroids** are anti-inflammatory medications available in inhaled, oral, and injectable forms (the U.S. Olympic Committee permits only inhaled forms). Different strengths of inhaled corticosteroids are available. For athletes whose symptoms tend to appear during a particular season (such as in the fall because of hay fever pollen), prophylactic use of a corticosteroid inhaler each morning and evening during that season often has a strong effect in preventing symptoms. Like the mast cell stabilizers, corticosteroids are primarily used to prevent symptoms and should not be used as a rescue medication. To minimize side effects, athletes should use the lowest concentration that optimizes lung function (Smith and LaBotz 1998).

Athletic trainers should be familiar with how to use an inhaler. The athlete should shake the medicine first. A spacer is often recommended to help guide the medicine to the airway. Commercial spacers are available, although a toilet paper roll works well (figure 8.3). The athlete then should exhale completely and take a slow, deep breath on inhalation. During inhalation, the athlete presses the inhaler and breathes the medicine deep into the lungs and holds the breath for at least 5 s. Make sure the head is tilted back slightly to aid airflow and medicine transport to the lungs (figure 8.4). When two puffs of medicine are prescribed, this process is repeated after at least a 1- to 2-min rest period.

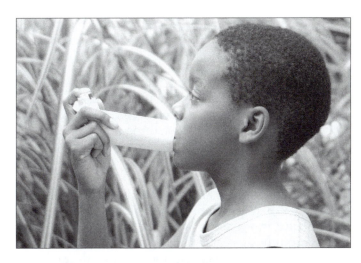

■ **Figure 8.3** A commercial spacer helps in the delivery of aerosolized medicine to the airway. In the absence of a commercial spacer, a toilet paper roll, used as shown, will also help.

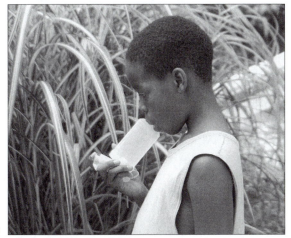

a

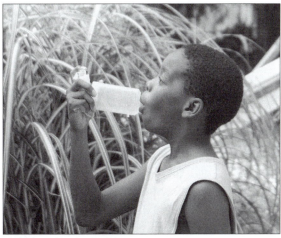

b

■ **Figure 8.4** Not even a commercial spacer will help in the delivery of aerosolized medicine if the athlete has the head in a downward tilted position *(a)*. The head should be in a slightly extended position to improve delivery of medicine to the airway *(b)*.

EIA That Is Unresponsive to Treatment

Some individuals continue to experience exercise-induced asthma even after they have adequately treated their baseline asthma and are essentially symptom free before exercise. Refer these athletes to physicians who can conduct appropriate exercise tests and more closely identify triggers for asthma attacks. Many times such testing will lead to use of other types of asthma medication and to further optimization of treatment that can maximize athletic performance. Pulmonary function testing pre- and postexercise permits evaluation for EIA as well as other disorders. A decrease of ≥10% in peak expiratory flow rate after exercise confirms a diagnosis of EIA. Though an exercise **bronchoprovocation test** can provide a specific diagnosis of EIA, a negative test does not rule out the diagnosis of asthma, as this test is specific only to exercise as a trigger. It may be necessary to use other triggers in bronchoprovocation testing—whether pharmacological (methacholine, histamine) or environmental (cold air)—to further evaluate an individual's propensity to wheeze or have reactive airways.

OTHER DIAGNOSTIC POSSIBILITIES

Not all athletes with exertional shortness of breath or cough suffer from EIA. Possible diagnoses include vocal cord dysfunction, gastroesophageal reflux, seasonal allergies, exercise-induced anaphylaxis, cholinergic urticaria, upper respiratory infections, influenza, or pneumonia.

■ Vocal cord dysfunction. If athletes develop symptoms of air flow obstruction that are not responsive to traditional treatment, advise them to be evaluated for **vocal cord dysfunction (VCD).** In this underdiagnosed condition, the vocal cords close during inspiration; VCD can mimic or complicate asthma. People who suffer from *both* asthma and VCD usually report a history of exercise-induced asthma that responds to neither traditional beta-agonist treatment nor any other medicinal treatment. Part (but not all) of the etiology, at least in many cases, appears to be psychological—athletes with VCD are often high-achieving perfectionists. It occurs more often among women than among men. When questioned in detail, the athlete reports difficulty with inspiration and difficulty in speaking while exercising. Often there appears to be an on/off switch—symptoms appear suddenly and disappear just as abruptly. Athletes with this condition may experience shortness of breath until they pass out from hyperventilation. Diagnosis often involves exercise provocation testing in which athletes exercise until symptoms appear. Pulmonary tests of symptomatic individuals show flattening of the inspiratory curve. Direct visualization of the vocal cords with flexible laryngoscopy before and after exercise can also aid diagnosis (Morris et al. 1999). Triggers for VCD include gastroesophageal reflux and postnasal drip (usually secondary to allergic rhinitis); treatment of the triggers helps ameliorate the VCD symptoms. Comprehensive treatment involves breathing and relaxation exercises, usually prescribed by a speech therapist, along with counseling to address potential psychological factors. Table 8.2 compares asthma and VCD.

■ Gastroesophageal reflux (GERD). GERD is a known precipitant for both asthma and VCD and should be suspected in either condition if symptoms are difficult to control with standard therapy. GERD may be clinically silent except for the symptoms associated with the asthma. Other symptoms to inquire about include heartburn, chest pain, a sour taste in the back of the mouth, and sometimes (when standard therapy is working) even emesis associated with or without exercise. If a history is consistent with this disorder, empiric treatment with some type of antacid may be necessary. If the history is negative but respiratory symptoms persist, the athlete should be referred to a physician. Further workup, including a barium swallow, may need to be pursued.

Table 8.2   Comparison of Vocal Cord Dysfunction (VCD) and Exercise-Induced Asthma

	VCD	EIA
Female preponderance	+	−
Chest tightness	+/−	+
Throat tightness	+	−
Stridor	+	−
Usual onset of symptoms after beginning exercise (min)	<5	>5-10
Recovery period (min)	5-10	15-60
Refractory period	−	+
Late-phase response	−	+
Response to beta-agonist	−	+

Tables 3 pp 66 reproduced, with permission, from Brugman, S.M., Simons, S.M.: Vocal cord dysfunction: Don't mistake it for asthma. The Physician Sportsmedicine 1998: 16(5): 63-85 © The McGraw-Hill Companies.

- Seasonal allergies. Common seasonal allergies, which can trigger both EIA and vocal cord dysfunction, are not unique to exercising individuals. Allergies often vary with the time of year: Grass and tree pollens are more abundant in the late spring and early summer, for example, whereas hay fever pollens are more common in the fall. Runny nose (rhinorrhea), sneezing, and itchy eyes are the classic symptoms. People with year-round symptoms may be allergic to dust mites or to mold (many people appear to have a general tendency toward allergies and suffer from several different ones). To avert major symptoms, people with seasonal allergies may avoid the environmental stimulus when possible; modify the time of year in which they exercise outdoors; and use corticosteroid nasal sprays, antihistamines, or both as needed. Athletes for whom standard treatments do not work may benefit by seeing an allergist who can test them to identify the offending agent; depending on the allergy, a desensitization program may be feasible.

- Exercise-induced anaphylaxis. You should be aware of the symptoms of **exercise-induced anaphylaxis,** which, although rare, can be dangerous. It is directly triggered by exercise, which leads to release of histamine and other trigger chemicals from mast cells. The condition is characterized by generalized skin itchiness (pruritis) with hives **(urticaria)** and a generalized warm feeling that may progress to swelling of the hands and face (angioedema), upper respiratory obstruction, and even cardiovascular collapse. The urticarial rash with this condition is characterized by large welts or wheals measuring 10 to 15 mm (about 3/8 in. to over 5/8 in.) in diameter. Some people are more susceptible to this condition shortly after they have eaten certain foods—shellfish and celery are most commonly implicated. First-line treatment is to stop exercising at the earliest hint of symptoms. Be certain that any athlete who has experienced exercise-induced anaphylaxis always carries and knows how to administer a subcutaneous dose of epinephrine (EpiPen®). Insist that such athletes always exercise with a partner and carry a mobile phone to contact emergency services. The parents of affected minor athletes must be informed of the risks of this problem. Unfortunately, acute episodes are often unpredictable and unresponsive to medical prophylaxis (Briner and Sheffer 1992).

Athletic trainers should be familiar with EpiPen use for treatment of any cause of anaphylaxis. At some institutions, an annual in-service is performed to refresh everybody working with athletes on how to use this device, seeing that it is not used frequently. This auto-injector device is very easy to use and is designed to inject a standard dose of epinephrine to abort the severe allergic response. The device comes with easy-to-read instructions, can be administered through clothing, and works very quickly. The epinephrine wears off within 20 min, and anybody who receives treatment with this device should be transported immediately to an emergency facility for further evaluation and treatment.

■ Cholinergic urticaria. A separate but related allergy to exercise is **cholinergic urticaria (CU),** characterized by small, diffuse lesions. People suffering from CU tend to have lesions every time they exercise, whereas athletes with exercise-induced anaphylaxis have more variable, intermittent symptoms. Wheezing commonly occurs with CU but not with anaphylaxis. Unlike exercise-induced anaphylaxis, CU may be triggered by temperature changes independent of exercise. Athletes with this condition often can be treated with antihistamines and do not usually need to take the same drastic precautions as those with exercise-induced anaphylaxis. Cholinergic urticaria is usually not serious but can be a significant nuisance if left untreated.

■ Upper respiratory infections. The common cold or **upper respiratory infection (URI)**—typically caused by a rhinovirus or some other respiratory virus—can diminish performance. Infection results in low-grade fevers, nasal congestion, or sore throat; sometimes there is a cough that, because it is caused by postnasal drip, is worse at night. Treatment for colds is usually symptomatic. Refer people to a physician for further evaluation if they have high fever (greater than 101.5° F) or a wet, productive cough—or if the most noticeable symptom is a constant cough, chest pain, severe malaise or fatigue, myalgia (muscle pain), or sore throat. Most often, an athlete with a viral URI can continue to exercise but may need to modify his practice schedule (and social calendar) to avoid weakening his immune systems. He should sleep as much as possible and drink large amounts of fluids (not coffee, pop, or other diuretics). Playability with the common cold is usually based on symptoms and the athlete's energy level. The athlete who feels that he is too sick to play should be held out of competition or practice until his malaise improves. A respiratory infection is considered a "lower" infection if it causes wheezing or shortness of breath. Pneumonia is also considered a lower respiratory infection (see below).

■ Influenza. Influenza is a viral respiratory illness resulting in severe myalgias, fatigue, sore throat, cough, and high fever. Patients often report they feel as if they were "run over by a truck." Diagnosis is usually made on history, with seasonal outbreaks in the winter months aiding in establishing the diagnosis. Treatment with antiviral medication may shorten the usual 5 to 7 d illness by 24 h if treatment is started within 48 h. An influenza vaccine is recommended for the elderly and any person suffering from chronic disease, especially cardiac or pulmonary problems, including asthma. The vaccine has variable effectiveness depending on the flu strain. As the athletic trainer, you may want to discuss with your athletes and team physicians the possibility of immunizing the entire team in hopes of preventing an outbreak during the competitive part of the season for athletes participating in winter and spring sports. Athletes with influenza will not feel up to practicing, let alone competing; for that reason, playability decisions are usually easily made.

■ Pneumonia. Often mistaken for a common cold, pneumonia is usually characterized by a deep, wet cough associated with fever. It may be caused by a virus or by bacteria. If an athlete exhibits a cough independent of exercise and has fever, chest pain, shortness of breath, or severe malaise, refer her to a physician. If the symptoms continue to appear suspicious even after a standard physical exam

For Further Information

Print Resources

McFadden, E.R., ed. 1999. *Exercise induced asthma.* New York: Marcel Dekker.

Rundell, K.W., R.L. Wilber, and R.F. Lemanske Jr., eds. 2002. *Exercise-induced asthma: Pathophysiology and treatment.* Champaign, IL: Human Kinetics.

Web Resources

National Jewish Medical and Research Center
www.nationaljewish.org/medfacts/induced.html
National Jewish Medical and Research Center is a respected private immunology research institution. Information on exercise-induced asthma, vocal cord dysfunction, and other respiratory ailments is available. The Web site features a search function.

National Heart, Lung, and Blood Institute
www.nhlbi.nih.gov/index.htm
The National Heart, Lung, and Blood Institute (NHLBI) Web site is searchable and provides information and health facts on a variety of respiratory conditions. The NHLBI is part of the National Institutes of Health (NIH).

National Library of Medicine and National Institutes of Health
www.nlm.nih.gov/medlineplus/
A searchable Web site sponsored by the National Institutes of Health and the National Library of Medicine. Extensive information is available on asthma, exercise-induced asthma, and a variety of respiratory conditions.

Anaphylaxis.com
www.anaphylaxis.com
Provides an excellent flash demonstration of how to use the EpiPen device.

National Collegiate Athletic Association
www1.ncaa.org/membership/ed_outreach/health-safety/drug_testing/banned_drugs
Includes NCAA drug-testing program information from the NCAA Committee on Competitive Safeguards and Medical Aspects of Sports.

U.S. Anti-Doping Agency (USADA)
www.usantidoping.org/prohibited_sub/list.asp
The USADA manages testing and adjudication for athletes involved in U.S. Olympic, Pan American, and Paralympic competitions. Check its Web site for the most up-to-date information on substances banned by the International Olympic Committee.

turns up nothing remarkable, encourage the individual to pursue further diagnostic testing, including a chest X ray, to establish an unambiguous diagnosis.

SUMMARY

1. *Identify the characteristics of exercise-induced asthma (EIA).*

Asthma is characterized by chronic airway obstruction secondary to inflammation and hyperresponsiveness to a variety of triggers or stimuli. Exercise-induced asthma (EIA) is an asthma attack *triggered by exercise*—the physical exam of people with EIA is often normal, with no more than an occasional wheeze provoked with forced expiration.

Exercise-induced asthma is common among athletes of all ages. Many athletic trainers, coaches, physical education teachers, and even primary physicians are tempted to turn a blind eye toward people with asthma as long as taking a couple of puffs on an inhaler seems to prevent emergencies. But you will do well to encourage athletes with asthma to aggressively pursue evaluation and treatment of their condition. The goal, which probably will require your intimate cooperation and participation, should be a comprehensive, proactive program to optimize lung function, health, and performance. Offending triggers should be thoroughly explored and treated prudently.

  2. *Discuss the triggers and symptoms of EIA.*

The symptoms of EIA may include wheezing, coughing, shortness of breath, or chest pain. The symptoms may occur during or immediately after exercise. Generally, the symptoms are most severe for a brief period (5-10 min) and resolve between 15 and 30 min after exercise. EIA usually has a gradual onset and gradual resolution, whereas some other causes of shortness of breath seem to have an on/off switch.

  The main factors that influence the degree of exercise-associated airway obstruction are the minute ventilation (the volume of air breathed each minute), the temperature and humidity of inspired air, and the athlete's baseline airway reactivity. Two theories have been proposed as the main cause of exercise-induced asthma: the water-loss theory and the heat-exchange theory. The water-loss theory is activated by high-intensity exercise, whereas the heat-exchange theory is activated by the rewarming of tissues following exercise. Although the mechanisms differ, each theory leads to the release of bronchial mediators that result in bronchospasm.

  3. *Describe the pharmacological and non-pharmacological treatment options for EIA.*

Non-pharmacological treatment of EIA includes modifying environmental triggers such as temperature or environment. Another standard non-pharmacological treatment is induction of a refractory period, which works in nearly half of people who experience EIA. If athletes commonly experience such a refractory period, have them warm up with an aerobic activity and then take 20 to 30 min to stretch. After this, they may proceed with the rest of practice or competition with reduced or even no asthmatic symptoms.

  Many different medications can prevent or at least ameliorate both ordinary asthma and exercise-induced asthma. The medications most often used to prevent EIA symptoms are beta-adrenergic agonists (stimulators), which are effective for approximately 90% of athletes with EIA. For patients who are symptomatic after a bout of exercise or because of some other trigger (such as a common cold or an allergy), beta-agonists are the treatment of choice due to their rapid bronchodilatory effect. Side effects include a fine tremor, jitteriness, and tachycardia. Alternative medications used in preventing EIA are the mast cell stabilizers. Mast cell stabilizers do not result in direct bronchodilation; they are used only prophylactically—not as rescue medications once acute symptoms have appeared.

  Athletes must first gain optimal control of their baseline asthma (i.e., asthma independent of exercise) before they can hope to control their exercise-related symptoms. Treatment of baseline asthma often starts with the two classes of medications—beta-adrenergic agonists and mast cell stabilizers. Like the mast cell stabilizers, corticosteroids are primarily used to prevent symptoms and should not be used as a rescue medication.

  4. *Identify other respiratory conditions that present with symptoms similar to those of EIA.*

If athletes do not respond to treatment, help them pursue a different diagnosis. Symptoms of some respiratory conditions can be quite serious, causing significant anxiety to both athletes and their families. Exercise-induced anaphylaxis, for example, can be life threatening. Other potential causes of respiratory problems include cholinergic urticaria, the common cold, seasonal allergies, pneumonia, and vocal cord dysfunction.

It may be necessary for a physician to supervise a broad diagnostic workup, including exercise provocation testing. Athletes and their families deserve to have a clear understanding of the nature and causes of respiratory problems. Such knowledge is not only reassuring, but it also permits the taking of appropriate measures to improve symptoms, thereby allowing the athletes to exercise with greater safety and success.

CHAPTER 9

Sexually Transmitted Diseases and Blood-Borne Infections

OBJECTIVES

Upon completion of this chapter the reader will be able to do the following:

1. Discuss the signs and symptoms associated with common bacterial, viral, and parasitic sexually transmitted diseases (STDs)

2. Explain the importance of latex condom use in reducing the spread of sexually transmitted diseases

3. Describe the transmission, treatment, and prevention of blood-borne viral infections including HIV (human immunodeficiency virus), HBV (hepatitis B virus), and HCV (hepatitis C virus)

4. Identify proper practice for health-care providers in adherence to universal precautions

Case Study

A 21-yr-old female basketball player comes to you for a 4-d history of abdominal pain. She has not had any nausea, vomiting, or diarrhea. She has no dysuria, urinary frequency, or nocturia. She reports that her pain is worse with exercise and sometimes when she is lying down. She has had some chills at night but not during the day. You send her to a physician later that day.

On exam at the doctor's office, she has a temperature of 37.3° C (99.1° F), blood pressure 112/72, pulse 64. The doctor's exam shows normal bowel sounds and moderate tenderness to deep palpation over the lower abdomen and especially over her bladder. When a pelvic exam is done, she has evidence of cervicitis, and the bimanual examination is extremely painful. Cultures for gonorrhea and chlamydia are obtained.

At the doctor's office she reveals that she has had four male sexual partners in her life and uses condoms on an intermittent basis. She has not had any unusual vaginal discharge.

Her laboratory findings reveal a normal urinalysis, a normal complete blood count, and an erythrocyte sedimentation rate (ESR) of 53 (normal up to 20). Her diagnosis is pelvic inflammatory disease (PID), and the physician tells her to inform her partner. He also warns the athlete that if any of the sexually transmitted disease (STD) tests are positive that he is required by law to report the result to the public health department. The public health department will contact the athlete so that they can inform her sexual partners. Because she is not vomiting, the physician gives her prescriptions for two antibiotics, ciprofloxacin (Cipro®) and metronidazole (Flagyl®) and warns her not to drink alcohol with the metronidazole because it will make her very ill and produce vomiting. The physician asks her if he can tell the diagnosis to you, the athletic trainer. She consents but says she doesn't want her coach to know. A few days later the physician reports to the athlete that the chlamydia test is positive and the gonorrhea test is negative. She returns to the physician 2 weeks later; the repeat chlamydia test is negative and her examination is normal.

SEXUALLY TRANSMITTED DISEASES

Athletes who are at risk for sexually transmitted diseases (STDs) are not always aware that they are at risk. As the athletic trainer, you should be knowledgeable about STDs because some athletes may prefer asking sensitive questions of someone they feel more familiar with than a physician they've never met. Other athletes may want to consult a physician about private matters, and the athletic trainer should facilitate this without questions. It may be appropriate to ask if the athlete's concern is anything that may affect his ability to play a sport. If not, respect the athlete's privacy. The athletic trainer must be aware that any rash or bumps on the genitalia might represent an STD. Any abdominal pain or urinary abnormalities (urinary frequency or painful urination) in either males or females may also represent an STD.

A number of photos illustrating the appearance of the more common STDs are included in this chapter so that the athletic trainer

- will more clearly understand physicians' notes;
- will be more prepared to answer the questions of a worried athlete who fears he may have an STD; and
- can give informed advice to athletes who seek him out for answers to their questions about sexual activity and its possible consequences.

Athletic training students who have not yet practiced their trade may think such information is so private that athletes will not consult them about it. Those

Terms and Definitions

acquired immunodeficiency syndrome (AIDS)—Advanced HIV infection characterized by the presence of opportunistic infection and lowered counts of helper T cells.

biohazard container—A plastic container into which are placed all nonsharp materials (e.g., bandages, rubber gloves) that have come into contact with body fluids.

CD 4 cells—The type of T cell specifically targeted by HIV.

cirrhosis—Liver disease typified by extreme fibrosis; scar tissue replaces normal cells, leading to decline of liver function.

fibrosis—Scarring (of the liver, in the context of this chapter).

hepatitis B virus (HBV)—Virus commonly spread by sexual intercourse, blood transfusion, or contaminated needles resulting in liver infection.

hepatitis C virus (HCV)—Virus spread by blood transfusion and possibly intercourse or contaminated needles resulting in liver infection.

human immunodeficiency virus (HIV)—A virus that selectively infects certain types of white blood cells (helper T cells) resulting in the disease AIDS.

human papilloma virus (HPV)—A virus that causes common warts on feet and hands, mucous membranes of anal and genital areas.

sharps container—A plastic container into which are placed all sharp items (e.g., needles, syringes, lancets) that have come into contact with body fluids.

subclinical—Not detectable, or producing no clinical manifestations (e.g., in the early stage of a disease).

T lymphocytes (T cells)—A type of white blood cell responsible for the cell-mediated immunity that is critical for fighting viral infections, fungal infections, and certain bacteria such as tuberculosis.

virulent—Able to cause severe disease or death in an infected person.

who have been working as ATCs, however, have learned by now that her trainer may be the only one whom a particular athlete will confide in. Sometimes athletes will show the trainer their skin lesions or genital lesions. Some are real extroverts, and others feel there is no one else they can trust. Even though the trainer won't be making the diagnosis, being aware of how common STDs look gives her a reasonable idea of what the athlete is dealing with and enables her to give informed advice to athletes who seek her counsel.

After discussing the most common STDs, we will discuss blood-borne infections. Blood-borne infections are rare in athletes, yet the possibility of contracting them may cause concern for athletes and their families, especially in sports where bleeding may occur.

Chlamydia

The most common sexually transmitted disease in the United States and in many countries in the world is infection with *Chlamydia trachomatis*. The rate of chlamydia infections continues to rise (figure 9.1). Chlamydia is an intracellular bacteria that is spread only by intimate contact through mucous membranes and is not transmitted by mouth-to-mouth contact.

Chlamydia is more likely to produce symptoms in males than in females, but about 50% of males are asymptomatic. If symptoms develop in either gender, they tend to do so 7 to 21 d after exposure. Men are likely to develop symptoms of urethritis, which are dysuria, increased frequency of urination, a watery discharge from the penis, or any combination of these. The disease may also cause inflammation of the rest of the male reproductive tract and can be responsible for epididymitis

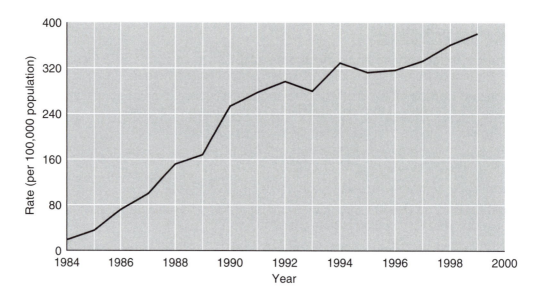

■ **Figure 9.1**   Chlamydia rates in selected U.S. cities (population > 200,000) have continued to rise.

and prostatitis. Women are more likely than men to be asymptomatic but can develop a discharge and lower abdominal pain due to inflammation of the cervix or the rest of the genital tract (uterus and ovaries). Irregular or heavy menstrual bleeding can also be a symptom of chlamydia (**menorrhagia** or **menometrorrhagia**).

Chlamydia is the leading cause of pelvic inflammatory disease (PID) in women, a problem associated with infertility later in life. In men, chlamydia can cause Reiter's syndrome, which is urethritis associated with arthritis and uveitis in the eye. To make the diagnosis of chlamydia, the physician inserts a small cotton swab into the urethra in men or the cervix in women; a newer test can diagnose it in urine by polymerase chain reaction (PCR). The patient must not urinate for 2 h before the test, and the urine specimen should be collected in the first 30 ml of urine during voiding.

Early diagnosis is particularly important in women because long-standing infections are associated with infertility. Neither men nor women should rely on symptoms to suspect chlamydia, as the infection can be indolent. A variety of antibiotics can successfully treat chlamydia infections, including the tetracyclines (of which doxycycline is the most common choice), erythromycin, and azithromycin (Zithromax®). A currently popular regimen is a one-time dose of 1,000 mg of azithromycin taken all at once on an empty stomach.

Gonorrhea

Gonorrhea is caused by an infection with the bacterium *Neisseria gonorrhoeae*. It commonly causes urethritis in the male and cervicitis in the female. The disease has a tendency to produce a copius white discharge in men and, like chlamydia, is more likely to be asymptomatic in women. Any symptoms produced tend to become apparent within 2 to 5 d after exposure, but they can occur anywhere between 1 and 14 d. Males may also have dysuria and polyuria. Females may have a vaginal discharge, dysuria, or intermenstrual bleeding. The infection may also cause menorrhagia. Gonorrhea can spread to the rest of the genital tract in both men and women and is another common cause of PID in women. In men, the disease has a tendency to produce a copious yellow discharge that is more opaque and less thick than semen and occasionally oozes from the penis.

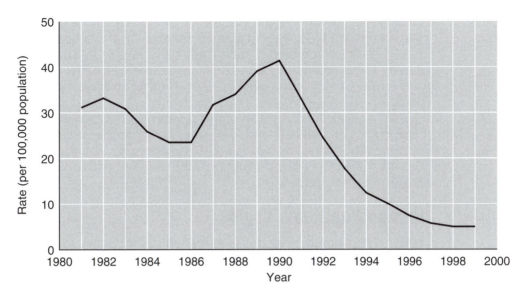

■ **Figure 9.2**   Rates of syphilis in selected U.S. cities (population > 200,000) have dropped after reaching a peak in 1990.

Like chlamydia, gonorrhea is more likely to be asymptomatic in women. When left untreated, it can spread to other areas of the body and may cause arthritis. Most untreated cases will resolve within 6 months. Gonorrhea is treated with a cephalosporin antibiotic.

Syphilis

Syphilis, caused by the bacterium *Treponema pallidum*, is a less common STD than gonorrhea and chlamydia in most parts of the world. Syphilis reached its peak incidence worldwide in 1990 and has gradually declined since that year. The dramatic increase in syphilis in the 1980s is thought to be linked with the rise in drug abuse (figure 9.2) and the common practice of exchanging sex for drugs, especially among users of crack cocaine.

Primary syphilis is usually seen as a chancre on the genitals or anus, but the chancre can be anywhere on the body. A chancre starts out as a papule that ulcerates. Secondary syphilis may produce a wide range of conditions. Early on a fever develops that may last for many weeks. Usually the patient also develops a rash that may appear on the hands and feet or over the entire body. The small spots can look like prickly heat rash, or larger lesions can resemble chicken pox. The rash lasts 2 to 6 weeks. It may look like measles, a drug-related rash, acne, or scabies. A syphilitic rash may mimic a variety of other infections. Usually the lymph nodes throughout the body become enlarged.

If secondary syphilis is untreated, tertiary syphilis develops as the disease spreads to the entire body, infecting bone, the liver, the heart, and the brain. Syphilis is easily treated with high-dose penicillin.

Genital Herpes

In addition to causing recurrent fever blisters on the lips and sores in wrestlers and other athletes who engage in sports requiring skin-to-skin contact, herpes simplex virus can cause lesions on the genitals and can be spread by sexual contact. In figure 9.3, the lesions appear as ulcers and may not have had a vesicular stage. Herpes simplex type I virus is usually the culprit in the first two scenarios, and type II virus is usually the cause of genital herpes. In many cases, however, type I causes sores on genitals and type II virus is isolated from the lips or mouth. The type of virus is more of a curiosity than a clinically important distinction. As with other herpes infections, antiviral medications can shorten the course of the outbreak and can be used prophylactically to prevent recurrences (see table 7.2 in chapter 7, page 107).

The most severe complication of herpes occurs when an infected mother gives birth during an outbreak and infects her baby. Herpes infections can be severe, and even deadly, for newborns. Surveillance of the pregnant mother and delivery by C-section if labor occurs during an outbreak can greatly reduce the risk of the baby acquiring the infection.

Human Papilloma Virus

Human papilloma virus (HPV) is related to the common wart viruses and causes warts on the genitals. The warts can be as small as 1 to 2 mm in diameter to large cauliflower-like lesions (figure 9.4). As with other warts, they can be difficult to treat, and treatments are often painful. HPV is most problematic in females because of its high association with cervical cancer. (The risk of a virginal woman getting cervical cancer is almost zero.)

No treatment is available to completely rid oneself of the virus, and worse yet, even if all the warts disappear, an infected person still carries the virus and can spread it to others. Any athlete who has "bumps" on the genitals needs a medical evaluation. If the bumps are caused by HPV, they need to be treated promptly, and the athlete's sexual partner(s) needs to be notified.

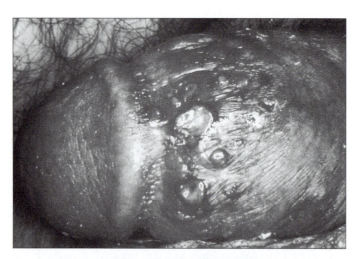

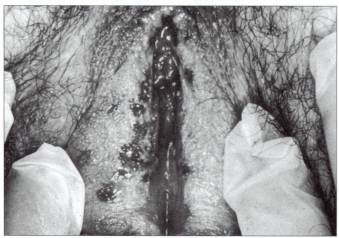

■ Figure 9.3   Genital herpes may cause tiny vesicles or as in these cases appear as painful ulcers in both the male and female.

Trichomoniasis

Trichomoniasis is an infection of the vagina or urethra caused by a small parasite, *Trichomonas vaginalis.* Infected men are usually asymptomatic. About 50% to 90% of infected women are symptomatic, with a new vaginal discharge the most common concern. The discharge is described as malodorous only about 10% of the time. Five to 12% of women have abdominal pain. The incubation period is 3 to 28 d. The diagnosis is made by an examination of some of the discharge under the microscope, where the flagellated protozoan is easy to identify. Once diagnosed, trichomoniasis is easily treated with an antibiotic (metronidazole).

Pubic Lice

Pubic lice *(Pediculosis pubis),* or *crabs,* are tiny lice that attach themselves to pubic

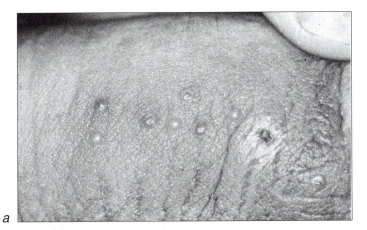

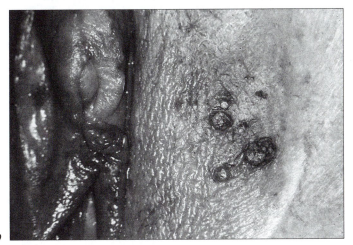

■ **Figure 9.4** *(a)* Small flat warts on the shaft of the penis and *(b)* on the labia majora.

Reprinted, by permission, from W.E. Stamm, H.H. Hansfield, and K.K. Holmes, 1980, *Multi-Media Medicine, Unit Five: Sexually Transmitted Disease, Part II* © American College of Physicians.

hair and feed on the blood of the host. About the size of a pinhead, they live for about 30 d but will die within 24 h when taken off the host. The major symptom is itching. Diagnosis is made by observation of lice or eggs on pubic hair. Pubic lice can be treated with over-the-counter shampoos such as those with pyrethrins (Rid) or primethrin (Nix), or a prescription shampoo with lindane (Kwell). Because the eggs can live for up to 6 d, it is important to launder clothing and bed linens concurrent with treatment.

Blood-Borne Infections

People can acquire HIV and the hepatitis viruses from sexual contact. Because of widespread concern about exposure to these infections from other types of contact, however, they are discussed later under the heading "Blood-Borne Viral Infections."

Prevention of Sexually Transmitted Diseases

Abstinence from any sexual activity is the most reliable way to prevent acquiring an STD. The next best method is to be totally monogamous with a sexual partner who is totally monogamous and always has been. All sexual behaviors with a partner carry some risk of transmission of an STD.

Condoms

Virtually all of the infections discussed in this chapter are transmitted sexually, and the chances of acquiring any infection from an infected partner are markedly reduced with the proper use of a latex condom. Even when condoms are used correctly, however, STDs can still occur. For example, a condom does not cover the base of the penis. The uncovered skin at the base of the penis will come into contact with the skin of the sexual partner. Herpes and HPV infections of the labia in women and base of the penis make transmission possible even with use of a latex condom. Athletes who have questions about condoms can consult Web sites on the subject. The shapes and sizes of condoms vary considerably, so if use has not been successful or if the condom breaks, a couple should try a different brand and possibly a different size.

Oral Sex

All of the STDs can be spread by oral-genital sex. The risk of transmission of blood-borne infections by oral sex is significantly less but is not zero. Any open sores in the mouth or genitals increase the risk of transmission. Herpes is easily spread by oral sex. Many couples are unaware that fever blisters are caused by the herpes virus and that the infection can be spread by oral contact to the genitals of a partner.

BLOOD-BORNE VIRAL INFECTIONS

Not long ago, blood on an athletic uniform was seen as a badge of courage. Athletes felt they were in combat and were proud to wear the blood of a competitor, or even their own blood. Not only was there no urgency to wash it off—some athletes intentionally left it on for effect. With the discovery of acquired immunodeficiency syndrome (AIDS) and its causative agent, human immunodeficiency virus (HIV), however, blood became more widely known as a source of infectious disease.

Although it was awareness of HIV that prompted the athletic community to examine how it handles blood spills, unvaccinated athletes are much more likely to acquire hepatitis B from blood exposure than they are to acquire HIV or any other virus. A variety of viruses cause blood-borne infections: The viruses live in blood and are transmitted through exposure of blood to an uninfected individual. Hepatitis A, by contrast, is food-borne—it is transmitted by the ingestion of infected food. The common blood-borne viral infections that are concerns to athletes are HIV, hepatitis B virus (HBV), and hepatitis C virus (HCV). These infections are also acquired from sexual contact, so they are considered sexually transmitted diseases as well. We review the symptoms and signs of each infection, along with information on how each infection is transmitted and treated.

Hepatitis B Virus

Because the medical community has been aware of the **hepatitis B virus (HBV)** for a very long time, it has a great deal of scientific data on this virus. Hepatitis B infects the liver and can make an individual very ill with fever, chills, loss of appetite, nausea, abdominal pain, jaundice, or any combination of these.

Of the three viruses we describe in this chapter, HBV is the most contagious, but it is not the most **virulent.** Despite this, HBV in the athletic setting is almost unknown.

Not everyone who is infected with HBV becomes ill. About half of infected individuals have **subclinical** HBV, which means the infection does not make them ill. Although some people become very ill with this infection, it rarely causes death. Two major problems are associated with HBV infections:

- In about 6% to 10% of infected adults, the virus remains in the liver and bloodstream because the immune system cannot kill all of the virus. These people become *carriers* of the virus: Their body fluids can infect other people at any time. Worldwide, an estimated 400 million people are carriers of HBV.

- About 5% of infected individuals develop chronic liver infection; and another 20% eventually die from liver cancer or cirrhosis, which tends to develop several decades after the original infection.

Transmission of HBV

HBV is present in an infected person's body fluids, especially blood, serum, semen, and vaginal secretions; it can be transmitted through any of these. It typically does not appear in urine or in feces unless these excretions contain blood. Although HBV may be present in low concentrations in other body fluids such as breast milk, tears, and sweat, these fluids as a rule are not involved in transmission of the disease. Saliva appears to be a source of transmission only via bites (as from a child in a daycare center), whereas kissing, performing cardiopulmonary resuscitation (CPR), and sharing of food do not appear to spread the virus. Carriers with open sores or cuts in their mouths potentially could transmit the virus under such circumstances.

People infected with HBV carry more virus particles in their blood and body fluids than do those infected with HCV or HIV (about 100 times more than HIV). The most common means of transmission is penile-vaginal sexual intercourse (about 40% of HBV infections worldwide occur through heterosexual intercourse). It can be transmitted through anal intercourse and oral-genital sex as well. People can acquire it from blood transfusions (but not in most industrialized nations, where blood is generally screened for HBV) and by sharing contaminated needles; babies may acquire HBV from their mothers during childbirth. Health-care workers can be infected with HBV through accidental exposure—such as infected blood splashing onto an abrasion, a small scratch, a burn, or even a minor rash, or onto a mucous membrane (mouth, nose, eyes). A few people appear to have acquired the virus by sharing toothbrushes or razors. There are reports that some people have acquired HBV through use of unsterilized tattoo needles, body-piercing tools, and acupuncture needles. HBV is not spread by casual physical contact, or by coughing or sneezing.

Because blood has the highest concentration of HBV, it is more infectious than other body fluids. Health-care workers who are stuck with needles from HBV-infected blood have a 2.5% chance of acquiring the infection. Some HBV carriers have in their blood a protein from the virus, the e antigen, whose presence makes the blood much more infectious. If a needle contains e antigen–positive blood, the person stuck with that needle has a 19% chance of acquiring the infection. Because their risk of acquiring the HBV infection is so high from needle sticks and other exposure to body fluids, all health-care workers are now required to receive the HBV vaccine series before working with patients.

In spite of the highly contagious nature of HBV, the relative frequency of bleeding and wounding in some sports, and the frequent physical contact in some sports, HBV transmission in the athletic setting is almost unknown. The only such incidence that has appeared in a published report occurred between Japanese sumo wrestlers. For an athlete shown to be an HBV carrier, the question of participation is controversial, especially in sports like wrestling or football, where bleeding episodes are frequent. The very small risk of transmission is further reduced in many countries by high vaccination rates among the competitors. Infectious-disease specialists and public health officials should be consulted in this case. In sports that involve little or no skin-to-skin contact and little or no bleeding, the athlete should be allowed to participate.

Treatment of HBV

Currently no effective treatment for acute, short-term HBV infection exists. People who carry the virus should abstain from alcohol or any other liver toxin to decrease their chances of sustaining liver damage.

Long-term infections may be treated with lamivudine (brand name Epivir-HBV®), essentially a lower dosage of an antiretroviral drug that was first used against HIV. In one study, lamivudine evoked significant improvement in 52% of people who took it for a 1-yr period; and 64% of recipients had a decrease in liver inflammation (Dienstag et al. 1999).

Fewer than half of people with HBV infection qualify for treatment with interferon alfa-2b because of the strict criteria used to select patients. (Note: These criteria are beyond the scope of this book.) Among those who qualify for treatment, about 40% experience significant long-term remission of viral infection. Patients who develop liver failure due to HBV need a liver transplant to survive.

Prevention of HBV Infection

The HBV vaccine is very effective, and all athletes should be vaccinated if they have not been already. The vaccine requires three injections—subsequent injections 1 month and 6 months after the first. Adverse effects are rare and mild. Avoiding high-risk behaviors—such as exposure to other people's body fluids, promiscuous sex, and sharing needles—will also help decrease an athlete's chances of acquiring the infection.

HIV Infection

When people began dying of a mysterious disease in the early 1980s, **human immunodeficiency virus (HIV)** caught the attention of the world. The disease became known as **AIDS (acquired immunodeficiency syndrome)** and is characterized by loss of immunity, including the inability to fight even common infections. It is associated with Kaposi's sarcoma, a cancer of the soft tissues that causes highly visible purplish skin lesions and is extremely rare among those with normal immunity.

During the first stage of infection, HIV infects the lymph nodes, which may enlarge much as they do with infectious mononucleosis. About 2 to 6 weeks after exposure, about half of newly infected people develop fever, chills, headache, and sore throat as with any common flulike illness. The other half of newly infected people experience no symptoms. Both groups then enter the second, asymptomatic stage of infection, which can last from months to several years, during which time HIV remains dormant in the body and only gradually begins destroying the immune system. The virus is not necessarily inactive during this stage; every day the body may produce billions of new virus particles that attack the body's immune system but without producing overt symptoms. HIV specifically targets a type of white blood cell called **T lymphocytes,** or simply **T cells.** There are several different kinds of T cells; the **CD 4 cells** are the ones specifically targeted by HIV. While B lymphocytes, another type of white blood cell, kill infectious agents by creating proteins (antibodies) that attack the microbes, T lymphocytes are responsible for the cell-mediated immunity that is critical for fighting viral infections, fungal infections, and certain bacteria such as tuberculosis. We cannot function without CD 4 cells and the immunity they provide. When the virus finally becomes virulent (the AIDS stage), the attack on the immune system begins to seriously compromise the body's ability to fight disease.

When people develop an immune-system deficiency caused by HIV, they may notice fatigue and weight loss; nutrients are not absorbed well, which may lead to diarrhea; the first sign may even be pneumonia. In a person with HIV infection, pneumonia is often caused by infectious agents that do not ordinarily cause pneumonia, such as the protozoan parasite *Pneumocystis carinii.* This parasite has long been known as a threat to patients who were immunocompromised from cancer chemotherapy, but before the discovery of AIDS, it had not been seen in any other group. People with HIV commonly exhibit fungal infections such as severe thrush, a yeast infection in the mouth and throat. As discussed in the case study, there are other causes of thrush, and presence of thrush does not mean a person is infected

Case Study

Kari is a 19-yr-old woman who presents to the doctor's office with a sore throat. She has white spots on her tonsils and white plaque on her cheeks and is worried that she has thrush and AIDS. She had one episode of oral sex 6 months ago, after a night of drinking alcohol. She has never had intercourse. The physician informs her that she probably has thrush and questions her further. She has asthma and uses an inhaler with corticosteroids. She reports that she has been using the inhaler more the past 2 weeks because of a cold and has not been rinsing her mouth out after each use. The physician tells her that this is the likely cause of her thrush. He treats her with an oral antifungal agent and asks her to rinse her mouth out after using the inhaler. A week later, she is asymptomatic.

with HIV. Virtually any infection may occur, and all infections are difficult to treat because of the weakened immune response.

Transmission of HIV

HIV is transmitted primarily in six ways: (1) through sexual intercourse of any kind (anal, vaginal, and oral, in descending order of hazard); (2) through sharing of needles (for drugs, e.g., anabolic steroids); (3) during childbirth, from an infected mother to her child; (4) through transfusion of blood or blood products infected with HIV (this method of transmission is almost unknown today in industrialized countries, where blood supplies are carefully screened); (5) by accidental exposure to HIV-infected blood through needle sticks; and (6) via breast milk from an infected mother to her infant child. HIV is not as easy to transmit as HBV. It is *not* transmitted by hugging or kissing (unless there is an open sore in the mouth) or other kinds of physical contact in which body fluids are not exchanged. There has never been a proven instance of HIV being transmitted during athletic competition. Even if health-care workers accidentally stick themselves with an HIV-infected needle, their chance of acquiring the infection is only 1 in 300.

HIV infection is identified by detection of blood-borne antibodies to the virus. The antibodies do not show up on tests, however, until about 6 months after the infection begins—which means that *a person may be infected, and able to transmit the virus to others, even after a negative antibody test.* Sexually active people who want to pursue a monogamous relationship cannot be confident of the safety of their sexual activity until a test appears negative at least 6 months after the last potential exposure to the virus.

Because bleeding occurs in some sports, there has been concern about the possibility of transmission from one competitor to another. As stated earlier, there has yet to be a confirmed case of HIV transmission through sport activities. The U.S. Centers for Disease Control (CDC) was not able to confirm one report that an Italian soccer player had acquired HIV during play. It appears that splashed blood is much less likely to transmit HIV than many people once feared. After a case of HIV transmission was alleged to have occurred from a bloody patient in a Baltimore emergency room, the CDC began a prospective study of splash

The National Football League's HIV Risk Formula

The National Football League (NFL) conducted a study to design a formula to determine the risk of HIV transmission during NFL competition. The league collected information from 11 NFL teams over 155 season games. Of the 575 observed bleeding injuries, 87.5% were abrasions and 12.5% were lacerations. The frequency of the bleeding injuries increased in association with games played on artificial surfaces and participating teams' having a losing season record. The probability of HIV transmission was calculated as follows (Brown et al. 1995, 272):

1. 1 infected player/200 players ×
2. 1 HIV transmission/300 exposures ×
3. 0.41 lacerated players/game per 45 players/game ×
4. 3.46 bleeding players/game ×
5. 3.46 bleeding players/game per 45 players/game = 1 HIV transmission per 85,647,821 game contacts

This study puts the risk of HIV transmission in the NFL during competition at 1 in 85 million contacts. It is the only study of its kind, and further research needs to be done to check the validity of the formula as well as to study other contact sports.

Reprinted, by permission, from T. Zeigler, 1996, *Management of bloodborne infections in sport: A practical guide for sports care providers and coaches* (Champaign, IL: Human Kinetics), 20.

injuries in health-care workers. After monitoring more than 1,000 exposures without evidence of transmission, the CDC concluded that the chance of transmission was too low for them to quantify. The National Football League (NFL) examined the number of bleeding episodes occurring in its sport and estimated that the risk of transmission is less than one transmission in a million games (see *The National Football League's HIV Risk Formula*, page 139). The exposure in sports is always from splashed blood—which carries much lower risk than a needle stick. Therefore, if the risk of exposure is very small in the health-care setting, it is minuscule in the athletic setting.

Because of the information presented in *The National Football League's HIV Risk Formula*, most sports' governing bodies do not forbid HIV-positive athletes to compete. Only boxing requires athletes to be tested for HIV and specifically excludes HIV-positive athletes from competing—a rule that has not been tested in U.S. courts.

Treatment of HIV

Medical researchers continue to develop drugs that are relatively effective against HIV. The most effective treatments as of early 2003 were "cocktails" of several different drugs, typically including two or more different nucleoside analogue reverse transcriptase inhibitors—for example, zidovudine (commonly called AZT, brand name Retrovir®) and didanosine (ddI, brand name Videx®)—and one or more protease inhibitors. An effective antiviral regimen can cause the number of viral particles in the blood to drop from 100,000 to 1,000 particles/ml within just a couple of weeks and to decrease even further in the following months. Because new drugs are constantly being tested and approved and new treatment regimens devised, it would be counterproductive to include discussion of HIV treatment in a book such as this. Any information we provide will probably be at least somewhat outdated by the time the book is printed. As of early 2003, a very good source of information about drug treatment regimens for HIV is a Web site sponsored in part by the U.S. Department of Health and Human Services (HHS). This site, at www.aidsinfo.nih.gov, remains up-to-date on the most recent federally approved treatment guidelines and also provides information about future and ongoing clinical trials of experimental treatments. A private site that provides information about clinical trials for HIV as well as for many other diseases, including HCV, is www.veritasmedicine.com.

HIV drugs are very expensive—at least $1,000US/month is a realistic cost just for the medicines and does not include charges from doctors or hospitals. These drugs are therefore not available to many people who are infected. Despite their effectiveness at preventing the HIV from multiplying, none of the products can eliminate all the viral particles from the body—in other words, none of the medications is curative. In fact, there is major debate about how to determine when to begin drug treatment. Because most of the drugs have serious side effects, some researchers believe it is best to delay treatment during the asymptomatic phase, in part because, once treatment begins, it should never be stopped—otherwise the virus will quickly rebound and become more virulent than ever, even if blood tests have not been able to detect any virus particles in the blood for several months before the end of treatment. Starting treatment sooner may also hasten the virus' apparently inexorable development of immunity to the drugs, leading to earlier manifestation of full-blown AIDS. On the other hand, very limited data suggest that very aggressive treatment, begun within just a few hours of infection (in those rare cases when people know precisely when they were exposed), *may* be successful in preventing AIDS altogether.

No matter what drugs people take to combat the virus, almost everyone infected with HIV eventually dies from the infection. Curiously, however, a very small number of people seem to have survived for many years with the infection; it is unclear why their immune systems are not destroyed by it.

Preventing HIV Infection

Because no HIV vaccine exists (or is likely to exist in the near future), the only way to avoid HIV infection is to avoid the behaviors that put a person at risk. For health-care workers, this means practicing universal precautions (see page 143). The vast majority of people can quite successfully avoid HIV infection by having only monogamous sex with a monogamous partner and by refraining from any other high-risk activity such as sharing needles. People who choose not to follow this advice should use a condom or latex barrier every time they engage in any kind of sexual activity (vaginal, oral, or anal) with any other person.

Hepatitis C

Hepatitis C virus (HCV) was discovered in 1989; by 1990 there were effective tests to detect the virus in blood. Unfortunately, before 1990 the virus had infected millions of people who had received infected blood transfusions or blood products. In developed countries, effective screening of blood products since 1990 has decreased the number of cases arising from such products to a minuscule level. Most of the four million HCV-positive people in the United States were infected before 1990. Today there are fewer than 30,000 new cases of infection in the United States each year. But because of the sometimes decades-long delay in manifestation of liver pathology, every year in the United States 8,000 to 10,000 deaths, and approximately 1,000 liver transplants, are attributable to HCV infection.

According to the World Health Organization, approximately 170 million people are infected worldwide—or nearly 3% of the world's population. The greatest prevalence is in Africa (5.3%), the eastern Mediterranean, and southeast Asia. About 1% of Europeans are infected, and a little less than 2% of people in the western hemisphere.

Initial symptoms of infection include diminished appetite, fever, muscle aches, fatigue, and sometimes jaundice. For an unknown reason, however, the large majority of people (about 75%) have subclinical cases at first—that is, they experience no symptoms.

The immune systems of about 15% to 20% of people infected with HCV succeed in banishing the virus from their bodies within a few months (note that these fortunate individuals do *not* remain immune to the virus—they can be reinfected later). The other 80% to 85% are chronically infected for the rest of their lives. Out of 100 chronically infected people, approximately 6 to 12 develop **cirrhosis** of the liver within about 20 yr, and as many as 12 more develop cirrhosis within 40 yr after infection. **Fibrosis** (scarring of the liver) typically precedes cirrhosis by a number of years. Each year, from 1% to 3% of people with HCV-induced cirrhosis develop liver cancer. HCV-induced cirrhosis is much more likely to develop in people who also are infected with HIV or HBV, and in people who consume alcohol; other risk factors for cirrhosis are being male and acquiring the virus at a relatively older age (older than 50). People who do not develop liver disease may experience no specific symptoms even over several decades, but they often have a diminished quality of life resulting from a variety of miscellaneous problems associated with less-than-optimal health. Because so many people infected with HCV experience no symptoms, in most cases infection is first identified during a routine blood test.

Transmission of HCV

HCV is quintessentially a blood-borne pathogen, present in body fluids other than blood only at very low levels. It is not particularly contagious in most social situations and appears to be transmitted only when blood of an infected person comes in contact with a portal to another person's bloodstream—through use of needles, via cuts and abrasions, and so on. At least in developed countries, transmission via tainted blood has been negligible since 1990.

Transmission occurs most often through use of nonsterile needles by intravenous drug users. It is estimated that about 90% of new intravenous drug users are infected with HCV within a year of beginning their habit. Estimates of the percentage of HCV cases acquired through sexual activity vary widely, from 6% up to 35%; the likelihood of acquiring the virus seems rather directly proportional to the number of different sexual partners a person has and is strongly enhanced if the infected person has a second infection such as genital herpes or HIV. A mother can transmit the virus to her child during childbirth (transmission rate is roughly 6%) but usually only if she has measurable levels of virus in her blood at the time of childbirth. In some parts of the world where donated organs are not routinely assayed for HCV, a large number of donated organs (up to 75% in one study) are infected with HCV and subsequently infect the recipient with the virus. Some people (as many as 4-10% of those who have the virus) acquire HCV while snorting cocaine—presumably because they share a straw with an infected person and the virus enters the bloodstream through tiny broken blood vessels in the nasal cavity. In theory, a person can acquire the virus from nonsterile needles used for body piercing or tattooing; but the incidence of the disease attributable to these activities is unknown.

HCV is not spread by breast-feeding. Mosquitoes do not appear able to transmit the virus, nor is it spread by everyday contacts such as sharing food, hugging, sneezing, and the like. The standard dogma among most experts is that it is not spread through kissing—yet people may be wise to avoid any activity in which an exchange of blood might be possible, as when they have an open sore or cut in the mouth.

It is important to note that a significant number of people with HCV have none of the risk factors mentioned here. Studies have estimated that as few as 5% or as many as 40% of HCV cases are of undiscovered origin. Though one might assume that many infected people are not honest about their past activities involving drugs and sex, nevertheless a significant number of cases remain whose mode of transmission is unknown.

Treatment of HCV

The most effective treatment as of early 2003 is a combination of intravenous interferon therapy with oral ribavirin (brand name Rebetol®). However, the treatment has strong side effects, is quite expensive, and is effective in fewer than half of treated patients; and the FDA has approved it only for people who have relapsed after treatment with interferon alone. The chances of a positive outcome from treatment are enhanced for women (vs. men), for individuals who do not yet have cirrhosis, for people younger than 40, for people with low levels of virus in their blood, and for those who are infected with HCV genotypes 2 or 3.

New drugs are under development, but for the indefinite future, the focus will be on preventing transmission.

Preventing HCV Infection

Preventing HCV transmission requires the same precautions as for the other blood-borne viruses. Health-care providers who adhere to universal precautions when handling blood or body secretions will greatly reduce the risk of acquiring HCV in the workplace. There is no HCV vaccine (but people who have liver disease caused by HCV are advised to be vaccinated for hepatitis A and hepatitis B).

Although athletes tend not to be among the population at most risk for acquiring HCV (intravenous drug users), you nevertheless should remain alert for possible cases. Athletes certainly are no less likely to be sexually promiscuous than other people, and promiscuity is a significant risk factor. Athletes from areas such as Africa and the eastern Mediterranean also have a greater likelihood of having HCV. Although HCV is not as contagious as hepatitis B and not as virulent as HIV, it is a serious threat that is not unlikely to be seen occasionally among even young athletes in western industrialized nations. By insisting that all participants in your sports program follow universal precautions against infectious diseases, you should easily be able to prevent transmission of HVC from an infected athlete.

Universal Precautions

Universal precautions refer to behaviors intended to prevent transmission of blood-borne pathogens, including use of personal protective equipment (PPE) to prevent exposure. In the health-care setting, PPE consists of gloves, gowns, laboratory coats, face masks, and eye protection. In the athletic setting, gloves are the primary item of PPE. It is important for health providers of athletes to know the universal precautions as well as other measures that will reduce the risk of transmission of blood-borne infections.

In the athletic setting, pre-event preparation is the first step in reducing the risk of transmission of blood-borne infections. See that all sports personnel know basic first aid and infection control:

- Before every practice or competition, all wounds in both athletes and medical personnel should be covered with an occlusive dressing (figure 9.5).
- Personnel (physicians, trainers, and the like) with extensive weeping dermatitis should refrain from direct care of athletes.
- Disposable gloves should always be available, and anyone who deals in any way with body fluids must wear gloves and know how to remove them properly (figure 9.6).
- Mouthpieces, resuscitation bags, or other ventilation devices should always be available.
- **Sharps containers** must be easily accessible and should be located as close as possible to the area where the sharps are being used. Sharps containers must be puncture resistant, leakproof, clearly labeled, and kept upright throughout use. They should be replaced routinely, closed when moved, and not allowed

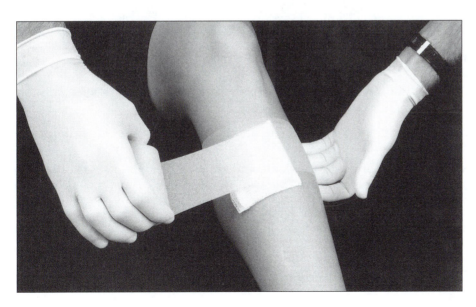

■ **Figure 9.5** Pre-event preparation to prevent blood-borne infection exposure includes covering wounds completely.

Reprinted, by permission, from T. Zeigler, 1996, *Management of bloodborne infections in sport: A practical guide for sports care providers and coaches* (Champaign, IL: Human Kinetics), 26.

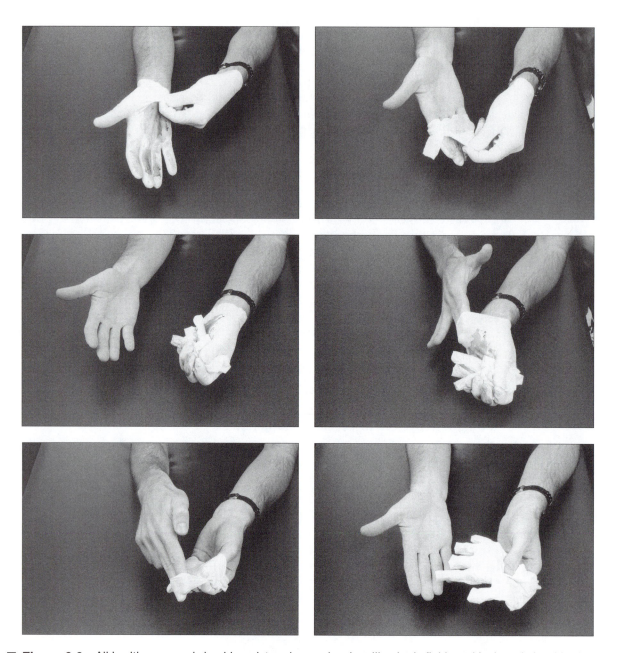

■ **Figure 9.6**   All health personnel should use latex gloves when handling body fluids and be knowledgeable about how to remove them properly.

Reprinted, by permission, from L.A. Cartwright and W.A. Pitney, 1999, *Athletic training for student assistants* (Champaign, IL: Human Kinetics), 36.

to overfill. Reusable sharps containers should never be opened, emptied, or cleaned by hand.

■ **Biohazard containers** must be available and easily accessible. These containers must be colored red and marked "biohazardous waste." They, too, should be leakproof and closable.

Follow these rules in general housekeeping:

■ Clean and decontaminate all equipment and environmental or work surfaces that have been contaminated with blood or potentially infectious materials.

For Further Information

Print Resources

Brown, L., D. Drotman, A. Chu, C. Brown, and D. Knowlan. 1995. Bleeding injuries in professional football: Estimating the risk of HIV transmission. *Annals of Internal Medicine* 122: 271-74.

Feigin, R.D., and J.D. Cherry. 1998. *Textbook of pediatric infectious disease,* 4th ed. Philadelphia: W.B. Saunders.

Gibson, R.J.C., and A. Mindel. 2001. Sexually transmitted infections. *British Medical Journal* 322: 1160-64.

Holmes, K.K., P. Mardh, P.F. Sparling, P.J. Wiesner, W. Cates, S.M. Lemon, and W.E. Stamm. 1990. *Sexually transmitted disease,* 2d ed. Boston: McGraw-Hill.

Hyde, J.S., and J.D. Delmater. 2000. *Understanding human sexuality,* 7th ed. Boston: McGraw-Hill.

Web Resources

Centers for Disease Control and Prevention
www.cdc.gov/nchstp/dstd/dstdp.html
The Centers for Diseases Control and Prevention in the United States provides this Web site on sexually transmitted diseases. It includes numerous links to statistics and slide shows on a variety of topics.

Avert
www.avert.org/usecond.htm
Avert is a United Kingdom–based organization for AIDS prevention. It provides this nicely designed Web site on condoms and their use.

Occupational Safety & Health Administration
www.osha.gov
A site dedicated to providing information from the Occupational Safety & Health Administration (OSHA) regarding workplace safety. Significant information is available regarding health-care work settings and blood-borne pathogens.

American College Health Association
www.acha.org
The American College Health Association (ACHA) serves as an advocate and leadership organization for issues surrounding college and university health. Several ACHA guideline reports are available online and frequently updated. The site provides many links to resources for sexual health issues.

- Immediately decontaminate work surfaces with an appropriate disinfectant as soon as they are contaminated; after any spill of blood or other potentially infectious materials; and at the end of each work shift, practice session, or competition in which such surfaces are used.

- Inspect and decontaminate on a regular basis reusable receptacles such as bins, pails, and cans that may be likely to become contaminated.

- Always use a mechanical means (such as tongs, forceps, or a brush and a dustpan) to pick up contaminated broken glassware. Never pick it up with the hands, even with gloves.

- Store or process reusable sharps in a way that ensures safe handling.

- Place all biohazardous waste in appropriately marked containers.

- If clothing becomes contaminated, remove it as quickly as possible and place it in the contaminated-laundry container for cleaning.

- Handle contaminated laundry as little as possible, with minimal contact even with gloved hands.

- Use appropriate PPE when handling contaminated laundry.

- Place contaminated laundry in leakproof labeled or color-coded containers before transporting it.

Commercial biohazard kits are available to assist with the care of contaminated areas, especially during travel. You can make your own biohazard kit, however, using these materials:

- Disposable paper towels or wipes
- Squirt bottle with 1:10 bleach-to-water solution or similar disinfectant
- Hydrogen peroxide to clean blood off uniforms
- Assorted sizes of latex gloves
- Disposable gauze pads
- Two cloth towels for containment of larger spills or larger wounds
- Red biohazard bag

Emphasize to athletes that they should never share razor blades, and see that they know the locations of sharps containers, biohazard containers, and contaminated-laundry containers. All athletes should be vaccinated against HBV. Remind athletes that they can acquire potentially deadly virus infections through sexual intimacy of all kinds—vaginal, anal, and oral; strongly advise them that, if they insist on being sexually active, they should use condoms and other appropriate latex barriers for *all* varieties of sexual intimacy.

SUMMARY

1. *Discuss the signs and symptoms associated with common bacterial, viral, and parasitic sexually transmitted diseases (STDs).*

This chapter has dealt with a number of sexually transmitted diseases that are bacterial, viral, and parasitic in origin. Although many are associated with discomfort, rashes or sores, and discharge, some may be present asymptomatically and not present for extended periods. The athletic trainer must be able to properly refer patients with questions concerning potential STDs to a physician immediately. Providing a trusting, nonjudgmental environment of care will facilitate this process. Though most STDs can be treated successfully, if left untreated some can have dire consequences, including fertility issues, possible cancers, and even death.

2. *Explain the importance of latex condom use in reducing the spread of sexually transmitted diseases.*

A person's chances of acquiring an STD infection from an infected partner are markedly reduced with the proper use of a latex condom. Even when condoms are used correctly, STDs can still occur. For example, the base of the penis is not covered by the condom. Herpes and HPV infections of the labia in women and base of the penis make transmission possible even with use of a latex condom.

3. *Describe the transmission, treatment, and prevention of blood-borne viral infections including HIV (human immunodeficiency virus), HBV (hepatitis B virus), and HCV (hepatitis C virus).*

This chapter has described the transmission, treatment, and prevention of blood-borne viral infections. Athletic trainers play a key role in educating patients about high-risk behaviors and protection from blood-borne pathogens. A variety of viruses cause blood-borne infections: The viruses live in blood and are transmitted through exposure of infected body fluids (blood, serum, semen, and vaginal secretions) to an uninfected individual. The common blood-borne viral infections that concern athletes are hepatitis B virus (HBV), human immunodeficiency virus

(HIV), and hepatitis C virus (HCV). Though an awareness of HIV prompted the athletic community to examine how it handles blood spills, unvaccinated athletes are much more likely to acquire HBV from blood exposure than they are to acquire HIV or any other virus. These infections are acquired from sexual contact, so they are also considered sexually transmitted diseases. People can also acquire them through the sharing of needles and other direct exposure to infected blood. All people should be vaccinated against HBV, in that the vaccine is safe and effective. Many research groups are seeking new treatments for HCV and HIV as well as the development of vaccines, but success in any of these areas appears to be many years away.

4. *Identify proper practice for health-care providers in adherence to universal precautions.*

Blood-borne infections are not a major threat to athletes if everyone involved in the athletic setting treats blood as a potential infectious agent and follows universal precautions. Universal precautions refer to behaviors intended to prevent transmission of blood-borne pathogens, including use of personal protective equipment (PPE) to prevent exposure. In the health-care setting, PPE consists of gloves, gowns, laboratory coats, face masks, and eye protection. In the athletic setting, gloves are the primary item of PPE. It is important for health providers of athletes to know the universal precautions to reduce the risk of transmission of blood-borne infections. These infections are a much more serious threat off the athletic field, especially for athletes who engage in high-risk behaviors.

CHAPTER 10

Common Infectious Diseases

OBJECTIVES

Upon completion of this chapter the reader will be able to do the following:

1. Describe the causes, treatment, and complications associated with bacterial and viral respiratory infections

2. Differentiate the signs and symptoms of influenza from those of the common cold

3. Discuss the cause, treatment, and complications associated with infectious mononucleosis

Common viral infections can frustrate the dedicated athlete. Whether it is the common cold, influenza, infectious mononucleosis, or a complication of a cold such as pneumonia or a middle-ear infection, viral infections can affect performance. This chapter will discuss some of the common infections that health providers may see in physically active individuals.

Case Study

Lisa is a 22-yr-old rower with a 4-d history of a sore throat and runny nose. She has an occasional cough. She asked to see the doctor for an antibiotic because that's what her doctor always prescribed for her when she was younger. She is sleeping well and has no vomiting or diarrhea. She does not have any myalgias (muscle aches). She had a mild headache when the illness started.

In the physician's office, further questioning reveals that Lisa has had a hoarse voice with this illness and nearly lost her voice 2 d ago. She had a few strep infections as a child but does not remember having one since elementary school. On examination, she does not have a fever. Her eardrums appear normal and her throat is also normal. Her cervical nodes are only slightly enlarged. Her larynx is slightly tender. Her chest is clear to auscultation and her heart sounds are normal.

The physician concludes from her laryngitis and runny nose that Lisa has a viral infection. He explains to her that an antibiotic does not kill viruses and that most colds last 10 to 14 d regardless of the treatment. He suggests a decongestant-antihistamine medication to help dry up her nose. He asks her to return if she has not improved in 5 to 7 d.

COMMON COLD

The common cold is familiar to everyone, even though the symptoms vary from virus to virus and person to person. A cold can be caused by one of more than a hundred rhinoviruses as well as a variety of coronaviruses, respiratory syncytial viruses, parainfluenza viruses, and adenoviruses.

There are so many viruses that cause the common cold that we can always get infected with one we have not had before. Most colds produce a mild headache, no fever, or a low-grade fever at the onset and eventually clear rhinorrhea (runny nose), sore throat, and a slight cough. They may cause a sore throat with inflammation of the pharynx (pharyngitis), tonsils (tonsillitis), or larynx (laryngitis). Throats can be very red and tonsils can become quite enlarged with viral syndromes. The common cold viruses rarely cause a rash. They may cause sinus congestion and sinus pain early in the course.

Treatments of the common cold are symptomatic. Anything that helps loosen the mucus in the nose may be helpful. A hot bath or shower may work the best. Medications that reduce the swelling of the mucous membranes in the nose and throat may provide relief; however, studies have failed to show efficacy. A decongestant such as pseudoephredrine may provide some relief without causing drowsiness. Popular medications often combine pseudoephredrine with an antihistamine that also may have some drying effect on the mucous membranes. About 50% of people get drowsy from over-the-counter antihistamines, but when combined with pseudoephedrine, which may increase energy, the net effect is often no drowsiness. Any analgesic such as acetaminophen, ibuprofen, or naproxen will help relieve any pain associated with a sore throat or headache. Many over-the-counter products contain an expectorant, such as guaifenesin. This chemical is designed to make a dry cough into a wet cough and assist with expectoration

---

Terms and Definitions

Epstein-Barr virus (EBV)—A herpes virus that causes infectious mononucleosis; it also is associated with Burkitt's lymphoma and certain nasopharyngeal cancers.

group A strep—The strain of *Streptococcus pyogenes* bacteria that causes streptococcal pharyngitis, rheumatic fever, and many skin infections.

Monospot test—A brand name of a laboratory exam that tests blood for antibodies to the Epstein-Barr virus; positive results usually indicate infectious mononucleosis, but other rarer diseases can also produce positive results. The generic name for this test is a heterophile antibody test.

pericardium—The membranous sac that surrounds the heart.

pharyngitis—Inflammation of the pharynx (back of the throat).

streptococcal pharyngitis—A sore and inflamed throat due to one strain of the *Streptococcus pyogenes* bacteria, usually group A; strep throat.

thrombocytopenia—A decrease in blood platelet count associated with decreased clotting ability.

(getting rid of mucus). Sometimes people find that a cough improves if they simply stop using the expectorant. Some cold medications contain a cough suppressant such as dextromethorphan (DM), which may cause mild drowsiness and is moderately effective. Some physicians may prescribe a low dose of a narcotic such as codeine, which is also an excellent cough suppressant but may cause stomach upset or drowsiness.

Complications of the Common Cold

Cold viruses cause inflammation of the mucosa in the nose and throat, and the swelling of the mucous membranes can alter the anatomy and normal physiology to allow bacteria a chance to multiply and cause problems. If a cold virus causes fever, it will usually do so in the first 2 to 3 d of the illness. If this is followed by a fever a week to 10 d later, especially with a worsening of symptoms, a bacterial complication should be suspected.

Otitis Media

A cold causes swelling of the eustachian tubes that drain and ventilate the middle ear, and this dysfunction can cause increased mucus production and negative pressure in the middle ear. The negative pressure encourages bacteria from the pharynx to invade the middle ear, causing an acute otitis media with a bulging, painful eardrum (see chapter 5).

Sinusitis

One of the most common complications associated with the common cold is bacterial sinusitis. This can be a difficult diagnosis in that its symptoms, sinus pain and inflammation of the sinuses, can also be caused by viral infections. Sinuses are openings in the skull in the maxillary area and frontal area that are lined with mucous membranes (figure 10.1). They serve to create resonance in our voices and decrease the weight of the skull.

As with other complications of cold viruses, diagnosis of bacterial sinusitis is related to the timing of symptoms. Sinus pain at the beginning of a cold is likely viral. If it occurs 10 to 14 d or later into a cold, it is more likely due to bacteria. The symptoms of bacterial sinusitis may include frontal headache or sinus pain, especially when bending forward or lying down; an increase in rhinorrhea; a change in color and consistency of the nasal discharge; a bloody nasal discharge;

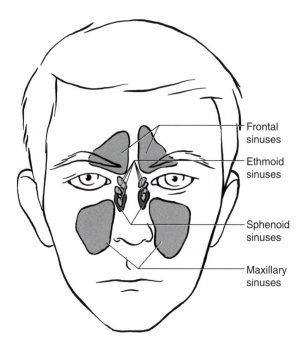

■ Figure 10.1 Location of the sinuses.

Labels on figure:
Frontal sinuses
Ethmoid sinuses
Sphenoid sinuses
Maxillary sinuses

cough; sore throat; and fever. Because many of the symptoms are similar to those of a cold, this diagnosis is challenging for even the most astute clinician. The only way to make the diagnosis with 100% certainty is to stick a needle in a sinus and culture the fluid from the sinus. Needless to say, this is not a common method to diagnose sinusitis. Some practitioners check X rays of the face, which are rather insensitive at diagnosing this problem. CAT scans of the sinuses are more sensitive but still not specific. This test tells the practitioner whether there is fluid in the sinuses or whether they look swollen. The usual practice is to treat the patient based on the timing of the symptoms and the number of symptoms that are consistent with a bacterial infection.

As with otitis media, the usual bacterial causes of sinus infection are bacteria that occur in the throat. Amoxicillin or trimethoprim-sulfa (Bactrim®, Septra®) is a reasonable first-line antibiotic for sinus infections, but numerous others will also work. Many practitioners also prescribe a corticosteroid nasal spray to reduce inflammation and swelling. Using decongestants with the antibiotic is more controversial in that they may dry the mucous membranes and make drainage more difficult, even though they may relieve the symptoms.

Pneumonia

When cold viruses irritate the lower respiratory tissues such as the bronchi, the usual mechanism that helps rid the lungs of mucus is impaired. This sets up the possibility of pneumonia resulting from bacteria in the throat that make their way into the lungs and multiply. Pneumonia produces high fever and a worsening cough. It may produce vomiting. It is associated with a productive cough (one that produces mucus, as opposed to a dry cough). On exam the patient may have an elevated respiratory rate (more than 30 breaths/min in an adult) and signs of respiratory distress. If a person is working harder to breathe, the skin above the collarbones or breastbone may sink in with inspiration. The muscles of breathing are working harder to generate a breath. If an examiner listens to the breath sounds in the area of the pneumonia, crackles (or rales) are often heard when the patient takes a breath in. Sometimes there is so much fluid in the lung in that area that there are no breath sounds or only diminished breath sounds. Most pneumonias that complicate a viral infection are caused by *Streptococcus pneumonia* (a.k.a. pneumococcus) and can be treated with any type of penicillin. Some pneumonias are not associated with a cold and do not make a person as ill as the pneuomococcal pneumonia. When a patient acquires a cough without a runny nose, the health provider should consider a community-acquired pneumonia (transferred by respiratory droplets in the community). Because the symptoms are milder, this type of pneumonia is often called walking pneumonia. Caused most often by *Mycoplasma pneumonia* and *Chlamydia trachomatis,* these infections are treated with antibiotics in the erythromycin or tetracycline family.

Sore Throats

As mentioned earlier, the common cold viruses may cause a sore throat because they can cause inflammation of the tissue in the throat **(pharyngitis),** including the tonsils (tonsillitis). Tonsillitis causes enlargement of the tonsils and sometimes a white or yellow exudate. The size of normal tonsils varies from person to person and is sometimes described using a numbering system to describe how much of the tonsil is visible. If no tonsillar tissue is seen, the score is 0; and if the tonsils touch each other, they are 4+ tonsils (figure 10.2). Strep throat, caused by *Streptococcus pyogenes,* is usually a disease of young childhood, decreasing in frequency through adolescence so that by adulthood it becomes a very uncommon cause of pharyngitis and tonsillitis. A common misconception holds that treatment with an antibiotic will make strep throat improve quickly. Treatment shortens symptoms by only 1 d at best, however. The main purpose of treatment of strep throat is to prevent rheumatic fever, an autoimmune disease that may cause permanent damage to heart tissue, including the heart valves. Rheumatic fever is associated with only one type of strep—group A. Many other types of strep can be cultured from the throat, but only type A is associated with rheumatic fever. Group C and group G strep may cause symptoms in adolescents and young adults, so most practitioners treat these with an antibiotic in hopes of making the patients feel better sooner.

Strep pharyngitis causes different symptoms compared to the common cold viruses. Strep causes a sore throat, fever, enlarged cervical lymph nodes, and a very inflamed throat and tonsils. It may cause a headache and stomachache. It may cause a characteristic rash that is very erythematous and has fine papules that make the skin feel like sandpaper. In the presence of the rash, this illness is sometimes called scarlet fever because of the degree of redness associated with this rash. If the rash appears only on the abdomen or upper thighs, it may be called a scarlatiniform rash, meaning it resembles scarlet fever. Strep pharyngitis does not cause a runny nose or cough (Bisno et al. 2002). So if a runny nose or cough is present, a strep infection is much less likely.

Features of **streptococcal pharyngitis** appear in *Common Symptoms of Streptococcal Pharyngitis,* page 154. It is important to realize that although these are indeed common symptoms, not every incidence of the disease will feature all of the symptoms. In the past, the only proof of a strep infection was a throat culture that grew that type of bacteria. The culture is created by touching the back of the throat with a cotton swab designed for bacterial cultures and then touching the swab to a culture plate in the laboratory to grow the bacteria out over 24 to 48 h. Fortunately, most physicians' offices have rapid strep tests, chemical tests that look for specific proteins on the **group A strep** bacterium. This test has reduced the time required to make the diagnosis. Because the rapid tests are not 100% sensitive, some offices still do a culture as well to be sure the rapid test has not missed a strep infection. Group A strep is universally sensitive to penicillin, and for those who are allergic to penicillin, erythromycin is the antibiotic of choice. Past studies have shown that if a patient does not take the antibiotic a full 10 d, risk of rheumatic fever increases. Although rheumatic fever is relatively rare, patients should complete the 10-d course.

Peritonsillar Abscess

Inflammation of the pharynx and tonsils may lead to cellulitis of the area around the tonsils and occasionally a peritonsillar abscess. This can be a complication of

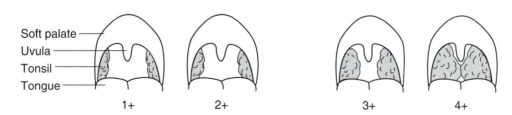

■ **Figure 10.2** Scoring system used for describing the degree of tonsillar enlargement.

Common Symptoms of Streptococcal Pharyngitis

- Sudden onset
- Sore throat
- Fever
- Headache
- Patchy exudates
- Moderate to severe tonsillar swelling*

- Lymphadenopathy*
- Scarlatiniform rash*
- Absence of runny nose*
- Absence of conjunctivitis
- Absence of cough

* = Most likely to be associated with strep.

strep pharyngitis or a viral pharyngitis. Unlike most sore throats with viruses, the abscess causes fever, and the patient may not be able to open the mouth very well due to the pain. If the back of the throat is visible, there is marked asymmetry of the two tonsils because an abscess pushes the tonsil medially toward the uvula (figure 10.3). If a true abscess has formed, it should be drained by an ear, nose, and throat specialist, and the patient usually requires admission to the hospital.

INFLUENZA

Influenza, or flu, describes a winter or early-spring viral infection associated with a group of respiratory viruses that cause a quite severe illness in susceptible individuals. This group of viruses, called influenza A and influenza B, are known for constantly trying to disguise themselves by changing their proteins to fool the human immune system. The change in proteins, called antigenic shift, is the reason why people who have had the flu previously can get it again. The viruses are named after the location where the most recent change was detected. For example, one strain of influenza A was called Taiwan because this new form was first detected in Taiwan.

Influenza causes high fever, cough, sore throat, headache, myalgias, and rhinorrhea. You should suspect influenza if the fever is high (>102° F) and the person is moderately ill and has muscle aches. Table 10.1 shows the symptoms of influenza compared to those of the common cold viruses. Flu rarely causes vomiting or diarrhea and should not be confused with the enteroviruses, or so-called "stomach

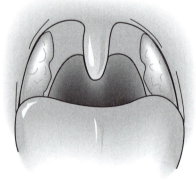
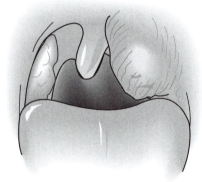

■ **Figure 10.3** When a peritonsillar abscess is present, the tonsil is shifted toward the uvula on the side of the peritonsillar abscess.

Table 10.1 Symptoms of Influenza Compared to Those of the Common Cold

Symptom	Cold	Influenza
Fever	Mild or absent	Always present and usually high → 102° F and above
Headache	Mild or absent	Present and moderate to severe
Sore throat	Mild	Moderate to severe
Muscle aches	Rare	Common, severe
Runny nose	Common	Occasional
Cough	Sometimes	Usually present and severe
Fatigue and weakness	Mild	Severe and persistent

Antibiotic Resistance

Bacteria throughout the world are becoming resistant to antibiotics. For example, all *Streptococcus pneumonia* were universally sensitive to amoxicillin. As of the early 2000s, some areas in the United States found 50% of strains isolated in bacteriology labs to be resistant to penicillin. The problem of resistance is thought to be a result of widespread antibiotic use. If antibiotics are used less frequently, antibiotic resistance will develop more slowly. As mentioned in the case study at the beginning of this chapter, practitioners used to routinely prescribe antibiotics for a cold "just in case" bacteria might be involved. It has become clear that this practice must stop, and the problem of resistance is the reason Lisa does not receive an antibiotic for her cold. In addition, there is no evidence that an antibiotic would help her symptoms at this stage of the illness.

flu." Influenza can make a person ill enough to miss several days of work or school and can keep an athlete from training for a week or more. Unlike other viruses, influenza can cause a fever for 4 to 5 d before subsiding (most viruses cause a fever for only 1 to 2 d). It is associated with all the same complications of common colds and is more likely to be associated with pneumonia.

Influenza is preventable with a vaccine that must be administered 6 to 8 weeks before exposure. It is highly effective and has a very low risk of any complications. About 1% of those vaccinated get a mild flulike illness. Antiviral medications for influenza are available, but they must be started in the first 48 h of the illness. Amantadine (Symmetrel®) and rimantadine (Flumadine®) are taken twice daily and have the same side effects as antihistamines—drowsiness and dry mouth. They are effective only against type A infections. The newer antivirals zanamivir (Relenza®) and oseltamivir (Tamiflu®) are more expensive but are effective against both type A and type B infections (Ison and Hayden 2001). Because of the prolonged detrimental effect flu can have on an athlete's season, all athletes participating in winter competitions should obtain vaccinations.

INFECTIOUS MONONUCLEOSIS

Few viral illnesses cause as much disability as infectious mononucleosis (IM). Athletes who are aware of this disease sometimes become anxious whenever they are fatigued that they have IM. They become especially concerned when they hear of a teammate or a classmate with the infection, because it has a reputation as being highly communicable. This section will help you answer athletes' many questions about IM and enable you to allay some of their fears. It will also help you determine which athletes should be referred for consultation and possibly blood work to diagnose the illness.

Case Study

A 17-yr-old high school football player approaches you with a 10-d history of sore throat, enlarged cervical glands, and fatigue. He has had little appetite and has lost 5 lb (2.3 kg). He has had mild intermittent abdominal pain, especially when he eats—and when he does eat, he feels full before he has eaten very much. He has continued to practice, although he feels quite tired and has found that when he gets home from practice, he falls asleep instead of doing homework. He has had trouble staying awake during class, which is unusual for him.

Recognizing that this is unusual for most viral infections, you consult the team physician, and the athlete is seen the same day in the doctor's office. The doctor's examination reveals an oral temperature of 99.5° F, blood pressure of 124/78, and a regular pulse of 76. His eyelids are slightly swollen. His tonsils and soft palate are quite red; he has very enlarged tonsils with copious exudate. His neck lymph nodes are tender, and his anterior cervical lymph nodes are very enlarged. His posterior neck reveals several palpable enlarged lymph nodes bilaterally.

His chest and heart exams are normal. Both liver and spleen are nonpalpable, although the upper left quadrant of his abdomen is tender to deep palpation. There is no rash, and the remainder of his exam is normal.

His rapid strep test is positive for group A beta hemolytic streptococcus bacteria. His white blood cell count is 11,500 (normal is roughly 5,000-10,000), with 22% reactive lymphocytes; his Monospot test is positive. Because he has no known drug allergies, the physician prescribes penicillin V at a dose of 500 mg, taken orally three times a day for 10 d. The doctor explains that the antibiotic may improve his symptoms somewhat but that most of his symptoms are probably from the infectious mononucleosis virus rather than from the strep bacteria. He strongly recommends that the athlete stop working out, get as much rest as possible, and take an afternoon nap whenever he feels the need. He also recommends that he try to eat frequent small meals to try to prevent further weight loss. He asks him to return to the office in 1 week.

The following week the athlete is feeling better, although he still requires naps after school and remains fatigued. At the doctor's office, his weight is down another 4 lb (1.8 kg). The facial swelling is gone. His throat reveals only mild exudate; his tonsils are still enlarged but are of normal color. His anterior cervical nodes are still enlarged but no longer tender, and they are smaller than they were the previous week. He still has some palpable posterior nodes, but they are less prominent. While both liver and spleen are still nonpalpable, he remains slightly tender to deep palpation. He wants to start working out and to play in this week's game in 5 d. Because he is only 2.5 weeks into his illness, and he still needs more sleep than usual, the team doc tells him that it is too early to allow him to return to play. He instructs him to return in 1 week for reevaluation.

The following week, the athlete reports that he no longer needs to nap after school. His appetite is normal, and his weight is up 5 lb (2.3 kg). His sore throat is gone. His throat appears normal, and his cervical lymph nodes are only mildly enlarged. His abdominal exam is normal.

Because he is feeling well 3.5 weeks into the illness, the physician gives him permission to start jogging and using an exercise bike. He asks the athlete to return in 4 or 5 d for reassessment.

He returns to the doctor's office at the 4-week mark and reports that he is a little tired after his workouts, but he wants to advance his workouts and start football practice. His exam is normal. The team physician discusses with his parents the controversy over returning to play, explaining that the risk of splenic rupture at this point is extremely low but not zero. With his parents' concurrence, he decides to allow him to return—and the athlete plays in the next game without incident.

Etiology and Symptoms

Infectious mononucleosis is caused by the **Epstein-Barr virus (EBV).** Although it can strike children of any age, symptoms are more severe in adolescents or young adults than in younger children. The virus infects many young children, especially those in families of lower socioeconomic status and those who live in close quarters. Approximately 80% to 90% of college freshmen have already been exposed to EBV and are immune. Unlike many viruses, IM is not very contagious and usually requires intimate contact for transmission. It is usually spread by saliva, which is why it is popularly known as the "kissing disease." It is spread by exchanging saliva by kissing or through sharing food or drink. Because the incubation period for EBV infection ranges from approximately 30 to 65 days, it is unusual to see more than one person with infectious mononucleosis on a team in one season.

The disease often begins with several days of preliminary symptoms: malaise, mild loss of appetite, low-grade fever, and perhaps headache. Because of the fairly long period of preliminary symptoms, many infected people do not seek medical care until they have been ill for 7 to 10 d.

Soon after the preliminary symptoms, almost all infected people develop a severe sore throat. More than 90% of people with IM experience fatigue, which is one of the most prominent symptoms. About 80% report loss of appetite, and about 40% experience headaches. Abdominal pain is common. Although swelling or puffiness of the eyelids is almost always present, sometimes it is noticed only by friends or family of the infected individuals, not by the infected people themselves. Examination of the throat typically reveals somewhat severe tonsillitis

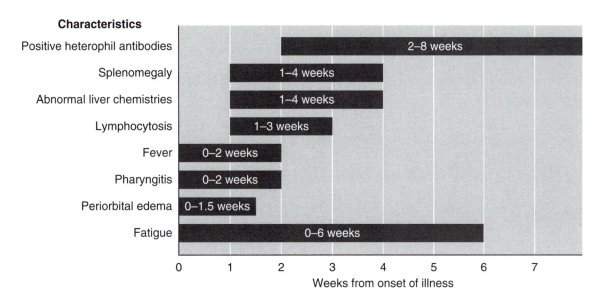

■ **Figure 10.4**   Infectious mononucleosis: Typical course of when symptoms and characteristics appear.

and pharyngitis, usually with copious exudate. Figure 10.4 describes the typical course of these symptoms. Group A strep infection accompanies about one in five cases of infectious mononucleosis.

The cervical lymph nodes are usually quite enlarged and tender. The degree of lymph node swelling and tenderness does not distinguish infectious mononucleosis from group A strep pharyngitis (strep throat). EBV infection typically also causes enlargement of the posterior lymph nodes; swollen posterior cervical lymph nodes provide a strong clue that the illness is due to EBV (figure 10.5). Some people also have enlarged lymph nodes in the armpits and groin. About 5% of IM patients have an enlarged liver that can be palpated on abdominal exam. Although everyone with IM has some enlargement of the spleen, only about half have a spleen that is palpable on physical examination—yet most people, even when the spleen is not palpable, have at least some tenderness in their upper left quadrant. About 5% of individuals with IM have a fine, raised rash, similar to that of measles. About 2% to 5% exhibit jaundice, the sclera of their eyes being somewhat yellow.

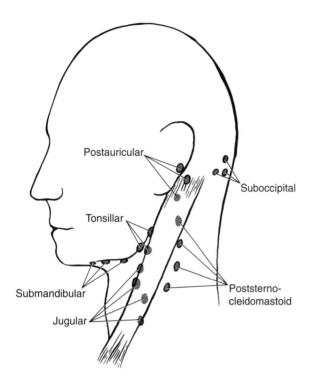

■ **Figure 10.5**   The location of the lymph nodes in the neck.

Blood smears of IM patients reveal a significant rise in the number of lymphocytes compared to normal. A small percentage of these have a lowered platelet count, and a small percentage exhibit **thrombocytopenia.** A small percentage also are mildly anemic. EBV is notorious for causing a large percentage of reactive lymphocytes (which in some laboratories were previously called atypical lymphocytes): Under the microscope these cells have a large nucleus and an increased number of granules in the cytoplasm (figure 10.6). Most laboratories perform a serologic test to look for heterophile antibodies. Commonly known as a **Monospot test,** this test uses sensitized red blood cells of sheep to detect the presence of specific antibodies that the body produces to fight EBV. Results are available in 5 min. Unfortunately, there is not always a significant rise in these antibodies with EBV infections until the second or third week of infection. Even 3 weeks into the illness, 10% to 15% of infected people exhibit no heterophile antibodies. Because college students with access to health-care services typically do not wait as long as high school students to seek treatment, depending on a Monospot test to diagnose IM

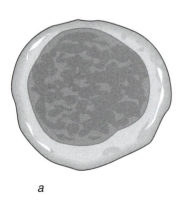

a

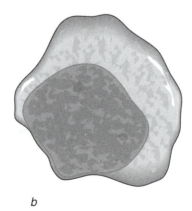

b

■ **Figure 10.6**   Normal lymphocytes in peripheral blood *(a)* are round and have very little cytoplasm. In reactive lymphocytes *(b)*, which indicate the presence of mononucleosis, note the variability in size, irregularity in shape, and increase in cytoplasm.

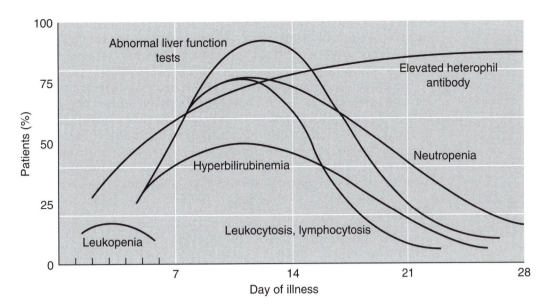

■ **Figure 10.7** Typical course of laboratory abnormalities observed in mononucleosis.

Reprinted, by permission, from S.C. Finch, 1969, Laboratory findings in infectious mononucleosis. In *Infectious mononucleosis*, edited by R.L. Carter and H.G. Penman (Oxford: Blackwell Scientific Publications).

is particularly inadequate with them. In a minority of cases, the Monospot never turns positive and there is uncertainty about the diagnosis. A few other viruses can cause a "mono-like" illness, with the most common imitator being cytomegalovirus (CMV). Occasionally a practitioner may order a test for the specific antibodies for EBV to make the diagnosis certain. Because EBV typically infects the liver, elevations of serum liver enzymes are very common. Figure 10.7 shows the typical course of the laboratory abnormalities.

Complications of Infectious Mononucleosis

Although they are rare, numerous potential complications of infectious mononucleosis exist. The decrease in platelets sometimes leads to severe nosebleeds, as well as bleeding from inflamed tonsils and throat. Lymph nodes may swell so much that they obstruct the airway. When this causes difficulty with breathing and swallowing, the patient is often treated with corticosteroids to prevent life-threatening obstruction that will require hospitalization for emergent intubation and mechanical ventilation.

The use of corticosteroids to reduce the duration and severity of general IM symptoms (other than difficulty breathing and swallowing) is controversial—studies on the effectiveness of corticosteroid therapy for IM have yielded mixed results. Furthermore, EBV is associated with Burkitt's lymphoma. Practitioners worry that use of a corticosteroid, which reduces immune response, might increase susceptibility to this rare type of cancer. The understanding of appropriate indications for use of corticosteroids in IM, other than to alleviate moderate to severe throat swelling, varies among practitioners. There is very little evidence that treatment with a corticosteroid will allow an athlete to return to a sport earlier than would occur without treatment.

The tonsillitis due to EBV may be associated with a secondary bacterial infection that can lead to a peritonsillar abscess. Rarely, EBV infects the **pericardium** or the heart muscle itself, or it may infect neural tissue and cause a variety of neuropathies, including an encephalitis that can produce cognitive deficits and changes in thought process. Occasionally an individual will hallucinate and exhibit psychotic behavior. It is not unusual, however, for EBV to affect mood in the absence of a clear indication of encephalitis. Many people with IM feel depressed—a special problem for anyone who already had symptoms of depression before the infection.

The most feared complication in athletes is rupture of the spleen, which can be life threatening. Because it filters the blood, the spleen is highly vascular. Injuring the spleen can cause massive bleeding that can lead to shock and, if untreated, to death. All the splenic ruptures reported in the medical literature have occurred in the first 3 weeks of IM—at least half being spontaneous, occurring without any trauma. The spleen can rupture with any Valsalva event—for example, such as during a bowel movement, sneezing, or coughing.

Treatment

The most important treatment for mono is rest, a prescription intense athletes find difficult to follow. Athletes must be reminded that without rest, the illness will be prolonged. Frequent small meals will help minimize weight loss and help the athlete recover more quickly. With a poor appetite and less exercise, athletes with mono tend to get constipated, so many practitioners recommend a stool softener.

Returning to Exercise

The course of IM is quite variable. Some people have a relatively mild course and are significantly ill for only 1 to 2 weeks. Typically, lingering fatigue keeps most athletes out of competition for at least 4 weeks. Some athletes, especially those in endurance events, take much longer—perhaps 2 to 3 months—to fully recover. Controversy surrounds the question of how to determine when athletes are ready to resume normal activities. Some researchers believe that avoiding contact sports for 4 weeks provides adequate rest for most infected athletes—a recommendation based largely on the fact that splenic ruptures generally occur within the first 3 weeks of the illness (Eichner 1996). Some practitioners believe that if the spleen is not palpable on examination, it is less vulnerable to rupture; yet neither laboratory nor clinical research has demonstrated any correlation between ruptures and the degree of spleen enlargement. Moreover, no scientific data suggest that a spleen that is normal in size or is decreasing in size is at lower risk of rupture.

Theoretically, however, the larger the spleen, the higher the risk of rupture (it's a bigger target). Few data exist on the range of normal splenic size; moreover, spleens are quite variable in shape among individuals. Splenic size can be measured by a variety of radiological methods including ultrasound, CT scans, and nuclear medicine studies. Plain radiographs are only a crude measure of splenic enlargement. Because ultrasound does not require exposure to ionizing radiation, some practitioners prefer this method to assess splenic size. Unpublished ultrasound studies at the University of Wisconsin demonstrated that virtually all patients with infectious mononucleosis have a significant degree of splenomegaly (Primos and Landry 1990) . These results confirmed previous studies that only about 50% of the enlarged spleens were palpable on physical exam. In the Wisconsin study, 50 healthy young adults had splenic ultrasounds. The mean splenic index (length × width × depth, divided by 27) for males was 18.9 ± 5.8 and for females was 13.7 ± 3.6. In the same study, 50 patients with infectious mononucleosis exhibited their maximal splenic index between week 2 and week 4 of the illness. The maximum mean splenic index was 44.36 ± 15.0, more than twice the normal size.

Questions of spleen size are moot in most cases, since many athletes feel so ill or fatigued for at least 4 weeks that they don't want to work out. The case study presented at the beginning of this chapter is typical in that the athlete needed at least 4 weeks to recover enough to begin workouts. Some health professionals

For Further Information

Print Resources

Bisno, A.L., M.A. Gerber, J.M. Gwaltney, E.L. Kaplan, and R.H. Schwartz. 2002. Practice guidelines for the diagnosis and management of Group A Streptococcal pharyngitis. *Clinical Infectious Diseases* 35: 113-25.

Eichner, E.R. 1996. Infectious mononucleosis: Recognizing the condition, "reactivating" the patient. *The Physician and Sportsmedicine* 24(4): 49-54.

Halstead, M.E., and D.T. Bernhardt. 2002. Common infections in the young athlete. *Pediatric Annals* 31(1): 42-48.

Ison, M.G., and F.G. Hayden. 2001. Therapeutic options for the management of influenza. *Current Opinion in Pharmacology* 1(5): 482-90.

Primos, W.A., and G.L. Landry. 1990. The course of splenomegaly in infectious mononucleosis. Presented before the Ambulatory Pediatric Association, Anaheim, CA.

Ressel, G. 2001. Principles of appropriate antibiotic use: Part IV. Acute pharyngitis. *American Family Physician* 64(5): 870-75.

Web Resources

Centers for Disease Control and Prevention
www.cdc.gov/ncidod/diseases/flu/
The Centers for Disease Control and Prevention Web site has useful information about influenza, including surveillance data on how frequently influenza is occurring in every state in the nation.

WebMD®
www.mywebmd.com
This site has medical advice about a variety of conditions and is especially helpful in describing treatment of the common cold and when a person should call a physician.

hold athletes out of participation for a minimum of 4 weeks regardless of their symptoms.

How do you handle athletes who say they are "feeling OK" and want to return to practice? The safest approach is first to check all symptoms. For example, an athlete says he feels fit enough to resume football practice after a bout with IM. Query him closely: Is his sore throat 100% gone? Are his lymph nodes completely back to normal size? Does he no longer need naps, and is he sleeping no more than usual? If the answer to any of these questions is no, tell him to rest for another week. By the end of that time, if he is back to normal in every way and his physician agrees, have him begin with light workouts—such as 20 min on an exercise bike followed by jogging for 1 or 2 mi (1.6 or 3.2 km). He may be amazed at how fatigued he feels after such a light workout. But if (or when) he can complete the light workout with little fatigue, gradually increase the exercise load until he is exercising for the length of a normal football practice but without the contact. Finally, let him begin weightlifting—with only light weights at first, seeing that weightlifting may involve Valsalva maneuvers that could be dangerous to the spleen. Once he has built up to lifting heavy weights with no problems, let him return to play if his physician agrees with that decision.

What if an athlete says she feels fine only a couple of weeks after the onset of the illness and appears completely normal in every way? The two most common approaches are

- to measure her spleen to be certain that it is not enlarged before permitting her to begin exercising again; or

- to insist that she rest a minimum of 4 weeks no matter what her symptoms do or do not show, as a precaution against rupturing the spleen and as a way to permit her immune system to recover fully.

Especially in view of the paucity of data that correlate spleen size with spleen rupture, we suggest the second approach. This is a judgment call in every case, and even capable practitioners disagree as to which approach is more appropriate.

SUMMARY

1. *Describe the causes, treatment, and complications associated with bacterial and viral respiratory infections.*

This chapter has dealt with a number of respiratory infections of both bacterial and viral origin. Athletes may come to you with a variety of respiratory signs and symptoms. Although most common respiratory infections respond to symptomatic care, occasional serious complications may develop. Athletic trainers must be able to make proper referrals to facilitate an appropriate course of care. Differentiating viral from bacterial infections is essential to preventing the inappropriate use of antibiotic medications. Care providers must take an active role in educating patients to the problems associated with overuse of antibiotics.

2. *Differentiate the signs and symptoms of influenza from those of the common cold.*

Influenza (flu) describes a winter or early-spring viral infection associated with a group of respiratory viruses that cause a quite severe illness in susceptible individuals. Influenza causes high fever, cough, sore throat, headache, myalgias, and rhinorrhea. You should suspect influenza if the fever is high (>102° F) and the person is moderately ill and has muscle aches. Fevers and headaches are usually mild or absent in the common cold, and muscle aches are rare. Influenza can make a person ill enough to miss several days of work or school and can keep an athlete from training for a week or more. Fatigue and weakness are severe with influenza, in contrast to the minor fatigue a person with a common cold experiences. Unlike other viruses, influenza can cause a fever for 4 to 5 d before subsiding (most viruses cause a fever for only 1-2 d). Influenza is preventable with a vaccine that must be administered 6 to 8 weeks before exposure. It is highly effective and has a very low risk of any complications; about 1% of those vaccinated get a mild flulike illness. Because influenza can have a detrimental effect on an athlete's season, vaccination is recommended for any athletes participating in winter competitions.

3. *Discuss the cause, treatment, and complications associated with infectious mononucleosis.*

Infectious mononucleosis (IM) is caused by the Epstein-Barr virus (EBV). Although it can strike children of any age, symptoms are more severe in adolescents or young adults than in younger children. Infectious mononucleosis is a relatively debilitating disease for active individuals. Despite its reputation, IM is not very contagious and usually requires intimate contact for transmission. It is usually spread by saliva, which is why it is popularly known as the "kissing disease." It is spread by exchanging saliva in kissing or through sharing food or drink.

As the athletic trainer, you must maintain a high degree of suspicion concerning any of the preliminary symptoms—malaise, mild loss of appetite, low-grade fever, and headache—so that the diagnosis can be made as early as possible, permitting the athlete to rest and recover more quickly. You need to watch the athlete carefully for excessive fatigue and weight loss. Referral to a physician is appropriate when the diagnosis is suspected or for reassurance of both the athlete and athletic trainer. The course of IM is quite variable. Some people have a relatively mild course and are significantly ill for only 1 to 2 weeks. Typically, lingering fatigue keeps most athletes out of competition for at least 4 weeks. Some athletes, especially those in endurance events, take much longer—perhaps 2 to 3 months—to fully recover. Although they are rare, numerous potential complications of IM exist. The primary concern for those who participate in sports is the potential of a ruptured spleen. This possibility is the reason that most sport authorities are conservative in permitting athletes with IM to return to practice.

PART III

NUTRITIONAL AND PHARMACO-LOGICAL CONCERNS

CHAPTER 11

Nutrition

OBJECTIVES

Upon completion of this chapter the reader will be able to do the following:

1. Differentiate the athletic diet from a typical American diet

2. Discuss the energy requirements for specific sport activities

3. Identify the recommended nutrient requirements for carbohydrates, fats, and proteins

4. Discuss the relationship between hydration and athletic performance

5. Explain how vitamins and minerals contribute to total nutrients

6. Explain the role of nutritional supplements

It would be wonderful if all athletes had a custom dietary prescription that would take into consideration their age, weight, resting metabolism, genetics, body type, and training conditions, as well as the demands of their particular sport. But this will not happen. Like it or not, you may be the default nutrition and diet counselor for the athletes you work with. Fortunately, some basic principles apply to most athletes. By helping your athletes follow these principles, you can set them on a path toward attaining a high level of general health and peak performance—and, in many cases, even gaining an edge over their competition.

Despite the advantages they can gain by following this sort of advice, many athletes will be looking for even more of an edge and will also turn to you for advice about "safe" nutritional supplements. This chapter reviews the effectiveness and side effects of the most common supplements. Potentially harmful supplements are discussed in chapter 14, "Drugs, Supplements, and the Athlete."

Case Study

An athlete seeks your help with her problem of fatigue; she is wondering if a vitamin or mineral deficiency may be the source of her problem. The athlete eats three meals a day and her weight has not changed over the last season. She admits, however, that she does not plan her meals to obtain nutritional balance, nor does she eat special pregame meals or follow any plan to replenish carbohydrates after practices or games. In addition, the athlete does not weigh herself before and after every practice, is not sure of the color of her urine, and drinks only when she is thirsty. What simple dietary advice would you give this athlete? How would you address the specific question she mentioned, that is, whether she may have vitamin or mineral deficiencies? How can you help her in terms of preventing dehydration as a potential contributor to her problem?

ATHLETIC DIETS VERSUS TYPICAL AMERICAN DIETS

Nutrition experts suggest that approximately 50% to 60% of a person's total calories should come from complex carbohydrates, 15% to 20% from protein, and 25% to 30% from fat. **Complex carbohydrates** consist of starches such as bread, pastas, and cereals; **simple carbohydrates** consist of sugars such as glucose, fructose, and galactose. The typical American eats too much fat, protein, and simple sugars and not enough complex carbohydrates—and certainly not enough vegetables and fruits.

Serious athletes have different requirements than do sedentary individuals or even "weekend warrior" athletes. Fluid lost as sweat during exercise requires serious athletes to consume more liquid on a regular basis, and athletes who exercise at least 2 h/d require a much higher intake of calories than other people—in particular, the athlete's diet requires higher levels of carbohydrate (up to 70% of the total calories) and protein to meet the energy demands such vigorous exercise requires.

ENERGY REQUIREMENTS

Energy requirements depend on age, body size, and resting metabolic rate—as well as the demands of the sport and the conditions under which a person trains. Long-distance swimmers, crew athletes, and triathletes, for example, clearly need

Terms and Definitions

adenosine triphosphate (ATP)—A nucleotide compound occurring in all cells where it represents energy storage in the form of phosphate bonds. To release energy, it is hydrolyzed to adenosine diphosphate (ADP) and a phosphate group.

beta-hydroxy-beta-methylbutyrate (HMB)—A metabolite of the amino acid leucine that is produced naturally in the body.

complex carbohydrates—Starches such as bread, pastas, and cereals.

free radicals—Chemicals containing one or more unpaired electrons that occur naturally in the body and play a role in numerous physiological reactions. The majority of these compounds are oxidants capable of oxidizing a range of biological molecules.

glycogen—A storage carbohydrate found mainly in the liver but also in muscle cells; consists of long chains of glucose. It is broken down during high-intensity exercise to provide glucose for energy.

recommended daily allowance (RDA)—The amount of a nutrient taken daily to prevent conditions associated with a deficiency. They are established with the goal of at least a 30% margin of safety to cover the nutritional needs of 97% of healthy Americans.

simple carbohydrates—Sugars such as those found in desserts, soda, candy, jelly, and the like.

more calories than baseball players and sprinters. Sports with the highest energy expenditure (as measured in kcal/min) include cross-country skiing, crew racing, swimming, and bicycle racing. Sports with lower energy expenditures include hammer throw, shot put, and discus throw. However, the mean caloric intake for both types of sports may be equal in that the throwers usually have a large body size and a relatively intense training regime.

Carbohydrates are the main fuel source for endurance performance as well as for short-duration, high-intensity exercise. Carbohydrate is stored in the liver and muscle as **glycogen,** and fatigue occurs when glycogen is depleted.

The basic chemical structure of carbohydrates is a chain of carbon atoms attached to hydrogen and oxygen atoms. Simple sugars such as glucose, fructose, and galactose have similar chemical makeup (each of these has a skeleton of six carbon atoms) and are termed *monosaccharides*. Glucose occurs naturally in some foods and is produced in the body as a result of the digestion of more-complex carbohydrates. Fructose is found in high quantities in fruit juices, whereas galactose is a milk sugar; both are converted in the body to glucose for energy metabolism. Sucrose, lactose, and maltose are disaccharides comprising two different sugar molecules. Polysaccharides, also called *complex carbohydrates*, contain three or more sugar molecules and for the most part are simply very long chains of glucose molecules. They are recommended as the basic fuel source for most exercising athletes. Sources of complex carbohydrates include the starches found in bread and pasta.

In high-intensity sports, there is a close association between activity levels and muscle glycogen concentration (Costill et al. 1988; Sherman et al. 1981). Athletes who do not replenish their glycogen stores will have less energy for practice in the days following. It is unclear exactly how much carbohydrate is needed in a given situation. Current recommendations are for approximately 8 to 10 g of carbohydrate per kilogram of body weight per day to maintain muscle glycogen in endurance athletes who train more than 90 min/d. It takes approximately 20 h to completely replenish carbohydrate stores in endurance athletes; note, however, that glycogen resynthesis appears to be 300% greater than basal levels when athletes ingest 2 g of carbohydrate per kilogram of body weight (about 3 oz per 100 lb body weight) *immediately after* exercise (Ivy 1991). Endurance athletes should therefore

Energy Nutrients Needed for Peak Performance

Relying on the food pyramid and your common sense may be all you need most of the time to keep your eating habits on track. At times, however, you may wonder if you're getting the right mix of energy-supplying nutrients (carbohydrate, fat, and protein) to perform up to your true potential. For this approach, keep in mind that the food you eat serves three basic needs: It supplies energy (measured in calories); supports the growth, maintenance, and repair of tissues; and helps regulate the body's metabolism.

Carbohydrate (About 60% of Total Calories)

- Training 1 h/d—3 g of carbohydrate per pound of body weight (6-7 g/kg)
- Training 2 h/d—4 g of carbohydrate per pound of body weight (8-9 g/kg)
- Training 3 h/d—5 g of carbohydrate per pound of body weight (10-11 g/kg)

Protein (About 15% to 20% of Total Calories)

- 0.55 to 0.75 g of protein per pound of body weight (1.2-1.7 g/kg)

Fat (at Least 20% of Total Calories)

- Approximately 0.5 g of fat per pound of body weight (1 g/kg)

Use the numbers you just derived to estimate your daily calorie needs: (grams of carbohydrate × 4 calories/gram) + (grams of protein × 4 calories/gram) + (grams of fat × 9 calories/gram) = estimated total daily calories.

Adapted, by permission, from S.G. Eberle, 2000, *Endurance sports nutrition* (Champaign, IL: Human Kinetics), 47.

eat a snack rich in carbohydrates within 30 min following an intense workout. Less carbohydrate is required for athletes participating in intermittent endurance activity, power sports, or sprinting events.

Certain carbohydrates can affect your energy level in different ways. Digestion rates are expressed as a *glycemic index*. Foods with a higher glycemic index release energy into the bloodstream rapidly, whereas foods with a moderate or low glycemic index release their energy more slowly. Consuming 30 to 75 g/h of high-glycemic-index carbohydrate in liquid or solid form when you exercise can minimize glycogen depletion associated with exercise.

After a long workout or competition, your depleted muscle glycogen stores must be replenished, especially if you will be exercising again within the next 8 h. Eat at least 50 g of high-glycemic-index carbohydrate just after exercise, and consume a total of at least 100 g of high-glycemic-index carbohydrate in the first 4 h afterward. Moderate-glycemic-index foods may be added for the next 18 to 20 h, with a goal of consuming at least 600 g of carbohydrate during the 24 h after an intense workout or competition (Kleiner 1997).

NUTRIENT REQUIREMENTS

A generally healthy athlete performs better than a generally unhealthy one, no matter how much carbohydrate energy he or she has available. Although obtaining adequate carbohydrate energy sources tends to be a short-term goal that can affect an athlete's performance, obtaining proper nutrients other than carbohydrates is a long-term process that affects current as well as future overall health. The negative effects of poor diet are subtle, however, and in many cases invisible until they manifest themselves decades into the future. It is therefore doubly important that athletes in your care "follow the rules" of adequate nutrition, no matter how they subjectively experience the apparent effects (or lack thereof) of their diets on sport performance.

Fluids

Although water is not technically a nutrient by some definitions, it is probably the single most important dietary component that can demonstrably affect sports performance. Many athletes practice and compete in a state of dehydration. Simply by being sure that your athletes are well hydrated, you can help them boost their performance significantly. Thirst is *not* an effective signal to measure fluid lost during workouts or competitions. By the time athletes are thirsty, they are already dehydrated—and dehydration contributes to poor performance and thermoregulatory dysfunction.

Educate your athletes to drink adequate amounts of fluids. Measuring their weight before and after exercise can help them estimate the amount of water they've lost. For every pound of weight lost during exercise, they should consume 16 oz of fluid (1.17 L for every kilogram of body weight lost). All athletes can meet their fluid needs by drinking water. For some ultraendurance sports, fluids that replenish lost carbohydrates and electrolytes may improve performance and delay fatigue. Because many such drinks are more palatable than plain water, you may recommend them to any athletes to boost the likelihood that they will remain hydrated. Because such drinks can cause nausea, cramping, and diarrhea in some individuals, athletes should experiment with these types of drinks in practice before using them in competition. Keep in mind that the higher the carbohydrate content of most flavored sports drinks, the more likely it is that athletes will experience gastrointestinal side effects—but individual response to these drinks vary.

In addition to the demands of their sport, some athletes have been known to drink caffeinated beverages on occasion or even imbibe in some beverages that contain alcohol. Both types of drinks can lead to further dehydration caused by their diuretic effect. Athletes must be educated regarding these potential side effects in hopes of avoiding further complications.

Protein

Many athletes mistakenly rely too much on high-carbohydrate diets, thereby failing to consume enough protein. Most athletes should consume about 2.4 oz of protein per 100 lb of body weight (1.5 g/kg of body weight) per day. Athletes on low-calorie, low-fat, or vegetarian diets are particularly susceptible to protein deficits. Low-calorie and low-fat diets often restrict fat, which tends to be associated with protein in many foods. Vegetarians must be careful that their protein sources are as high in protein quality as those from animal products. Proteins from milk products and eggs contain all eight of the essential amino acids (the building blocks of proteins) our bodies need. Proteins from most plant products lack one or more of these essential amino acids, however, and therefore by themselves are not nutritionally adequate. Athletes obtaining protein solely from plant sources should be sure that they consume both grains (rice, bread, tortillas, and the like) and beans or lentils on the same day to obtain complete protein. Other protein sources include soy milk and other soy products such as tofu.

People who engage in resistance training have higher protein requirements than other athletes because their training leads to muscle hypertrophy—that is, they create a lot of new muscle tissue (see table 11.1). Endurance athletes, however, often need more protein per kilogram of their body weight because the energy demands of their endurance sport actually require protein utilization for energy. Resistance athletes such as weightlifters and bodybuilders actually consume and need more

Table 11.1   General Nutritional Guidelines for Differing Athletic Levels

Type of conditioning	Percentage of calories attained from specific nutritional source		
	Complex carbohydrates	Protein	Fat
Average adult	50-60%	15-20%	25-30%
Endurance athletes	Up to 70%	15-20%	15-20%
Athletes in resistance training	50-60%	30-40%	15-20%

Table 11.1 lists the approximate percentage of calories that should be consumed from three major energy sources (complex carbohydrates, protein, and fat) by differing levels and intensities of athletes. (The exact number of calories required will vary by size of the athlete and length and intensity of the workout.)

absolute protein in grams because of their increased size baseline compared to many of these endurance athletes (Clark 1996).

Fat

The popular press exalts the idea of no-fat and low-fat diets, as do some athletes. Yet dietary fat is important. It carries fat-soluble vitamins, makes food taste better, and serves as a concentrated fuel source; in addition, certain kinds of fat—the essential fatty acids—are so important that we would die without them in our diets. Trained people oxidize more fat and less carbohydrate than untrained individuals, thus sparing the glycogen stores that are so important for sustained performance. Athletes in training ought to watch their fat intake like anyone else to be sure that they don't overindulge; but because they are less susceptible to the deleterious health effects of fat than most people, they probably should avoid low-fat diets unless they are directed to such diets by a health professional.

Vitamins and Minerals

Most athletes eating a balanced diet ingest adequate vitamins and minerals for activities of daily living and exercise. Observation suggests, however, that few young people actually eat a genuinely balanced diet as defined by the food pyramid (how many of the athletes you know *really* eat five full servings of veggies or fruits every day?) (figure 11.1). Consuming vitamins above the recommended daily allowance has not been shown to improve performance, and large doses of some fat-soluble vitamins (A, D, and K) and some of the B vitamins may be toxic. Nutrient deficiencies, on the other hand, can lead to undetectable compromises in overall health, which can compromise performance. Advise your athletes to go heavy on fruits; green, red, and yellow vegetables; and milk products. However, given that some athletes may have poor diets even when in heavy training, one daily multivitamin tablet with minerals may be a good idea just to maintain optimal health and development. No evidence shows that additional micronutrients such as magnesium, zinc, or copper enhance performance or are deficient in athletes.

Antioxidants

Recent evidence shows that exercise leads to production of **free radicals.** This has increased the interest in so-called *free-radical scavengers* as supplements. The most widely known free-radical scavenger vitamins, more frequently known as antioxidants, are alpha-tocopherol (vitamin E), ascorbic acid (vitamin C), and beta-carotene (precursor of vitamin A). Studies of the effects of antioxidant supplementation have had mixed results. It is not clear that these compounds are helpful, and some research suggests that megadoses of vitamin C and beta-carotene may have deleterious side effects.

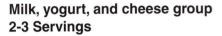
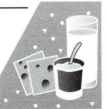
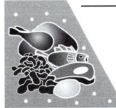
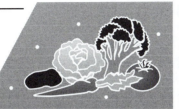

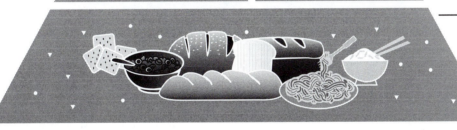

**Fats, oils, and sweets
Use sparingly**

**Milk, yogurt, and cheese group
2-3 Servings**

**Meat, poultry, fish, dry beans,
eggs, and nuts group
2-3 Servings**

**Vegetable group
3-5 servings**

**Fruit group
2-3 Servings**

**Bread, cereal,
rice, and
pasta group
6-11
Servings**

■ **Figure 11.1** Food pyramid.

Source: United States Departments of Agriculture and Health and Human Services.

Quick Vegetarian Snacks and Meals

- Whole-grain pancakes
- Whole-grain muffins or cookies
- Graham crackers, rice cakes, whole-grain crackers, tortillas
- Instant macaroni and cheese, couscous with lentils, polenta, or mashed potatoes
- Instant brown rice or other grains
- Bagels or whole-grain bread with nut butter
- Oatmeal or cold cereal with milk
- Dried fruit—raisins, apricots, dates, figs, papayas, apples
- Frozen juice bar
- Bean taco, burrito, or enchilada
- Lentil or split-pea soup

- Fruit shakes or smoothies
- Low-fat cottage cheese
- Yogurt (dairy or soy)
- Canned beans, vegetarian chili
- Ethnic frozen meals—Mexican, Chinese, Thai, or others
- Tofu hot dogs
- Veggie burgers
- Quick mixes of tabouli, hummus, refried beans, black beans
- Roasted soy nuts or other nuts
- Vegetable pizza

Reprinted, by permission, from S.G. Eberle, 2000, *Endurance sports nutrition* (Champaign, IL: Human Kinetics), 170.

Table 11.2   Potential Causes of Iron Deficiency

Inadequate supply	Blood loss	Life stage
Iron-deficient diet	Menstruation	Childhood
	Pregnancy	Adolescence
	Bleeding	Pregnancy
	Gastrointestinal bleeding	

Iron

The nutrients most often deficient in athletes' diets are iron and calcium. Iron functions as an integral part of hemoglobin, myoglobin, and enzymes that control oxygen transport and energy metabolism. Inadequate iron stores can affect performance through development of iron-deficiency anemia. There is considerable debate as to whether iron deficiency *without* associated anemia results in decreased performance. Experimental evidence demonstrates that lack of iron hinders the ability of skeletal muscle to utilize oxygen and generate adenosine triphosphate (ATP; discussed later in chapter); yet research has not consistently shown that isolated iron deficiency (without anemia) actually hurts athletic performance.

Iron deficiency occurs most often when there is inadequate iron in the diet (vegetarians) or blood loss (menstruating women, gastrointestinal bleeding), as well as when iron requirements are elevated (during adolescence or pregnancy) (table 11.2). Caffeine can also inhibit the absorption of iron and should be avoided for 2 h before and after taking iron supplements or eating foods high in iron.

When an athlete complains of fatigue, lack of energy, or decreased performance, first rule out chronic dehydration, overtraining, and sleep problems. In women, blood loss during the menstrual cycle can also lead to iron-deficiency anemia. If the person is consuming plenty of fluids and getting adequate sleep, have him or her assessed by a physician for iron-deficiency anemia. Athletes exhibiting iron deficiency without anemia should look for other causes of their symptoms, including overtraining, depression, or some other medical explanation.

Treatment of iron-deficiency anemia requires iron supplementation. The usual starting supplement is ferrous sulfate in a dosage of 3 to 6 mg of elemental iron per kilogram of body weight (1.4-2.8 mg/lb body weight) per day, divided among two or three doses. For adults, this typically comes to about 300 mg taken three times daily. Some nutritionists suggest that people take ascorbic acid (vitamin C) along with the iron to increase iron absorption. For isolated iron deficiency without anemia, the usual supplement is 300 mg ferrous sulfate once daily, with increased dosage as needed.

Calcium

Calcium plays an integral role in intracellular homeostasis and in determining bone density. Poor calcium intake is the single biggest predictor of low bone mineral density in young people and largely determines who may develop osteoporosis later in life. If adolescent or young adult women do not engage in weight-bearing physical activity, or if they have inadequate gonadal hormones (estrogen and progesterone), they may have increased risk for osteoporosis later in life.

Many athletes obtain less calcium than the amount recommended by the National Academy of Science's Food and Nutrition Board. Without a diet heavy in dairy foods, it is difficult to match the standards. Calcium supplementation increases bone mineral density in children, but the positive effects persist only if the supplementation continues into adulthood. Calcium supplementation is also correlated with bone mineralization in adults. Adequate calcium intake is around 1,500 mg/d for active athletes. Because an 8-oz glass of milk contains only 200 mg of calcium, many athletes need calcium supplements. Other sources of calcium may include calcium-fortified foods such as orange juice. Calcium carbonate is readily absorbed and inexpensive. Remind athletes taking calcium carbonate supplements to take them *with meals*—and to be sure to get adequate vitamin D, which increases absorption of calcium. Calcium supplements and iron supplements should not be taken at the same time, because calcium interferes with absorption of iron.

Calcium Sources*

1 c milk	3 c broccoli
1 c fortified soy milk or rice milk	1 1/2 c canned baked beans
1 c yogurt	1/2 c soy nuts
1 1/2 oz cheese	11 dried figs
1 c tofu (made with calcium sulfate)	3 tbsp sesame seeds
1 1/2 c cooked dark leafy greens—kale, collard, turnip greens	4 oz canned salmon or sardines (with bones)
1 1/2 c cooked bok choy	1 c fortified orange juice
	Fortified breakfast cereals (varies)

* = Contains at least 300 mg per serving.

Adapted, by permission, from S.G. Eberle, 2000, *Endurance sports nutrition* (Champaign, IL: Human Kinetics), 169.

Chromium

Chromium is a trace element believed to be deficient in some diets. It serves as a cofactor for insulin, helping it to bind receptor tissue and enhancing its actions. The body releases chromium from its stores in response to a rise in blood insulin. Chromium is found in many foods, including brewer's yeast, nuts, asparagus, prunes, mushrooms, wine, and beer. Intestinal absorption of inorganic chromium is only about 0.5% to 2%. In most supplements, picolinic acid is added to the trivalent form of chromium to make it more bioavailable. Because so little is known about trace element supplementation, there is no **recommended daily allowance (RDA)** for chromium. Daily intake of 50 to 200 µg is generally believed to be safe and adequate. Although some evidence exists that active athletes have increased excretion of chromium, it is not clear that athletes need higher levels of chromium in their diets.

Chromium is sometimes advertised as a fat burner. Hypothetically, by enhancing the action of insulin, chromium might be expected to help increase muscle mass, decrease tissue breakdown, and decrease fat deposition. Supplement manufacturers sometimes make such claims—but they are based largely on a single study on football players. Other studies have been unable to demonstrate that chromium is a fat burner.

Current research does not provide enough evidence to endorse the use of chromium for fat loss or weight loss in either athletes or untrained people. Side effects of chromium supplementation are not well known, but anecdotal reports suggest that some side effects are damaging. Moreover, excessive chromium levels may interfere with the body's absorption and metabolism of iron.

PREGAME MEALS

You can have a profound effect on athletes' performance by educating them about pregame meals. The effect of pregame meals on performance and overall health can even make the difference between winning and losing.

Although the meal that immediately precedes a game can supply the athlete's body with energy, it cannot supply *all* the energy for the event. Athletes can significantly increase glycogen storage by eating the correct foods for several days before the event. The pregame meal itself does not cause large increases in muscle glycogen, but a well-planned meal can provide an extra edge of energy, help avoid hunger during the event, ensure adequate hydration, provide a relatively empty stomach at game time, and prevent gastrointestinal upset or other adverse reactions to food.

Although people vary widely in their tastes and in their responses to various foods, here are some basic guidelines you can give your athletes about their last meal before a competition:

- Drink plenty of fluids (but not soda pop or coffee) with the pregame meal. Remember: Prehydration prevents dehydration.

- Allow enough time for digestion. Eat your meal at least 3 h before the event.

- Choose a meal that's high in complex carbohydrates. These are easy to digest and can help your body maintain steady supplies of blood glucose during the competition.

- If you commonly have problems with gas-producing foods such as raw vegetables, fruits, or beans, avoid those foods in your pregame meal. Avoid any other foods that have a history of causing problems such as flatus, cramps, and diarrhea.

- Consume only moderate amounts of protein and fat, because your body digests these more slowly than it digests carbohydrates.

- Restrict simple sugars such as candy bars and sodas. Sweets can cause rapid swings in blood sugar levels, resulting in low blood sugar and less energy at game time.

- Avoid caffeine. Caffeine stimulates the body to increase urine output, which can contribute to dehydration.

COMMON NUTRITIONAL SUPPLEMENTS

Athletes are always looking for ways to improve their performance, and some will do anything to succeed. Use of nutritional supplements to enhance performance appears to be on the rise. Because many are advertised as "herbal" or "natural," athletes often consider them to be harmless. Most of the supplements are readily available and do not require a prescription.

Case Study

John is attending his first practice as a freshman high school football player. It is a hot August day, and about an hour into the practice, he develops a stomachache and has to leave practice to go to the restroom. He has a loose bowel movement and gets some relief from his pain. In another 15 to 20 min, he has to leave the field again because of abdominal pain and the urge to have another bowel movement. After the third trip to the bathroom, his coach suggests that he shower and go home.

Before he goes in, you ask him if he has eaten anything different, and his response is no. When you ask him about any supplements, he tells you that he purchased a new amino acid supplement and took extra this morning for his first workout. You ask him to stop taking it temporarily and to bring the bottle in to you. You tell him that he probably took more than his stomach and bowels can digest. The next day, he reveals that he took four times the recommended dosage, hoping that a larger amount would help his performance.

It is common for athletes to think that, if a small amount of a supplement is helpful, more will work better. As in John's case at the beginning of this chapter, few people think about side effects. A survey of a large number of college athletes revealed significant use of amino acid supplements and creatine. The nutritional supplement market is largely unregulated—producers of supplements promote benefits supported by little or no scientific evidence. The most popular supplements are those that claim to build muscle, improve endurance, or reduce body fat. Many athletes spend significant sums of money on supplements for whose effectiveness there is no clear evidence.

Creatine

Creatine is produced primarily by a joint effort between the kidneys and the liver, at a rate of 1 to 2 g/d, from the precursors glycine and arginine. Although there are numerous food sources of creatine, most dietary creatine comes from meats. Creatine is stored in the muscle and is a source of energy and muscle. It has been known since the 1920s and, unlike other supplements, has received a lot of attention from research labs.

Function of Creatine in the Body

The energy that cells use to drive virtually all of their functions (including muscle movement) derives from removal of a phosphate ion from **ATP (adenosine triphosphate)**. The resulting ADP (adenosine diphosphate) must be rephosphorylated—that is, it must be given another phosphate ion—back to ATP before it can once again provide energy to the cell. Resting muscle cells contain sufficient ATP to fuel perhaps a 1- to 3-s burst of high-intensity effort. For high-intensity effort that lasts a few seconds longer than that, the cells must rephosphorylate the ADP immediately—and they do that through a small reserve of creatine phosphate, which donates the extra phosphate ion to ADP to reconstitute ATP. After 5 to 10 s of maximum muscle effort, the creatine phosphate reserves are diminished—and the muscle cells begin to utilize anaerobic glycolysis to produce ATP. After a minute or two (depending on the individual), the heart and blood vessels begin to increase oxygen delivery to exercising muscles—and aerobic metabolism (known widely as the *Krebs citric acid cycle*) takes over.

Think of creatine as a battery that can be quickly recharged. Within a few seconds after cells have used most of their store of creatine phosphate, they are able to rephosphorylate creatine—and the creatine phosphate is once again available to donate phosphate to ADP and fuel another several-second burst of energy.

Higher levels of creatine in muscle cells can increase the availability of creatine phosphate, enabling it to produce more ATP. An average adult has about 120 g of creatine in his or her muscle cells, each day losing and reacquiring about 2 g. About half of the 2-g turnover is replaced through the diet, and about half is synthesized within the body.

For very short-term, high-intensity activities that call for only a few seconds of maximum power (e.g., sprinting, jerking a weight bar, swinging a baseball bat, starting a new football play every minute or so), additional levels of creatine obtained through supplements appear to increase strength. Creatine monohydrate has been available as a nutritional supplement and potential ergogenic aid since the early 1990s and is probably the most popular supplement among football players and athletes in strength sports.

Dosage

Most studies that have demonstrated creatine's efficacy used a loading dose of 20 g/d for 5 d, followed by maintenance doses of 2 to 5 g/d. It is not clear that a loading dose is necessary, however, and many athletes simply start on a maintenance dose. Creatine is better absorbed if taken with a source of glucose or some other sugar. Because its uptake in muscle occurs more readily during exercise, athletes often take it shortly before exercise.

Efficacy

Not all athletes will benefit from creatine supplementation. Some athletes already have high concentrations of creatine in their muscles, but there is no way to determine the levels without a painful and expensive muscle biopsy. Theoretically, individuals with the lowest natural concentrations of creatine in muscle will benefit most from supplementation.

There have been many studies of creatine as an ergogenic aid. Although manufacturers of creatine sometimes make broad claims for it—that it increases weight and strength as well as endurance—the bulk of the research shows that it can be effective for some people who need extra strength in quick bursts, as described previously. It does appear to stimulate weight gain in muscle tissues, but thus far there is no way of knowing if the gain results from an increase in muscle fibers or simply from higher water content in existing muscle cells. Creatine does *not* appear to help in endurance events and may even decrease performance in such events (possibly because of weight gain that creates more work for the athlete).

Side Effects

Because creatine has not been used for very long, we know of few long-term side effects. It appears to be well tolerated in the majority of young people who take it. Nausea, diarrhea, dizziness, and weakness are occasionally reported, usually associated with dosages greater than 5 g/d; the frequency of these complaints is unknown.

A few athletes report muscle soreness when they use creatine, although the reasons for this have not been established. There is usually some immediate weight gain, which makes some people feel uncomfortable. For muscle cells to remove creatine from the bloodstream, they must remove water along with it. Because the body therefore has lower levels of available free water, it is very important for athletes to drink extra water when using creatine as a supplement—especially if they are training in warm weather, which already increases the need for extra water. Creatine is metabolized to creatinine and excreted by the kidneys, and because exogenous creatine increases the load on the kidneys, many researchers are concerned about chronic stress to the kidneys. Currently there are two reports in the literature of athletes who developed renal failure while using creatine as a supplement. Further evaluation of these athletes revealed that their kidney function was borderline before they began taking creatine, and their kidney failure reversed once they stopped using the supplement.

No evidence exists that creatine is harmful to a person with healthy kidneys. Yet there will be no hard data on long-term use for several more decades. The *possibility* exists that long-term use could damage the kidneys. You may want to caution athletes that, although creatine appears to be safe for use by athletes who need short-term bursts of strength, its long-term side effects are unknown. It is also wise to caution anyone taking over-the-counter dietary supplements that the FDA does not regulate their purity. In past years there have been occasional instances of serious complications and even deaths among people who took supplements that contained potentially life-threatening impurities. Anyone taking such supplements should do so with the knowledge that there is a small but real chance that serious complications may result.

Proteins and Amino Acids

Current research shows that some athletes may benefit by ingesting 50% to 125% more protein than the current recommended daily allowance of 0.8 g/kg of body weight per day. Very athletic individuals who are building muscle would potentially benefit by ingesting up to 2.0 to 2.5 g/kg/d; the RDA for endurance athletes is about 1.2 to 1.4 g/kg/d. There is no evidence that protein intake above these levels has an ergogenic effect, in spite of claims to the contrary by supplement manufacturers. Although 8 of the 20 amino acids are essential—that is, the body cannot synthesize them and therefore must obtain them through the diet—most balanced diets have more than enough to meet the day-to-day needs of even the most active athletes.

Some supplement manufacturers suggest that supplementing certain amino acids may trigger the body to produce higher levels of other useful substances. For example, increased intake of the precursors of creatine (arginine, methionine, and glycine) might increase the production of creatine. These claims, however, have no scientific basis. Intravenous arginine has been shown to stimulate the release of growth hormone, both alone and in combination with lysine, but there is no evidence that oral supplementation of these amino acids results in any increase in growth hormone levels.

Adverse effects of high protein and amino acid intake seem to be mild and uncommon. There has been concern about the risk of kidney damage, but the concern is probably overstated. Oral amino acid supplements may cause stomach upset and diarrhea caused by increased osmotic load; the side effects are dose-dependent and vary among individuals.

Most athletes consume adequate protein in their diets. For most athletes, using protein or amino acid supplements is simply an expensive way to consume additional calories. If athletes insist that they need extra protein, remind them of the relatively inexpensive sources of protein on supermarket shelves—such as powdered milk, egg or soy protein powder, or most kinds of instant breakfast drinks. Food-based sources of amino acids are also readily available (see *Amino Acids: Food Versus Pills*, p. 180).

Carnitine

Carnitine is not an amino acid but does bear resemblance to amino acids and is usually grouped under this heading. L-Carnitine is the chemically active form of carnitine, and the body uses it to transport long-chain fatty acids to the mitochondria in the cells, where it is burned for energy. It is synthesized in the body from the essential amino acids lysine and methionine. Carnitine is present in meats and other animal foods, so vegetarians or vegans may want to consider supplementing with carnitine. About 95% of the carnitine in the body is in muscle. It is a component of several enzymes involved in fatty acid metabolism—an important source of energy as exercise increases in length or intensity.

Studies on carnitine and athletic performance have shown mixed results. Theoretically, carnitine should be helpful for endurance exercise, but the most recent studies have not shown any ergogenic effect. Carnitine appears to cause few side effects, but large doses cause diarrhea. You probably should discourage athletes from using carnitine until more information is available.

Beta-Hydroxy-Beta-Methylbutyrate (HMB)

Beta-hydroxy-beta-methylbutyrate (HMB) is a metabolite of leucine and one of the essential branch-chain amino acids. It is found in citrus fruits, catfish, and breast milk. Many advocates of nutritional supplements believe that high HMB levels decrease protein breakdown. Research on animals suggests an anabolic

Amino Acids: Food Versus Pills

Bodybuilders commonly spend a lot of money on special amino acid supplements that claim to provide more energy, stamina, and muscle mass. These athletes could have gotten more amino acids if they'd spent that money on wholesome foods. This chart shows the amounts of two popular amino acids, arginine and leucine, that occur naturally in food and how they compare to the amounts found in commercial supplements.

Amount	Arginine (mg)	Leucine (mg)
Food		
2 egg whites	380	600
1 c skim milk	350	950
4 oz chicken breast (1 small)	2,100	2,650
6 oz tuna (1 can)	2,700	3,700
Supplement		
1 serving TwinLab® Amino Fuel®	85	320
1 serving Ultimate Nutrition® Amino Gold®	350	1,260
1 serving Nature's Best Amino Acids	440	1,300

When compared according to milligrams of amino acid per 25 g of protein, the supplements are very expensive sources of protein.

Equivalent of 25 g protein	Arginine/ 25 g protein	Leucine/ 25 g protein	Cost
3 c skim milk	1,050	2,850	$0.60
2/3 can (4 oz) tuna	1,800	2,400	$0.80
3 oz chicken breast	1,600	2,000	$0.65
7 egg whites	2,650	4,200	$0.75
24 pills TwinLab Amino Fuel	1,020	3,840	$2.80
27 pills Ultimate Nutrition Amino Gold	1,050	3,780	$2.60
18 pills Nature's Best Amino Acids	1,320	3,900	$1.80

Adapted, by permission, from N. Clark, 1997, *Nancy Clark's sports nutrition guidebook,* 2nd ed. (Champaign, IL: Human Kinetics),142.

effect. Few researchers have studied the effect of HMB supplements in humans. At least two studies have pointed to a dose-dependent ergogenic effect: Individuals receiving higher doses of HMB gained more muscle mass and demonstrated greater strength gains; but some scientists believe there were serious methodological weaknesses in the studies, not the least of which was that they were not double-blind (in a double-blind study, neither researchers nor athletes know who is getting the supplement and who is getting a placebo).

No side effects were reported with HMB in these limited studies. This supplement is too new for us to know if it is effective or safe; we believe you should discourage athletes from using it until much more extensive research data have demonstrated not only that it is harmless but that it actually works.

For Further Information

Print Resources

Benardot, D. 2000. *Nutrition for serious athletes.* Champaign, IL: Human Kinetics.

Eberle, S.G. 2000. *Endurance sports nutrition.* Champaign, IL: Human Kinetics.

Manore, M., and J. Thompson. 2000. *Sport nutrition for health and performance.* Champaign, IL: Human Kinetics.

Web Resources

American Dietetic Association
www.eatright.org
A professional organization Web site that provides information and resources on a variety of nutrition topics.

Nutrition.Gov
www.nutrition.gov
A federal government–sponsored Web resource that provides information to the public regarding all aspects of food safety and dietary guidelines. Offers several links to current publications and research.

SUMMARY

1. *Differentiate the athletic diet from a typical American diet.*

Nutrition experts suggest that approximately 50% to 60% of a person's total calories should come from complex carbohydrates, 15% to 20% from protein, and 25% to 30% from fat. The typical American eats too much fat, protein, and simple sugars and not enough complex carbohydrates—and certainly not enough vegetables and fruits. Athletes have different nutritional requirements when compared to sedentary people or even moderately active people. Fluid lost as sweat during exercise requires serious athletes to consume more liquid on a regular basis, and athletes who exercise at least 2 h/d require a much higher intake of calories than other people—in particular, the athlete's diet requires higher levels of carbohydrate (up to 70% of the total calories) to meet the energy demands that such vigorous exercise requires.

2. *Discuss the energy requirements for specific sport activities.*

Energy requirements depend on age, body size, and resting metabolic rate—as well as the demands of the sport and conditions under which a person trains. Long-distance swimmers, crew athletes, and triathletes, for example, clearly need more calories than baseball players and sprinters. Sports with the highest energy expenditure (as measured in kcal/min) include cross-country skiing, crew racing, swimming, and bicycle racing. Sports with lower energy expenditures include the hammer throw, shot put, and discus throw. However, the mean caloric intake for both types of sports may be equal in that the throwers usually have a large body size and a relatively intense training regime.

3. *Identify the recommended nutrient requirements for carbohydrates, fats, and proteins.*

The negative effects of poor diet are subtle and in many cases invisible until they manifest themselves decades into the future. Carbohydrates make up 60% (more for athletes) of the overall diet and are the main fuel source for endurance performance as well as for short-duration, high-intensity exercise. Carbohydrate is stored in the liver and in muscle as glycogen, and fatigue occurs when glycogen is depleted. In high-intensity sports, there is a close association between activity levels and muscle glycogen concentration. If glycogen stores are not replenished, athletes will have less energy for practice in the days following. Current recommendations for carbohydrate intake are approximately 8 to 10 g of carbohydrate per kilogram of body weight per day to maintain muscle glycogen in endurance athletes who train more than 90 min/d. While it takes approximately 20 h to completely replenish carbohydrate stores in endurance athletes, glycogen resynthesis appears to be greater than basal levels when athletes consume carbohydrate immediately following exercise. Endurance athletes should therefore eat a snack rich in carbohydrates immediately following an intense workout. Less carbohydrate is required for athletes participating in intermittent endurance activity, power sports, or sprinting events.

Dietary fat is important and should comprise 25% to 30% of the overall diet. It carries fat-soluble vitamins, makes food taste better, and serves as a concentrated fuel source. Trained people oxidize more fat and less carbohydrate than untrained individuals, thus sparing glycogen stores. Athletes in training ought to watch their fat intake like anyone else, to be sure that they don't overindulge; but because they are less susceptible to the deleterious health effects of fat than most people, they probably should avoid low-fat diets unless they are directed to such diets by a health professional.

Protein should account for 15% to 20% of the diet. Yet many athletes mistakenly rely too much on high-carbohydrate diets, thereby failing to consume enough protein. Most athletes should consume about 2.4 oz of protein per 100 lb of body weight (1.5 g/kg of body weight) per day. Athletes on low-calorie, low-fat, or vegetarian diets are particularly susceptible to protein deficits. People who engage in resistance training have higher protein requirements than other athletes because their training leads to muscle hypertrophy—that is, they create a lot of new muscle tissue.

4. *Discuss the relationship between hydration and athletic performance.*

Although water is not technically a nutrient by some definitions, it is probably the single most important dietary component that can demonstrably affect sports performance. Many athletes practice and compete in a state of dehydration; simply staying hydrated can boost their performance significantly. Thirst is *not* an effective signal to measure fluid lost during workouts or competitions. By the time athletes are thirsty, they are already dehydrated—and dehydration contributes to poor performance and thermoregulatory dysfunction. All athletes can meet their fluid needs by drinking water. For some ultraendurance sports, fluids that replenish lost carbohydrates and electrolytes may improve performance and delay fatigue. Because many such drinks are more palatable than plain water, you may recommend them to any athletes to boost the likelihood that they will remain hydrated. However, because such drinks can cause nausea, cramping, and diarrhea in some individuals, athletes should try these types of drinks in practice before using them in competition.

5. *Explain how vitamins and minerals contribute to total nutrients.*

Athletes eating a balanced diet will ingest adequate vitamins and minerals for activities of daily living and exercise. Observation suggests, however, that few young people actually eat a genuinely balanced diet (how many of the athletes you know *really* eat five full servings of veggies or fruits every day?). Consuming vitamins and minerals above the recommended daily allowance has not been shown to improve performance, but nutrient deficiencies can lead to undetectable compromises in overall health, which can compromise performance. Athletes should be encouraged to consume a diet rich in fruits; green, red, and yellow vegetables; and milk products. However, given the poor diets of even athletes in training, a daily vitamin tablet with minerals may be a good idea just to maintain optimal health and development. Deficiencies in iron and calcium in particular can have detrimental effects on the training athlete.

6. *Explain the role of nutritional supplements.*

Athletes eating a proper diet and training appropriately may ask for advice in terms of nutritional supplements in hopes of gaining an edge over their competition. Some supplements are relatively safe and may improve strength in the laboratory setting for the short term. Other supplements are relatively safe but have not been found to improve performance. How performance in the lab translates to performance in competition may vary with the type of sport (i.e., a long-distance runner is not going to improve with a large increase in muscle mass resulting from associated weight gain) and type of supplement used. Creatine can have positive effects for short-term, high-intensity activities in terms of increasing strength. It does appear to be well tolerated by many individuals; however, because the long-term side effects of this supplement are unclear, we are not willing to endorse its use and feel athletes should discuss possible use with their physicians. Protein and amino acid supplements are also well tolerated but have even less data supporting their use as a performance enhancement. Because most athletes consume enough protein in their regular diet, there is really no reason for them to consume these expensive supplements. Further information and investigation is required before any other supplements for enhancing performance can be recommended.

CHAPTER 12

Weight Control

OBJECTIVES

Upon completion of this chapter the reader will be able to do the following:

1. Discuss the concept of ideal body weight

2. Explain the roles of body composition and body mass index in weight control

3. Describe the diagnostic criteria for identifying an eating disorder as compared to disordered eating patterns

4. Explain the common features of a screening program to identify unhealthy eating patterns for patients with weight-management questions

5. Discuss issues common to athletes who desire to gain weight

Athletes often engage in unhealthy weight-management practices in hopes of improving their performance. Weight loss or gain may benefit an athlete, depending on the sport—yet the strategy employed to reach weight goals may compromise not only the athletes' performance but even their short- and long-term health.

Case Study

A collegiate freshman crew athlete weighs 137 lb (62.3 kg). She is considering dropping to the lightweight boat, which would require that she lose 7 lb (3.2 kg). Her body fat, measured by skinfold calipers, is 18%. As a distance runner her sophomore year in high school, she was diagnosed with anorexia nervosa. You must consider several issues before approving this athlete's plan: (1) How difficult is it for her to maintain a weight of 137 lb (62.3 kg)? (2) What has been her highest and lowest weight in the last 2 yr? (3) How anxious is she about being weighed? (4) Is the athlete having regular menses? (5) Does the team have a specific plan for setting weight targets during the year?

IDEAL BODY WEIGHT

Ideal body weight is a term that is overused by the popular media as well as many dietitians, physicians, coaches, athletic trainers, exercise physiologists, insurance companies, and athletes themselves. Ideal body weight is not the same for everybody of a given height and frame: Clearly, the ideal body weight for a 6-ft (183-cm) nose tackle differs from that of a distance runner of the same height. *The ideal body weight for athletes is the weight and body composition they can maintain in a healthy manner and that enables them to perform at their best.*

Having said that there is no single ideal body weight for a person of a given height, we nevertheless ought to provide you (for the record) with the following rough formula that many health professionals use—rightly or wrongly—to determine ideal body weight:

For women, allow 100 lb (45.5 kg) for the first 5 ft (152 cm) of height and add 5 lb (2.3 kg) for every inch (2.5 cm) taller than 5 ft (152 cm). For men, allow 106 (48 kg) lb for the first 5 ft (152 cm) of height and add 6 lb (2.7 kg) for every inch (2.5 cm) taller than 5 ft (152 cm). For both men and women, allow 10% on either side of the calculated ideal body weight to account for differing body frame sizes.

Your best use of the concept of ideal body weight will probably be in casual conversations with athletes. For serious consideration of issues regarding weight versus height, there are better measures to use, and we will discuss these next.

BODY COMPOSITION

Scientists by and large no longer use standards of "ideal weight." Most agree that the best current measure of normal weight and body composition is **body mass index (BMI)**—defined as a person's weight in kilograms divided by his or her height in meters squared. For example, a person who weighs 55 kg (about 121 lb) and is 165 cm, or 1.65 m, tall (about 5'5") would have a BMI of 55 kg/2.72 m^2, or about 20.2 kg/m^2 (the square of 1.65 m = 1.65 m × 1.65 m = 2.72 m^2). In generally accepted practice, BMIs of 25.0 to 29.9 kg/m^2 define overweight, whereas a BMI greater than 30.0 kg/m^2 indicates obesity. *In adults, BMI strongly correlates with total body fat.*

For adolescent males, normal body fat is 10% to 20%. For adolescent females, the range is 17% to 25%. A percentage body fat of less than 8% in men and 15% in

Terms and Definitions

anorexia nervosa—An eating disorder, seen mostly in young women, characterized by pathological fear of weight gain and accompanied by excessive weight loss via severe dieting or starvation.

body mass index (BMI)—A measure of body composition, equal to an individual's weight in kilograms divided by the square of the height in meters.

bulimia nervosa—An eating disorder, seen mostly in young women, characterized by compulsive over-eating followed by self-induced vomiting, use of laxatives, or use of diuretics to prevent weight gain.

women is considered lean. Greater than 25% fat for men and 32% for women is considered obese.

There are several different ways to calculate percent body fat. Skinfold thickness, measured using calipers, is the most common method. Formulas vary according to the number of sites measured and the person's gender. An inherent problem with skinfold measurement is its dependence on the skill and experience of the operator. Moreover, results are less accurate for extremely lean or obese individuals. Even in the most skilled hands, skinfold measurement is usually accurate to only about 3%.

Other methods not as commonly used for calculating percent body fat include electrical impedance, dual-energy X-ray absorptiometry, and measurement of total body water. Although these techniques are highly accurate, cost and availability limit their usefulness.

The most accurate determination of percent body fat measures hydrostatic weight. The accuracy of this technique, however, is partly dependent on the athlete's ability to remain calm underwater with only residual amounts of air remaining in the lungs. Claustrophobia or inordinate fear of water usually precludes use of this technique.

WEIGHT-LOSS ISSUES

Athletes participating in sports where appearance or "making weight" are important sometimes engage in unhealthy weight-control practices. In figure skating, gymnastics, cheerleading, and ballet, judges often give subjective scores that are based at least in part on a very slender physical appearance. Wrestling, lightweight crew, weight-class football, and horse racing have rules against active competition unless athletes are under a certain weight. Unfortunately, participants in these activities sometimes turn to extreme weight-loss practices such as overexercising, restricting calories, recurrent vomiting, spitting, or using medications (laxatives, diet pills, nicotine). When athletes in these sports use rapid dehydration (utilizing saunas, steam baths, and rubber suits) to "make weight" below an acceptable limit, the result, in rare cases, can be sudden death. A more sensible and safer approach is simply to eat a few hundred (with emphasis on *few*) less calories a day than the athlete requires until the desired weight is reached. At that point, the caloric requirement can be computed based on the new body weight and can be used to help the athlete "budget" what he eats. Figure 12.1 illustrates clearly how to calculate daily caloric needs.

Eating Disorders

The incidence of eating disorders among athletes appears to be no different from that of the general population. Fortunately, more athletes suffer from disordered eating rather than from the more serious psychological eating disorders. Most athletes

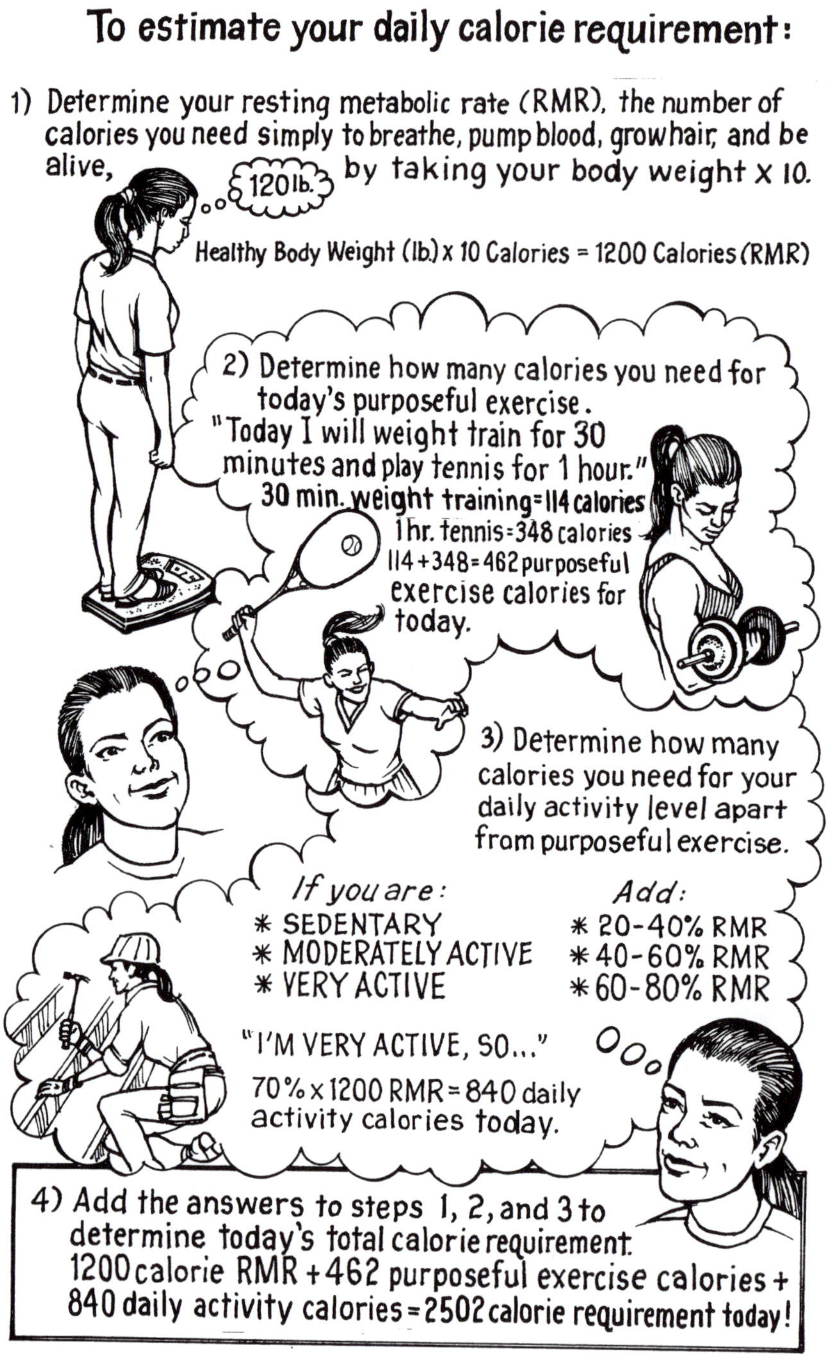

To estimate your daily calorie requirement:

1) Determine your resting metabolic rate (RMR), the number of calories you need simply to breathe, pump blood, grow hair, and be alive, _120 lb._ by taking your body weight x 10.

Healthy Body Weight (lb.) x 10 Calories = 1200 Calories (RMR)

2) Determine how many calories you need for today's purposeful exercise.
"Today I will weight train for 30 minutes and play tennis for 1 hour."
30 min. weight training = 114 calories
1 hr. tennis = 348 calories
114 + 348 = 462 purposeful exercise calories for today.

3) Determine how many calories you need for your daily activity level apart from purposeful exercise.

If you are:
* SEDENTARY
* MODERATELY ACTIVE
* VERY ACTIVE

Add:
* 20-40% RMR
* 40-60% RMR
* 60-80% RMR

"I'M VERY ACTIVE, SO..."
70% x 1200 RMR = 840 daily activity calories today.

4) Add the answers to steps 1, 2, and 3 to determine today's total calorie requirement.
1200 calorie RMR + 462 purposeful exercise calories + 840 daily activity calories = 2502 calorie requirement today!

■ **Figure 12.1** If your athletes are concerned about how many calories they should consume to supply adequate energy for their activities, the method pictured above will enable them to find out.

Reprinted, by permission, from N. Clark, 1997, *Nancy Clark's sports nutrition guidebook*, 2nd ed. (Champaign, IL: Human Kinetics), 261.

using unhealthy weight-loss techniques do not meet the official parameters for **anorexia nervosa** or **bulimia nervosa,** as defined by the *Diagnostic and Statistical Manual of Mental Disorders,* 4th ed. (DSM-IV; APA 1994). Two retrospective surveys of female collegiate athletes reported a 32% and 62% incidence of unhealthy weight-control methods (Rosen et al. 1986; Rosen and Hough 1988).

The use of only one unhealthy weight-control method does not establish the diagnosis of anorexia or bulimia nervosa. Among high school wrestlers polled in one study (Oppliger et al. 1993), 21% had fasted more than 24 h, 16% had used diuretics, and almost 10% had induced vomiting at least once a week.

If you are in a position to do so, screen your athletes for potential problems at the beginning of a season; early recognition, education, and treatment may prevent individual and team complications. A subtle approach looking at the overall nutritional health of a team helps you avoid singling out athletes who may at present have problems or have a history of eating disorders. A good way to start is to look at an athlete's energy levels, performance, and personal goals. Amenorrhea can be a significant clue to potential problems in females in that it often results from negative energy balance. Obtain a dietary history from the previous 24 to 72 h to look for imbalances (e.g., lack of fat or minerals) that can affect performance. Finally, focus on individuals' perceptions of their body image; history of eating disorders and family; and coaches' or teammates' concern about possible eating disorders in the past. If you identify a problem, refer the athlete to his primary care provider, the team physician, or a psychologist for further assessment. It is important that you work closely

Table 12.1   Effects of Dehydration and Starvation on Health and Performance

Organ system	Effect
Endocrine	Growth retardation Decreased testosterone Amenorrhea Osteoporosis
Neuromuscular	Decreased strength and power Decreased endurance Decreased short-term sprinting speed
Psychological	Decreased school performance Depression and mood swings
Fluid and electrolytes	Decreased plasma volume and renal blood flow Electrolyte abnormalities → cardiac dysfunction
Thermoregulation	Susceptibility to hyperthermia

Adapted, by permission, from V.A. Perriello, 1995, "Health and weight control management among wrestlers: A proposed program for high school athletes," *Virginia Medical Quarterly* 122: 179-185.

with the psychologist and that you permit the athlete to continue participating in his sport as long as participation will not compromise physical health.

Although few athletes suffer true anorexia or bulimia, athletes tend to develop disordered eating patterns for unique reasons. Prolonged periods of dieting, frequent weight fluctuations, sudden increases in training volume, and traumatic events such as injury or loss of a coach appeared to trigger disordered eating practices among elite Norwegian athletes (Sundgot-Borgen 1994).

Dehydration

Within weight-class sports, athletes who can dehydrate themselves to make weight often feel they can maximize their competitive advantage over athletes who naturally weigh less and therefore have less muscle power. Concerns about the consequences of short-term fluid restriction as a means of making weight were brought to a head with the ultimate deaths of three collegiate wrestlers in 1997—each was using dehydration to lose weight in an attempt to qualify for a particular weight class (Centers for Disease Control and Prevention 1998).

Table 12.1 lists the negative effects of both starvation and fluid restriction. Chronic starvation and fluid restriction can very seriously affect multiple organ systems. Though the most direct consequence of acute, severe dehydration is death, even modest dehydration or starvation can compromise both athletic performance and the long-term health of an athlete. You must help athletes take these facts into consideration when they contemplate restricting their weight for performance reasons.

Treatment Guidelines

The best nutritional education for athletes involves a team approach of health-care professionals, including athletic trainers, nutritionists, psychologists, and physicians. Unfortunately, this ideal situation is rare. Depending on your position and responsibilities, you may be the one to identify community resources for helping athletes who have difficulty with weight management. Educating coaches, athletes, parents, and administrators can help prevent future problems.

The American College of Sports Medicine has developed a six-part program to educate wrestlers about the dangers associated with weight loss attained through cyclical calorie and fluid restriction (see *Six-Part Program to Educate Wrestlers About the Dangers of Cyclical Calorie and Fluid Restriction*, page 190). Following the three deaths in 1997, the NCAA established new guidelines, adding a 7-lb (3.2 kg) weight allowance to each weight class, prohibiting use of drugs or environmental conditions to dehydrate, establishing a weigh-in time 2 h before competition, and establishing a permanent

Six-Part Program to Educate Wrestlers About the Dangers of Cyclical Calorie and Fluid Restriction

1. Educate coaches and wrestlers about the adverse consequences of prolonged fasting and dehydration on physical performance and health.
2. Discourage the use of rubber suits, steam rooms, hot boxes, saunas, laxatives, and diuretics for making weight.
3. Adopt new state or national governing body legislation that schedules weigh-ins immediately before competition.
4. Schedule daily weigh-ins before and after practice to monitor weight loss and dehydration.
5. Assess body composition at the start of each season: Males 16 yr and younger with body fat below 7%, or over 16 yr with body fat below 5%, need medical clearance before competition.
6. Emphasize consistent proper nutrition.

Adapted from Oppliger et al. 1996, ix-xii.

healthy weight class for each wrestler early in the season. Similar guidelines have been adopted at the high school level and could be used in other weight-restricted sports (Oppliger et al. 1995). Only through education and implementation of similar recommendations and rule changes will sports with weight restrictions (e.g., wrestling, crew) or those that implicitly prohibit reasonable amounts of body fat (e.g., gymnastics, long-distance running, ballet) become healthier and safer.

WEIGHT-GAIN ISSUES

Some athletes attempt to gain weight in hopes of improving strength for power sports such as football, bodybuilding, and powerlifting. On the Internet and in bodybuilding and conditioning magazines, advertisements abound for supplements claiming to help athletes increase strength, improve performance, and gain weight. Some athletes even turn to illicit performance-enhancing substances for similar purposes. In most cases, there has been insufficient research to support or reject claims that such substances, whether legal or illegal, can fulfill their promises. Yet the potential for side effects, both known and unknown—not to mention ethical concerns—demands that intelligent people steer clear of these substances until many more years of research have proved their safety and efficacy. Pharmaceutical companies spend hundreds of millions of dollars in research and development for each prescription drug they release, yet some of these drugs exhibit dangerous side effects years after their release, in spite of many published research papers that earlier suggested they were safe. Many of the commonly used supplements have never been studied in terms of potential benefit or risk; in addition, there is no guarantee as to their purity in many instances. You will do well to encourage athletes to achieve their goals, whatever they are, through proper exercise, strength training, and diet. The simple use of a supplement is unlikely to result in any positive effect if the athlete is not making the necessary sacrifices in terms of exercise and nutritional regimen. Chapter 11 gave you more detailed information on these issues.

To gain weight, athletes obviously must consume more calories than they burn. The extra calories may come from an extra serving of milk, an extra snack, or larger portions of meals (see table 12.2). Athletes who consistently ingest extra calories, especially if the focus is on extra protein and carbohydrate, will increase their muscle mass. Yet this will happen *only* if they participate in the correct conditioning program. Too often, athletes—especially high school students—look for

Table 12.2 Sample Weight Gain Menus

The trick to gaining weight is to consistently eat larger-than-normal portions, three meals per day, plus one or two snacks. These sample menus suggest healthful high-calorie, carbohydrate-rich sports meals.

	Approximate calories		Approximate calories
Breakfast			
16 oz orange juice	200	2 c pineapple juice	280
6 pancakes	600	1 c granola	500
1/4 c syrup	200	1/4 c raisins	120
1 pat margarine	50	2 c low-fat milk	200
8 oz low-fat milk	100	1 large banana	130
Total	1,150	Total	1,230
Lunch			
4 slices hefty bread	400	1 7-in pita pocket	240
1 6.5-oz can tuna	200	6-oz turkey breast	300
4 Tbsp lite mayo	150	2 Tbsp lite mayo	80
1 bowl lentil soup	250	2 c apple juice	250
2 c low-fat milk	200	1 c fruit yogurt	250
2 oatmeal cookies	150	1 large muffin	300
Total	1,350	Total	1,420
Dinner			
1 medium cheese pizza	1,400	1 breast chicken	300
2 c lemonade	200	2 large potatoes	400
Total	1,600	2 pats margarine	100
		1 c peas	100
		2 biscuits	300
		2 Tbsp honey	100
		2 c low-fat milk	200
		Total	1,500
Snacks			
2 slices hearty bread	200	2 bagels	440
2 Tbsp peanut butter	200	3 oz lite cheese	260
3 Tbsp jelly	150	2 c crangrape juice	340
1-1/2 c low-fat milk	150	Total	1,040
2 Tbsp chocolate powder	100		
Total	800		

Day's total: 4,900 calories	Day's total: 5,190 calories
60% carbohydrate (745 g)	65% carbohydrate (830 g)
15% protein (193 g)	15% protein (180 g)
25% fat (121 g)	20% fat (123 g)

Reprinted, by permission, from N. Clark, 1997, *Nancy Clark's sports nutrition guidebook,* 2nd ed. (Champaign, IL: Human Kinetics), 295.

shortcuts such as supplements that theoretically permit them to avoid time in the weight room. You must educate your athletes about what is legitimately required for them to gain muscle mass and increase performance.

SUMMARY

1. *Discuss the concept of ideal body weight.*

Athletes sometimes attempt to either lose weight or gain weight through use of potentially dangerous techniques. Ideal body weight is not the same for everybody of a given height and frame: Clearly, the ideal body weight for a 6-ft nose tackle

For Further Information

Print Resources

American College of Sports Medicine, American Dietetics Association, and Dietitians of Canada. December 2000. Joint position statement on nutrition and athletic performance. *Medicine and Science in Sports and Exercise* 32(12): 2130-45.

Oppliger, R.A., G.L. Landry, S.W. Foster, and A.C. Lambrecht. 1993. Bulimic behaviors among interscholastic wrestlers: A statewide survey. *Pediatrics* 91: 826-31. Available online at www.acsm-msse.org

Roemmich, J.N., and W.E. Sinning. 1997. Weight loss and wrestling training: Effects on growth related hormones. *Journal of Applied Physiology* 82:1760-64.

Web Resources

The Weight-control Information Network (WIN)
www.niddk.nih.gov/health/nutrit/nutrit.htm
The Weight-control Information Network (WIN) is a national service of the National Institute of Diabetes and Digestive and Kidney Diseases (NIDDK) of the National Institutes of Health. WIN was established in 1994 to raise awareness and provide up-to-date, science-based information on obesity, physical activity, weight control, and related nutritional issues.

American College of Sports Medicine
www.acsm.org/publications/positionstands.htm
December 2001 position stand on appropriate intervention strategies for weight loss and prevention of weight regain for adults.

differs from that of a distance runner of the same height. *The ideal body weight for athletes is the weight and body composition they can maintain in a healthy manner and that enables them to perform at their best.* Whether athletes are trying to lose or gain weight, they should do so under the direction of health professionals, and their strategies should rely on scientific principles of healthy diet and exercise.

2. *Explain the roles of body composition and body mass index in weight control.*

The best current measure of normal weight and body composition is body mass index (BMI), defined as a person's weight in kilograms divided by his or her height in meters squared. In generally accepted practice, BMIs of 25.0 to 29.9 kg/m^2 define overweight, while a BMI greater than 30.0 kg/m^2 indicates obesity. *In adults, BMI strongly correlates with total body fat.*

There are several different ways to calculate percent body fat. Measuring skinfold thickness using calipers is the most common method. Formulas vary according to the number of sites measured and the person's gender. For adolescent males, normal body fat is 10% to 20%. For adolescent females, the range is 17% to 25%. A percentage body fat less than 8% in men and 15% in women is considered lean; greater than 25% fat for men and 32% for women is considered obese.

BMI and body composition incorporate far more realistic measures to assist with weight control than scale weight alone. Judicious use of these measurements can assist patients in determining their current status and provide measures for healthy weight control under the guidance of a health professional.

3. *Describe the diagnostic criteria for identifying an eating disorder as compared to disordered eating patterns.*

The incidence of eating disorders among athletes appears to be no different from that of the general population. Fortunately, more athletes suffer from disordered eating rather than from the more serious psychological eating disorders. Most athletes using unhealthy weight-loss techniques do not meet the official parameters for anorexia or bulimia nervosa, as defined by the *Diagnostic and Statistical Manual of Mental Disorders,* 4th ed. (DSM-IV). Two retrospective surveys of female collegiate athletes reported a 32% and 62% incidence of unhealthy weight-control methods.

Although few athletes suffer true anorexia or bulimia, athletes tend to develop disordered eating patterns for unique reasons. Prolonged periods of dieting, frequent weight fluctuations, sudden increases in training volume, and traumatic events can trigger disordered eating practices.

4. *Explain the common features of a screening program to identify unhealthy eating patterns for patients with weight-management questions.*

If possible, health-care professionals should screen athletes for potential problems at the beginning of a season; early recognition, education, and treatment may prevent individual and team complications. Looking at the overall nutritional health of a team helps you avoid singling out individuals who may at present have problems or have a history of eating disorders. When dealing with an individual athlete, the athlete's energy levels, performance, and personal goals can be indicators of diet-related problems. Amenorrhea can be a significant clue to potential problems in females, as it often results from negative energy balance. A dietary history from the previous 24 to 72 h may reveal imbalances (e.g., lack of fat or minerals) that can affect performance. Finally, focus on athletes' perceptions of their body image; history of eating disorders and family; and coaches' or teammates' previous concerns about possible eating disorders. If you identify a problem, refer the athlete to his or her primary care provider, the team physician, or a psychologist for further assessment. Working closely with the psychologist and permitting the athlete to continue participating (as long as physical health is not compromised) will contribute to a positive outcome.

5. *Discuss issues common to athletes who desire to gain weight.*

Athletes often attempt to gain weight in hopes of improving strength for power sports such as football, bodybuilding, and powerlifting. Countless supplements claiming to help athletes increase strength, improve performance, and gain weight are available at many nutritional outlets, or online from less-than-reputable companies. Some athletes even turn to illicit performance-enhancing substances. The potential for side effects, both known and unknown—not to mention ethical concerns—demands that athletes steer clear of these substances until many more years of research have proved their safety and efficacy. Many of the commonly used supplements have never been studied in terms of potential benefit or risk; in addition, there is no guarantee as to their purity in many instances.

Encourage athletes to achieve their goals, whatever they are, through proper exercise, strength training, and diet. The simple use of a supplement is unlikely to result in any positive effect if the athlete is not making the necessary sacrifices in terms of exercise and nutritional regimen. To gain weight, athletes must consume more calories than they burn. The extra calories may come from an extra serving of milk, an extra snack, or larger portions of meals. Athletes who consistently ingest extra calories, especially if the focus is on extra protein and carbohydrate, will increase their muscle mass if they participate in the correct conditioning program.

CHAPTER 13

Nonsteroidal Anti-Inflammatory Drugs

OBJECTIVES

Upon completion of this chapter the reader will be able to do the following:

1. Explain the mechanism of action for non-steroidal anti-inflammatory drugs (NSAIDs)

2. Describe the therapeutic effects and side effects of NSAID use

3. Identify possible drug interactions associated with NSAIDs

Nonsteroidal anti-inflammatory drugs (NSAIDs) are the most commonly used medications for musculoskeletal, rheumatologic, and other painful conditions. Both over-the-counter and prescription forms of these medications are available in the United States. It is estimated that more than 70 million NSAID prescriptions and more than 30 billion over-the-counter NSAID products are sold annually. In addition to anti-inflammatory effects, NSAIDs have **antipyretic, analgesic,** and **antiplatelet** properties. The most commonly used NSAIDs have a high **therapeutic index,** meaning that they are unlikely to have serious side effects even when used in high doses. However, since NSAIDs are so ubiquitous, you need to be aware of the indications for their use, their mechanisms of action, and their possible side effects.

Case Study

A 19-yr-old gymnast sprains her ankle and has significant swelling, pain, and limitation in her range of motion 3 d after the injury. She asks you if it is OK for her to use ibuprofen to help in her recovery. You discuss the pros and cons of using the medication, its proper dosing, and its side effects—information the athlete must be told before your team physician will approve her using it. The gymnast calls 3 d later with significant abdominal pain in the epigastric area; she questions whether the medication may have caused the pain. After reviewing other possible causes of abdominal pain, you discuss the situation with the team physician, who recommends discontinuing the ibuprofen. The athlete's abdominal pain resolves over the next 48 h. After further discussion with the athlete about use of NSAIDs, you suggest that she try other medications in the future.

NSAIDs vary widely in terms of chemical classification, absorption, duration of action, mechanism of action, and side effects. They are used primarily to treat pain and inflammation and to reduce fever, and many people at risk for heart attacks or strokes use low doses of aspirin, the most common NSAID, to inhibit clotting. This chapter focuses on the mechanisms of action and potential side effects of the common NSAIDs and highlights differences where they are significant.

MECHANISM OF ACTION

The major mechanism of action of most NSAIDs is inhibition of cyclooxygenase, an important enzyme responsible for the synthesis of prostaglandins from arachidonic acid. Prostaglandins are chiefly responsible for the inflammatory response; they also enhance renal blood flow, help prevent acid damage to the stomach mucosa, and support the clotting function of platelets. And they produce pain. According to current knowledge, there are two forms of cyclooxygenase. Whereas **cyclooxygenase-1 (COX-1)** is seemingly ubiquitous and omnipresent in the tissues mentioned, **cyclooxygenase-2 (COX-2)** is induced or expressed more in times of inflammation. Both enzymes promote inflammation and fever, and both produce pain. COX-1, however, does more: It synthesizes prostaglandins that protect gastrointestinal mucosa, enhance blood flow to the kidneys, and inhibit platelets. Aspirin, ibuprofen, naproxen, and other traditional NSAIDs inhibit both enzymes. But it is clearly preferable to inhibit only the action of cyclooxygenase-2 (COX-2) while permitting COX-1 to function normally (figure 13.1).

Researchers have developed inhibitors specific for COX-2; because these substances have less reported effect on COX-1, they also have fewer effects on renal blood flow, gastric protection, or platelet activity. Two commonly used selective

COX-2 inhibitors recently released in the United States include celecoxib (brand name Celebrex®) and rofecoxib (brand name Vioxx®).

CLASSIFICATION

Therapeutic and side-effect profiles vary among the different classes of NSAIDs (table 13.1); responses among individuals also vary, both therapeutically and with regard to toxicity. The classification and descriptions of the medications discussed here relate to their chemical classification. The majority of NSAIDs are metabolized by the liver and bind to proteins in the blood. For most NSAIDs the elimination half-life is relatively short (<6 h), with therapeutic effects lasting as long as the drug itself. Drugs that are dosed on a one-time-per-day recommendation have a longer half-life than drugs dosed four times daily. Drugs with a longer half-life take longer to produce a desired action

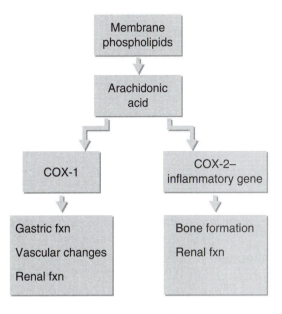

■ **Figure 13.1** Metabolism of arachidonic acid starts with the COX-1 and COX-2 specific enzymes. The COX-2 gene is preferentially expressed at sites of inflammation. Inhibition of this gene is more specific for inflammation and therefore has potential for fewer side effects if used properly.

and take longer to eliminate, which results in longer-acting side effects as well. Most of these medications are eliminated by the kidney. A few of the medications are available without a prescription, including ibuprofen, naproxen, and aspirin. Because of their increased side effects, most other NSAIDs must be obtained with a prescription.

Table 13.1   NSAID Characteristics

Classification	Time of peak response	Typical dose	Side effects (unique)	Common trade names
Salicylates				
Aspirin (OTC)	4-5 h	80-325 mg/d*		
Salsalate	3-4 d	1,500 mg BID	Edema	Disalcid®
Indoles				
Etodolac	1-2 h	400 mg TID		Lodine®
Indomethacin	3-5 d	25 mg TID	Psychosis	Indocin®
Sulindac	2-5 d	200 mg BID	Diarrhea	Clinoril®
Tolmetin	3-7 d	200-600 mg TID		Tolectin®
Proprionic acid				
Ibuprofen (OTC)	30 min-24 h	400-800 mg QID		Motrin®, Advil®
Naproxen (OTC)	2 h-2 d	500 mg BID	Headache	Anaprox®, Naprelan®, Naprosyn®
Ketoprofen (OTC)	6 h	100 mg TID	Tinnitus	Orudis®
Enolic acid				
Piroxicam	1 month	20 mg QD	Edema	Feldene®

*Typical dose used to prevent stroke and heart attacks: QD = one time daily; BID = two times daily; TID = three times daily; QID = four times daily.

Terms and Definitions

analgesic—An agent that reduces pain without causing loss of consciousness.

antiplatelet—A substance that inhibits action of platelets in the blood and hence inhibits clotting.

antipyretic—An agent that relieves or reduces fever.

cyclooxygenase-1 (COX-1)—An important enzyme present in most human tissues; responsible for converting arachidonic acid to terminal prostaglandins, the hormones that promote the inflammatory process. COX-1 is involved in many other physiologic autoregulation processes.

cyclooxygenase-2 (COX-2)—Same function as COX-1 and present in smaller amounts in tissues. It is only responsible for inflammation, but its role in the inflammatory process is larger than that of COX-1.

nonsteroidal anti-inflammatory drug (NSAID)—Any medication that blocks inflammation and is not chemically related to a corticosteroid (e.g., ibuprofen).

therapeutic index—A measure of the margin of safety of a drug. It is sometimes defined as the TD50/ED50, where TD50 is the dose of a drug that produces a toxic endpoint in 50% of the population and the ED50 is the dose of a drug that produces a therapeutic endpoint in 50% of the population. A high therapeutic index means that serious side effects are unlikely even at high doses.

Salicyclates such as aspirin, salsalate (brand name Disalcid), and diflunisal (brand name Dolobid®) are not used as commonly as some other drugs because they can inhibit platelet aggregation (i.e., increase bleeding) and precipitate bronchospasms (severely in some individuals).

Indoles include indomethacin (brand name Indocin), sulindac (brand name Clinoril), and tolmetin (brand name Tolectin). Indomethacin, which is sometimes thought to prevent myositis ossificans (calcium deposits at an injured area), is a potent inhibitor of cyclooxygenase and is frequently associated with gastrointestinal and renal side effects.

The most commonly used and safest of the over-the-counter NSAIDs are the propionic acid derivatives such as ibuprofen (brand names Motrin, Advil), naproxen (brand names Naprosyn, Aleve®), and ketoprofen (brand names Orudis, Oruvail®). Although these medications are usually well tolerated, athletes should be aware of their potential side effects.

THERAPEUTIC EFFECTS

A host of placebo-controlled studies have shown that NSAIDs significantly alleviate postoperative pain and pain associated with musculoskeletal injury. Although these drugs are commonly used to treat swelling and inflammation, research in these areas has been limited by the subjective measures of improvement. Many people use these medications in attempts to prevent delayed-onset muscle soreness and damage associated with conditioning. Research studies have demonstrated improvement in early decreased pain, early improved motion, and earlier return to activity. The benefits of most NSAIDs are thought to be secondary to early pain control, which leads to the ability to regain motion earlier and earlier starting of physiotherapy. The benefits in most injuries are unrelated to their anti-inflammatory properties.

Remind athletes who feel they must take NSAIDs that, as is true with most pain medications, these drugs work much better if they are taken at the first sign of pain or swelling. Athletes who take their NSAID as prescribed will have much greater success in quelling inflammation and pain than if they simply take a dose or two of medication when they can no longer stand the pain. On the other hand, some physicians prefer that injured athletes wait 2 or 3 d before taking NSAIDs to permit the body to take advantage of the natural healing processes inherent in swelling and inflammation and production of scar tissue. Acetaminophen, an over-the-counter nonsteroidal pain reliever, can be recommended for pain relief in these situations because it has no anti-inflammatory properties and therefore has no risk of impairing the healing process. In addition, as athletes get older and suffer from degenerative joint disease and require more chronic pain therapy, acetaminophen should be the pain reliever of first choice because of its better side-effect profile with chronic use.

Although selective COX-2 inhibitors can produce the same side effects as standard NSAIDs, the incidence of those side effects is much lower than with standard NSAIDs. These agents are generally used in patients with a history of peptic ulcer disease, renal disease, or platelet dysfunction, *whether or not* such problems are associated with use of traditional NSAIDs. The very high cost of COX-2 inhibitors currently limits widespread use of these medications.

SIDE EFFECTS

Most side effects related to the use of NSAIDs are quite rare. However, athletes sometimes take a higher-than-recommended dose (believing that "more is better") without supervision and may be predisposed to increasing their risk of side effects.

Dyspepsia, or indigestion, is the most frequently reported side effect from commonly used NSAIDs. Although the abdominal pain related to NSAID use usually stems from altered prostaglandin synthesis in the stomach lining and may not be alleviated with food, it is generally recommended that people take NSAIDs with food rather than on an empty stomach. A more serious but rare gastrointestinal side effect associated with NSAIDs is peptic ulcer disease—and, even more seriously, perforation of the stomach lining or massive gastrointestinal bleeding. Peptic ulcer disease usually causes more severe pain than does dyspepsia, and it may be associated with a change in stool color (from brown to black) resulting from the presence of oxidized blood. Although current research has identified no clear safety procedures to ameliorate gastrointestinal side effects, one study of patients at risk for peptic ulcer disease found that antacids used in conjunction with NSAIDs lessened the side effects. Risk factors for ulcer disease related to NSAID use include age >60 yr, previous history of ulcers, concomitant use of other NSAIDs, and higher NSAID dosing. Another consideration involved in who may be at risk includes duration of therapy, with one meta-analysis suggesting that shorter duration of use increases the risk more than longer duration of use (Gabriel et al. 1991).

The other major, if infrequent, problem of NSAIDs stems from their effects on the kidneys. Prostaglandins enhance renal blood flow and kidney filtration. Because NSAIDs may significantly inhibit these functions of prostaglandins, on rare occasions their use leads to acute renal failure, electrolyte abnormalities, generalized swelling (edema), and hypertension. In fact, any athlete who takes NSAIDs regularly for more than 6 months should be screened for early signs of kidney pathology. Dehydration (often a problem in athletes) may exacerbate the renal effects. People at risk for renal side effects include athletes with preexisting renal disease and individuals with hypertension.

Dermatologic reactions, including increased sensitivity to sunlight (photosensitivity), are quite common but are usually not serious. Athletes may find that they sunburn more easily when taking an NSAID.

Allergies to NSAIDs are not uncommon, the most frequent symptom being shortness of breath. Asthmatics are more prone to exhibit severe allergic reactions to NSAIDs—and serious allergy to one such drug is likely to indicate allergies to other NSAIDs as well. Athletes with asthma should avoid NSAIDs if possible, although most will be able to take an NSAID safely.

Most people are aware now that use of aspirin or other salicylates (e.g., salsalate) increases the chances that children or teens who have chicken pox or influenza will develop Reye's syndrome. Therefore, aspirin is not recommended as an antipyretic for children or adolescents who are suffering from a febrile illness.

Because NSAIDs tend to inhibit blood clotting, athletes should avoid their use as appropriate—for instance, athletes prone to nosebleeds or those who for various reasons may have reduced clotting mechanisms. With COX-2 inhibitors having less effect on bleeding problems, their use is recommended for athletes with postoperative pain or dental pain where bleeding may be of concern. Acetaminophen would also be recommended for these situations.

DRUG INTERACTIONS

You are most likely to see drug interactions in older athletes, in that young people rarely take the medications mentioned in this section. Because NSAIDs may reduce blood flow to the kidneys, they sometimes interfere with the action of diuretics. They also can decrease the elimination of lithium (brand names Carbolith®, Duralith®, Eskalith®) and methotrexate (brand names Amethopetrin®, Folex®, Rheumatrex®). NSAIDs do not interact with alcohol (or vice versa); it is safe to drink in moderation while taking NSAIDs.

NSAIDs sometimes increase blood pressure in patients with hypertension. NSAIDs interfere with and diminish the antihypertensive effects of diuretics, beta-

For Further Information

Print Resources

Brooks, P.M., and R.O. Day. 1991. Nonsteroidal antiinflammatory drugs—differences and similarities. *New England Journal of Medicine* 324(24): 1716-25.

Reents, S. 2000. *Sport and exercise pharmacology.* Champaign, IL: Human Kinetics. Discusses how commonly used medications can affect performance.

Tseng, C.C., and M.M. Wolfe. 2000. Nonsteroidal anti-inflammatory drugs. *Medical Clinics of North America* 84(5): 1329-44.

Web Resources

National Library of Medicine/National Institutes of Health
www.nlm.nih.gov/medlineplus/
A searchable Web site maintained by the National Library of Medicine and National Institutes of Health. Offers significant information on NSAIDs.

National Institute of Diabetes, Digestive and Kidney Disease
www.niddk.nih.gov/health/digest/summary/nsaids/
Information from the National Institute of Diabetes, Digestive and Kidney Disease (NIDDK), a division of the National Institutes of Health, regarding NSAIDs and peptic ulcers.

Arthritis Foundation
www.arthritis.org/conditions/drugguide/gutcheck.asp
A patient information article describing how to avoid stomach-related problems with NSAIDS.
www.arthritis.org/conditions/drugguide/chart_nsaids.asp
An extensive guide to the names, dosage, uses, and precautions associated with several classes of anti-inflammatory medication.

adrenergic receptor antagonists (beta-blockers), and angiotensin-converting enzyme (ACE) inhibitors. Be sure that athletes who take drugs to treat high blood pressure are aware that NSAIDs may counter the effect of their medications; urge them to have a physician monitor the interactions of the hypertension medications and NSAIDs.

The anticlotting effect of some NSAIDs can be a major problem. As it is estimated that 16,000 Americans die each year of NSAID-related gastrointestinal bleeding (Singh and Triadafilopoulos 1999), it is vitally important that people know when they should *not* take such medications. Anyone who takes Coumadin or any other blood thinner should avoid NSAIDs unless the drugs are prescribed by a physician and the reactions carefully monitored. Aspirin is unique among NSAIDs in that its anticlotting effects last for several days, compared to only a few hours with most other NSAIDs. This effect, however, is quite positive for some people: The now-common practice of taking an aspirin every other day has probably saved many thousands of lives of older people who otherwise may have suffered a stroke or a heart attack caused by clogged arteries.

SUMMARY

1. *Explain the mechanism of action for nonsteroidal anti-inflammatory drugs (NSAIDs).*

The major mechanism of action of most NSAIDs is inhibition of cyclooxygenase, an important enzyme responsible for the synthesis of prostaglandins from arachidonic acid. Prostaglandins are chiefly responsible for the inflammatory response, and they produce pain. There are two forms of cyclooxygenase: cyclooxygenase-1 (COX-1) and cyclooxygenase-2 (COX-2). Both enzymes promote inflammation and fever, and both produce pain. COX-1, however, is also responsible for protecting the mucosa of the stomach, enhancing blood flow to the kidneys, and inhibiting platelets. Although traditional NSAIDs (such as aspirin and ibuprofen) inhibit both enzymes, it is preferable to inhibit only the action of cyclooxygenase-2 (COX-2) while permitting COX-1 to function normally.

2. *Describe the therapeutic effects and side effects of NSAID use.*

NSAIDs significantly alleviate postoperative pain and pain associated with musculoskeletal injury. Although these drugs are commonly used to treat swelling and inflammation, research in these areas has been limited by the subjective measures of improvement. Many people use these medications in attempts to prevent delayed-onset muscle soreness and damage associated with conditioning. Research studies have demonstrated improvement in early decreased pain, early improved motion, and earlier return to activity. The benefits of most NSAIDs are thought to be secondary to early pain control, which leads to the ability to regain motion earlier and earlier starting of physiotherapy.

Dyspepsia, or indigestion, is the most frequently reported side effect from NSAID use. Although the pain usually stems from altered prostaglandin synthesis in the stomach lining and may not be alleviated with food, it is generally recommended that people take NSAIDs with food rather than on an empty stomach. Peptic ulcer disease is a more serious but rare gastrointestinal side effect associated with NSAID use. Even more serious is potential perforation of the stomach lining or massive gastrointestinal bleeding. Though current research has identified no clear safety procedures to ameliorate gastrointestinal side effects, one study of patients at risk for peptic ulcer disease found that antacids used in conjunction with NSAIDs lessened the side effects. COX-2 inhibitors can produce the same side effects as standard NSAIDs; however, the incidence of those side effects is much lower than with standard NSAIDs.

Less-frequent side effects are seen in the kidney and associated with prostaglandins' role of enhancing renal blood flow and kidney filtration. Because NSAIDs may significantly inhibit these functions of prostaglandins, on rare occasions their use leads to acute renal failure, electrolyte abnormalities, generalized swelling (edema), and hypertension. Dehydration (often a problem in athletes) may exacerbate the renal effects.

3. *Identify possible drug interactions associated with NSAIDs.*

As with all medications, patients must be aware of possible drug interactions associated with NSAID use. Most of the potential medications for interaction are more common to older physically active individuals as opposed to younger athletes. NSAIDS may interfere with the effectiveness of diuretics and hypertensive medications. Patients taking these medications need to review carefully potential NSAID side effects with their physician. Any patient who takes NSAIDs regularly for more than 6 months should be screened for early signs of kidney pathology.

CHAPTER 14

Drugs, Supplements, and the Athlete

OBJECTIVES

Upon completion of this chapter the reader will be able to do the following:

1. Identify various drugs and supplements as performance-enhancing (ergogenic), restorative, or recreational

2. Access current U.S. Olympic Committee and National Collegiate Athletic Association (NCAA) information on which drugs and substances are banned

3. Recognize the side effects and potential dangers of using anabolic steroids and human growth hormone

4. Identify the signs of drug dependence and the risks associated with alcohol abuse

5. Explain current regulatory issues surrounding herbal supplements

6. Recognize the potential dangers of using herbal supplements

Some of the most important advances in medicine have occurred with the discovery of new drugs to treat diseases. Some of these drugs not only treat disease but may also be used to enhance performance. Some may impair performance. Because of the publicity surrounding athletes who get into trouble with alcohol or street drugs, some people incorrectly think of the issue of drugs in sports in only these terms.

Performance-enhancing drugs such as anabolic steroids, growth hormone, and erythropoietin are used more frequently by athletes than nonathletes, but athletes use recreational drugs such as alcohol, marijuana, and cocaine at about the same rate as does the general population. Most drugs used to enhance performance not only provide an unfair advantage in competition, but their side effects can range in seriousness from mere annoyance to death. Athletes who are becoming dependent on alcohol or another drug usually exhibit social or physical problems in addition to declining athletic performance. In addition, in an effort to boost performance with herbal supplements—which most people assume are safe—some athletes have caused serious permanent damage to their health, or have even died. This chapter discusses these complex issues with an emphasis on how drugs affect athletic performance.

Case Study

A very muscular 17-yr-old lineman arrives at football camp, having gained 25 lb (11.4 kg) over the summer. His face looks puffy and his acne has become much worse since you saw him last spring. When you ask about his workouts this summer, he reports great gains in all of his strength tests. He says he feels great. You heard he got in a fight this summer and was arrested. A teammate has confided in you that the athlete is isolating himself and is a "maniac" in the weight room.

Because you suspect use of anabolic-androgenic steroids, you arrange to visit with this young man on a couple of occasions on unrelated issues. During a recent private meeting with him, you tell him that people are concerned about him—and, promising strict confidentiality, you ask if he has been using anabolic steroids. He admits to use and says he is trying to quit for the season but that he can't stand the depression when he stops. He says he has not used any needles to inject drugs. He reluctantly agrees to talk to a physician who is a specialist in addiction and to start an antidepressant medication. You also refer him to a dietitian, who can help him maintain his weight and strength as much as possible while he is stopping his steroids.

OVERVIEW

Although some substances fit into more than one group, drugs are often separated into three categories as they relate to sports:

■ Drugs that are used to potentially improve athletic performance are called performance-enhancing, or **ergogenic,** drugs. Though anabolic-androgenic steroids are probably the most publicized performance-enhancing drugs, a long list of other substances potentially fit into that category as well. The intent of the use is unclear in some cases, and some people use drugs not just to enhance performance but also to provide a "high." For example, amphetamines provide a high and also can increase endurance.

■ Restorative drugs are used to treat injuries or illnesses and are not very controversial. They are called restorative because they are intended to restore sick athletes to a healthier state. The only group in this category that is occasionally controversial is the analgesics; since they block pain, they can be overused or

Terms and Definitions

acromegaly—Abnormal enlargement of the jaw, nose, fingers, and toes.

anabolic—Stimulating the biosynthesis of tissue.

anabolic steroids—Name for synthetic derivative of male sex hormone, testosterone.

androgenic—Causing masculine characteristics.

dehydroepiandrosterone (DHEA)—A steroid compound synthesized from cholesterol and with mild androgenic properties. In the body, it is converted to testosterone, a more potent androgen.

doping—Use of performance-enhancing drugs.

ergogenic—Any substance taken or used for the purpose of improving performance.

erythropoietin—Hormone that stimulates the bone marrow to make more red blood cells; high-altitude exercise leads to greater synthesis of erythropoietin in the kidneys.

gigantism—Excessive growth in the long bones as well as in specific body parts.

gynecomastia—Development of breast tissue in males.

high-density lipoprotein (HDL)—The so-called "good" cholesterol.

hirsutism—Excessive hairiness; in women, it usually manifests as an adult male pattern of hair distribution.

tetrahydrocannabinol (THC)—The primary active ingredient in marijuana.

U.S. Anti-Doping Agency (USADA)—Organization dedicated to the elimination of doping in sport.

abused. For example, both short- and long-acting local anesthetics (e.g., lidocaine and bupivacaine) can block pain sufficiently that athletes might compete whose injuries should prevent them from doing so.

■ Recreational drugs alter moods and are usually used to provide a high or euphoria. This group includes alcohol, marijuana, amphetamines, cocaine, hallucinogens, and many others. Athletes appear to use recreational drugs at about the same frequency as the general population.

Most of the athletic community's interest in drugs has revolved around use of performance-enhancing substances. Olympic athletes began using stimulants in the 1950s, and these drugs appeared responsible for deaths of several cyclists a few years later. From the 1960s to the present, many male and female athletes have used anabolic steroids. The deaths that occurred from stimulant abuse led to the interest in drug testing and the desire to prevent use of ergogenic drugs. Because of widespread abuse of other types of drugs, such as depressants and hallucinogens, sports' governing agencies also are proactive in banning substances that have no positive effect on performance. The purposes behind such regulations often stem from athletes' roles as character models within our society, and from the desire to raise the general level of behavior and ethics among all athletes as well as those who look up to athletes.

ERGOGENIC DRUGS

In international competition, use of performance-enhancing drugs is called **doping.** The International Olympic Committee (IOC) defines doping as "the administration of or use by a competing athlete of any substance foreign to the body or any physiologic substance taken in abnormal quantity or taken by an abnormal route of entry into the body with the sole intention of increasing in an artificial and unfair manner his or her performance in competition. When necessity demands medical treatment with any substance which, because of its nature, dosage, or application, is able to boost the athlete's performance in competition in an artificial and unfair manner, this too is regarded as doping" (Voy and Deeter 1991, p. 5). The list of drugs whose use is considered to be doping at the international level is extensive. Note that other governing bodies use lists different from that of the IOC. Many drugs are controversial; usage that is considered doping in one sport may not be in another. Some venues also ban the social or personal use of illicit drugs. The decision to ban a drug is sometimes made on the basis of politics rather than science.

Some prohibitions are difficult to enforce: Some of the newer substances are difficult to detect by traditional drug-testing methods, and the use of growth hormone or any other injectable protein is virtually impossible to detect by current methods. The IOC discourages use of alcohol and marijuana but does not require testing for those drugs. On the other hand, the National Collegiate Athletic Association (NCAA) bans marijuana use and assays for it during standard tests. It is very important that athletes and those who work with athletes remain current on which organizations ban which drugs, to ensure that athletes do not inadvertently ingest a banned substance (see chapter 15). Many lists of banned substances appear on the World Wide Web, and many organizations have toll-free numbers for athletes to call with questions about medications. For a list of the substances currently banned by the NCAA, along with details of its rules about drug use, check its Web site at www.ncaa.org/sports_sciences/drugtesting/banned_list.html.

Figure 14.1 lists drugs banned by the International Olympic Committee as of mid-2000. The **U.S. Anti-Doping Agency (USADA)** manages testing and adjudication for athletes involved in U.S. Olympic, Pan American, and Paralympic competitions. Check its Web site for the most up-to-date information on substances banned by the International Olympic Committee: www.usantidoping.org/prohibited_sub/list.asp.

Anabolic Drugs

Anabolic drugs are used in sport to increase muscle mass, strength, and speed. Although anabolic steroids have been extensively used and studied, other substances such as DHEA and androstenedione are also commonly used and will be discussed in this chapter.

Anabolic Steroids

Anabolic steroids are probably more appropriately called anabolic-androgenic steroids because all the substances in this category are both **anabolic** (they stimulate the building of tissue) and **androgenic** (they are masculinizing). Examples are two popular oral supplements, androstenedione and dehydroepiandrosterone (DHEA). Athletes take these steroids, either by mouth or by injection, for their anabolic effects. A popular practice known as stacking entails simultaneous use of two or more steroids and may include both oral and injected steroids. This method has no scientific basis, and its benefits to an athlete are little more than urban legend.

Potential Benefits   The most recent research shows that anabolic steroids improve strength and muscle mass. Along with a proper diet (including an adequate amount of protein) and an intense strength-training program, steroids can increase an athlete's lean body mass as well as strength. Anabolic steroids also have psychological effects, leading those who take them to become more aggressive—a clearly desirable effect in a few sports but quite undesirable in most contexts. There is tremendous individual variability in the effects of anabolic steroids.

Damaging Side Effects   Anabolic steroids exhibit a long list of adverse effects (table 14.1). They can produce unacceptable levels of aggressiveness, both on and off the

I. Prohibited classes of substances

A. Stimulants

Examples of prohibited substances:

Amineptine, amiphenazole, amphetamines, bromantan, caffeine (concentration in urine >12 μg/ml), carphedon, cocaine, ephedrines (>5 μg/ml for cathine, >10 μg/ml for ephedrine and methylphedrine, >25 μg/ml for phenyl propanolamine and pseudoephedrine), fencamfamin, mesocarb, pentetrazol, pipradrol, salbutamol, salmeterol, terbutaline (last three permitted only if taken via inhaler by asthmatic athlete with written notification from physcian), and related substances.

Note: All imidazole preparations are acceptable for topical use. Vasoconstrictors may be administered with local anesthetic agents. Topical preparations (e.g., nasal, ophthalmological, rectal) of adrenaline and phenylephrine are permitted.

B. Narcotics

Examples of prohibited substances:

Buprenorphine, dextromoramide, diamorphine (heroin), methadone, morphine, pentazocine, pethidine, and related substances.

Note: Codeine, dextromethorphan, dextropropoxyphene, dihydrocodeine, diphenoxylate, ethylmorphine, pholcodine, propoxyphene, and tramadol are permitted.

C. Anabolic agents

Examples of prohibited substances:

1. Anabolic androgenic steroids

   a. Clostebol, fluoxymesterone, metandienone, metenolone, nandrolone, 19-norandrostenediol, 19-norandrostenedione, oxandrolone, stanozolol, and related substances.

   b. Androstenediol, androstenedione, dehydroepiandrosterone (DHEA), dihydrotestosterone, testosterone,* and related substances.

   Evidence obtained from metabolic profiles and/or isotopic ratio measurements may be used to draw definitive conclusions.

   *Testosterone (T) to epitestosterone (E) ratio >6:1 in the urine constitutes an offense unless there is evidence that this ratio is due to a physiological or pathological condition—e.g., low epitestosterone excretion, androgen-producing tumor, or enzyme deficiencies. In the case of T:E > 6, it is mandatory that the relevant medical authority conducts an investigation before the sample is declared positive. A full report will be written and will include a review of previous tests, subsequent tests, and any results of endocrine investigations. If previous tests are not available, the athlete should be tested unannounced at least once per month for three months. The results of these investigations should be included in the report. Failure to cooperate in the investigations will result in declaring the sample positive.

2. Beta-2 agonists

   Bambuterol, clenbuterol, fenoterol, formoterol, reproterol, salbutamol (urine concentration >1 μg/ml is considered a positive), salmeterol, terbutaline (the last three are acceptable only if by inhalation), and related substances.

D. Diuretics

Examples of prohibited substances:

Acetazolamide, bumetanide, chlortalidone, etacrynic acid, furosemide, hydrochlorothiazide, mannitol (prohibited by intravenous injection), mersalyl, spironolactone, triamterene, and related substances.

E. Peptide hormones, mimetics, and analogs

Prohibited substances include the following examples and their analogs and mimetics, as well as their releasing factors and analogs of the releasing factors:

Chorionic gonadotrophin (hCG) prohibited in males only, pituitary and synthetic gonadotrophins (LH) prohibited in males only, corticotrophins (ACTH, tetracosactide), growth hormone (hGH), insulin-like growth factor (IGF-1), erythropoietin (EPO). Insulin is permitted only to treat athletes with certified insulin-dependent diabetes. The presence of an abnormal concentration of an endogenous hormone in class E or its diagnostic marker(s) in the urine, constitutes an offense unless it has been proven to be due to a physiological or pathological condition.

(continued)

■ **Figure 14.1** Drugs banned by the International Olympic Committee as of mid-2000.

Adapted from USADA, 2003. Available: www.usantidoping.org.

II. Prohibited methods

The following procedures are prohibited:

Blood doping; administering artificial oxygen carriers or plasma expanders; pharmacological, chemical, and physical manipulation.

Classes of prohibited substances in certain circumstances:

A. Alcohol

Where the rules of a responsible authority so provide, tests will be conducted for ethanol.

B. Cannabinoids

Where the rules of a responsible authority so provide, tests will be conducted for cannabinoids (e.g., marijuana, hashish). At the Olympic Games, tests will be conducted for cannabinoids. THC concentration in urine >15 μg/ml constitutes doping.

C. Local anesthetics

Injectable local anesthetics are permitted under the following conditions:

a. Bupivacaine, lidocaine, mepivacaine, procaine, and related substances can be used, but not cocaine. Vasoconstrictor agents may be used in conjunction with local anesthetics.

b. Only local or intra-articular injections may be administered.

c. Only when medically justified.

Where the rules of a responsible authority so provide, notification of administration may be necessary.

D. Glucocorticosteroids

The systemic use of glucocorticosteroids is prohibited when administered orally, rectally, or by intravenous or intramuscular injection.

E. Beta-blockers

Examples of prohibited substances:

Acebutolol, alprenolol, atenolol, labetalol, metoprolol, nadolol, oxprenolol, propranolol, sotalol, and related substances.

Where the rules of a responsible authority so provide, tests will be conducted for beta-blockers.

IV. Out-of-competition testing

Unless specifically requested by the responsible authority, out-of-competition testing is directed solely at prohibited substances in class IC (anabolic agents), ID (diuretics), IE (peptide hormones, mimetics, and analogs), and II (prohibited methods).

Examples of prohibited substances:

Note: This is not an exhaustive list of prohibited substances. Many substances that do not appear on this list are considered prohibited under the term "and related substances." Athletes must ensure that any medicine, supplement, over-the-counter preparation, or any other substance they use does not contain any prohibited substance.

A. Stimulants

Amineptine, amfepramone, amiphenazole, amphetamine, bambuterol, bramantan, caffeine, carphedon, cathine, cocaine, cropropamide, crotethamide, ephedrine, etamivan, etilamphetamine, etilefrine, fencamfamin, fenetylline, fenfluramine, formoterol, heptaminol, mefenorex, mephentermine, mesocarb, methamphetamine, methoxyphenamine, methylenedioxyamphetamine, methylephedrine, methylphenidate, nikethamide, norfenfluramine, parahydroxyamphetamine, pemoline, pentetrazol, phendimetrazine, phentermine, phenylephrine, phenylpropanolamine, pholedrine, pipradrol, prolintane, propylhexedrine, pseudoephedrine, reproterol, salbutamol, salmeterol, selegiline, strychnine, terbutaline.

B. Narcotics

Buprenorphine, dextromoramide, diamorphine (heroin), hydrocodone, methadone, morphine, pentazocine, pethidine.

C. Anabolic agents

Androstenediol, androstenedione, bambuterol, boldenone, clenbuterol, clostebol, danazol, dehydrochlormethyltestosterone, dehydroepiandrosterone (DHEA), dihydrotestosterone, drostanolone, fenoterol, fluoxymesterone, formebolone, formoterol, gestrinone, mesterolone, metandienone, metenolone, methandriol, methyltestosterone, mibolerone, nandrolone, 19-norandrostenediol, 19-norandrostenedione, norethandrolone, oxandrolone, oxymesterone, oxymetholone, reproterol, salbutamol, salmeterol, stanozolol, terbualine, testosterone, trenbolone.

■ **Figure 14.1** *(continued)*

D. Diuretics

Acetazolamide, bendroflumethiazide, bumetanide, canrenone, chlortalidone, ethacrynic acid, furosemide, hydrochlorothiazide, indapamide, mannitol (by intravenous injection), mersalyl, spironolactone, triamterene.

E. Masking agents

Bromantan, diuretics (see above), epitestosterone, probenecid.

F. Peptide hormones, mimetics, and analogs.

ACTH, erythropoietin (EPO), hCG (prohibited in males only), hGH, insulin, LH (prohibited in males only), clomiphene (prohibited in males only), cyclofenil (prohibited in males only), tamoxifen (prohibited in males only).

G. Beta-blockers

Acebutolol, alprenolol, atenolol, betaxolol, bisoprolol, bunolol, carteolol, celiprolol, esmolol, labetalol, levobunolol, metipranolol, metoprolol, nadolol, oxprenolol, pindolol, propranolol, sotalol, timolol.

■ **Figure 14.1** *(continued)*

playing field. They can be toxic to the liver, causing damage to liver cells as well as blockage of bile (cholestasis), and are associated with a variety of liver tumors, including cancer. Anabolic steroids are associated with permanent pattern baldness in both men and women who are genetically susceptible. They can greatly worsen acne in susceptible people and increase hair growth, especially in females. In the adolescent who may still be growing, they can cause premature cessation of bone growth. During use, anabolic steroids cause fluid retention that can create swelling (edema) of the skin and soft tissue, especially in the face. Some of the most profound side effects occur in the reproductive system. Males who take anabolic steroids experience shrinkage of their testicles and are temporarily sterile because of a low sperm count. These compounds stimulate the prostate gland, which becomes enlarged; sometimes the enlargement obstructs the urinary tract, causing difficulty urinating. Anabolic steroids are also associated with cancer of the prostate and (rarely) of the kidney. In some males, estrogenic metabolites of anabolic steroids produce breast tissue (a condition called **gynecomastia**) that does not subside with disuse.

When withdrawing from use of anabolic steroids, some males become impotent. In females, the permanent side effects can be quite dramatic. Females who use anabolic steroids can be masculinized—they develop a deep voice and excessive body hair **(hirsutism),** as well as an enlarged clitoris. Anabolic steroids usually disrupt the menstrual cycle and make a woman temporarily infertile.

Anabolic steroids have significant adverse effects on the cardiovascular system, increasing total serum cholesterol and profoundly lowering levels of **high-density lipoproteins (HDLs),** the "good" cholesterol. These changes may make a person more susceptible to hardening of the arteries. Anabolic steroids also increase blood pressure, probably because of their propensity to cause fluid retention. Their use can lead to mood swings, and even to hallucinations and psychosis. One of the most profound side effects is depression, which occurs during withdrawal from use. Evidence is increasing, moreover, that anabolic steroids have a significant addictive potential.

No hard data are available concerning the frequency of side effects. In general, most of the mild side effects are common, whereas the more severe and life-threatening effects are rare. In males, the side effects appear reversible except for male pattern baldness, tumors, and gynecomastia. In females, pattern baldness, tumors, and the masculinizing effects are permanent. Most sports' governing bodies ban use of anabolic steroids.

Dehydroepiandrosterone (DHEA)

Dehydroepiandrosterone (DHEA) is a precursor to both estrogen and testosterone—in the latter case, the body converts DHEA to androstenedione, which is

Table 14.1   Ergogenic Aids, Uses, and Potential Side Effects

Drug/Supplement	Ergogenic use	Potential side effects

Anabolic-androgenic steroids
  Dehydroepiandrosterone
  (DHEA)*
  Androstenedione (andro)
	Improve strength and muscle mass	General changes
		  Unacceptable levels of aggression
		  Liver toxicity
		  Liver tumors, including cancer
		  Male pattern baldness (men and women)
		  Hirsutism in women (increased hair growth)
		  Deepening of the voice in women
		  Fluid retention (general edema)
		  Premature cessation of bone growth in
		    adolescents
		  Gynecomastia (breast tissue development in
		    males)
		Psychological changes
		  Mood swings
		  Psychosis
		  Depression with withdrawal
		  Increasing evidence of addictive nature of
		    steroids
		Reproductive changes
		  Shrinkage of testicles in men
		  Low sperm count in men
		  Possible cancers of the prostate and
		    kidneys
		  Enlargement of the prostate
		  Enlargement of the clitoris in women
		  Disruption of the menstrual cycle
		  Temporary infertility
		Cardiovascular changes
		  Elevated blood pressure with fluid retention
		  Elevated cholesterol with decrease of HDL
		    (good cholesterol)
		  Possible elevated susceptibility to
		    arteriosclerosis

Human growth hormone
  (HGH)
	Improves strength and muscle mass	Gigantism and acromegaly
		May cause weakness of proximal muscle
		  groups
		Associated with damage to cardiac muscle
		Enlargement of organs (liver and spleen)
		Osteoporosis
		Sexual dysfunction
		Diabetes mellitus with prolonged use

Erythropoietin/Blood doping	Increases blood count by reintroduction of red blood cells or use of hormone (erythropoietin) to stimulate production of red blood cells Increases oxygen capacity of blood during endurance events	Heart attack Stroke (risk increases with dehydration) Increased blood pressure (can lead to heart failure and leakage of fluid into lungs)

Drug/Supplement	Ergogenic use	Potential side effects
Stimulants		
Amphetamines	Decrease a sense of fatigue	Appetite suppression Anxiousness Agitation Cardiac arrhythmia and failure Addiction Depression and fatigue with withdrawal
Cocaine	Greater recreational use than ergogenic; may be used for euphoria, to decrease sense of fatigue	Greater effect on mental processing than amphetamines Problematic purity Cardiac arrhythmia Anxiousness, insomnia, restlessness, and anxiety Toxic psychosis; hallucinations, paranoia, and delusions
Caffeine	Enhances performance in endurance events	Mild stimulant effect possible cardiac arrythmia Gastrointestinal upset (diarrhea, vomiting) Mild diuretic (increased risk of dehydration) Possibly elevated blood pressure Possible cardiac arrhythmia Headaches, drowsiness, irritability, and lethargy with withdrawal
Depressants		
Alcohol	Not a true ergogenic; athletes may use it to calm themselves before or after competition Social drug	Impaired reactions and judgment Reduced hand-eye coordination Impaired balance Diuretic effects (increasing risk of dehydration) Many side effects with chronic use: damage to heart muscle, damage to arteries, reduced sexual performance, damage to the liver, increased risk of stomach ulcers, and damage to parts of the brain Significant social implications: unwanted sexual contact, assaults, increased motor vehicle accidents, accidental death
Marijuana⁺	Not a true ergogenic; athletes may use it to calm themselves before or after competition Social drug	Potentially sedation or excitement Adverse effect on coordination Decreased blood pressure Decreased depth of breathing Altered perceptions Impaired depth perception Impaired memory with chronic use Amotivational syndrome
Beta-andrenergic blockers for endurance sport	Used to decrease heart and blood pressure Desirable in sports that require steady control, such as archery and shooting	Adverse effect for endurance sport

* = DHEA and androstenedione are precursors to the sex hormones estrogen and testosterone; many long-term risks have not been directly linked specifically to these substances. However, because both substances significantly increase the levels of testosterone and estrogen, it is safe to assume they would mimic the known potential effects of elevating these substances.

⁺ = Marijuana may have legitimate medicinal uses for the treatment of glaucoma and reducing the detrimental effects of chemotherapy.

Case Study

Since taking anabolic steroids as a college football player, Jeff had always noticed that he had breast tissue. As months and years passed, it seemed that the tissue was getting more prominent and more tender. At the age of 32, Jeff consulted a plastic surgeon to have the tissue removed. After a battle with his health-insurance company, which argued that this was cosmetic surgery, Jeff finally got insurance coverage for the surgery and had the tissue removed through small incisions under his nipples.

converted to testosterone. DHEA is itself a natural, mildly androgenic hormone produced in the adrenal glands; as a nutritional supplement, it is readily available in pharmacies and health food stores. Endogenous DHEA levels decline naturally with age.

Potential Benefits   Through supplementation, people can maintain or increase their DHEA levels to those of a younger person. A single 100-mg oral dose of DHEA can raise testosterone levels in the blood by over 300% within 1 h. Manufacturers even claim that DHEA can reverse the natural aging process: It is touted as a wonder drug to lengthen lives, prevent heart disease, melt fat, and stimulate libido. *Such claims are based on scant research data at best and often on no scientific data at all.* Several studies have suggested that DHEA supplements can lead to rapid growth of muscle fiber and significant gains in strength; a double-blind study (in which neither athletes nor researchers knew who was getting DHEA and who was taking a placebo), however, found no significant increases in body weight or lean mass in athletes who took 400 mg DHEA per day for 4 weeks (Welle et al. 1990).

Potential Damaging Side Effects   Because supplementary use of DHEA is a relatively recent phenomenon, scientists know little about long-term side effects. Because it is a precursor to the sex hormones, it is reasonable to assume that exogenous supplements may produce the same side effects as would ingestion of the pure anabolic sex hormones. At doses over 100 mg/d, estrogen can cause growth of breast tissue (gynecomastia) in men; and testosterone can cause growth of facial hair (hirsutism) in women. Raising testosterone levels can also produce much more dangerous side effects associated with the other anabolic steroids such as elevated levels of low-density lipoproteins (LDLs, or so-called "bad" cholesterol) and lowered levels of HDLs.

We believe you should discourage adolescents from using DHEA because of the potential for side effects (the substance is completely illegal in Australia). College-level athletes or athletes involved in international competition have an additional concern besides side effects: DHEA will cause a positive drug test for anabolic steroids and is banned by both the NCAA and the IOC (see table 14.2).

Androstenedione

Synthesized in the testes, ovaries, and in the adrenal cortex, androstenedione is a natural, immediate precursor to the sex hormones testosterone and estrone (a potent estrogen). Like DHEA, androstenedione is itself a mild androgen. And as with DHEA, few scientific studies support the numerous claims manufacturers make about the supplement. One recent study showed that 300 mg of androstenedione a day significantly boosted levels of serum testosterone—but it also increased serum estrogen levels in the young men who were subjects in the study. If estrogen rises, gynecomastia may be a common side effect in males who take this compound as a supplement. It is not clear whether the rise in serum testosterone is sustained long enough to make a difference in the weight room.

Table 14.2   Urinary Concentrations Requiring Report of Findings for Specific Substances*

Substance	Reportable concentrations
Caffeine	>12 µg/ml
Carboxy-THC	>15 µg/ml
Cathine	>5 µg/ml
Ephedrine	>10 µg/ml
Epitestosterone	>200 µg/ml
Methylephedrine	>10 µg/ml
Morphine	>1 µg/ml
19-norandrosterone in males	>2 µg/ml
19-norandrosterone in females	>5 µg/ml
Phenylpropanolamine	>25 µg/ml
Pseudoephedrine	>25 µg/ml
Salbutamol as stimulant	>100 µg/ml
Salbutamol as anabolic agent	>1,000 µg/ml
Testosterone/Epitestosterone ratio	>6

*For urinary concentrations of these substances above the levels shown here, the IOC requires laboratories to report their findings.

Reprinted from IOC, 2002. Available: http://multimedia.olympic.org/pdf/en_report_542.pdf.

Research data suggest that androstenedione lowers serum concentrations of high-density lipoproteins, putting individuals at risk of cardiovascular disease. Research has also linked high levels of androstenedione with cancer of the prostate and of the pancreas. As with DHEA, many other long-term risks are ambiguously linked specifically to this substance; but because androstenedione significantly increases testosterone and estrogen levels, it is tentatively safe to assume that potential side effects of androstenedione would parallel the known potential effects of elevated testosterone, estrogen, or both. In males, such side effects can include enlarged breasts, shrinkage of the testes, premature baldness, enlarged prostate, reduced sperm count, and increased aggression. In females, they can include menstrual irregularity, hirsutism, and general masculinization. For both males and females, potential side effects of elevated sex hormones include damage to the kidneys, the liver or both; cessation of long bone growth in adolescents; severe acne; and increased risk of cardiovascular disease.

Urge athletes to avoid this compound. If health warnings are not sufficient to persuade athletes to keep away from androstenedione, remind them that it is banned by the National Collegiate Athletic Association, the National Football League, and the International Olympic Committee.

Peptide Hormones

The two most common peptide hormones that are used by athletes to enhance performance are growth hormone and erythropoietin. Because these are virtually identical to the naturally occurring hormones, they are virtually undetectable by any drug test, including blood tests.

Human Growth Hormone

Although human growth hormone appears to affect the growth of nearly every organ and tissue in the body, its effects on strength and acquisition of body mass have not been well studied. Athletes use growth hormone for the same reasons they use anabolic steroids: Growth hormone is anabolic and helps build muscle, and may actually speed repair of injured tissue. It stimulates the mobilization of lipids from fat tissue and increases their use for energy. It also stimulates the synthesis of collagen, an important connective tissue protein. HGH is administered only by needle and is given subcutaneously or intramuscularly on a daily basis.

Because growth hormone affects all the organs in the body, it has significant adverse affects. When taken in excess, it produces all of the signs of **gigantism,** including **acromegaly** (enlargement of the nose, jaw, fingers, and toes). It may cause weakness in the proximal muscles (those that are closer to the body, such as in the thighs and upper arms). Exogenous growth hormone is associated with damage to the heart muscle. It tends to cause enlargement of several organs, including the liver and spleen. It can cause osteoporosis and is associated with sexual dysfunction. Prolonged use of growth hormone may lead to the development of diabetes mellitus. Although there is currently no assay to detect use of growth hormone by athletes, both the NCAA and the IOC forbid its use.

Erythropoietin and Blood Doping

The more red blood cells a person has available in the bloodstream, the more oxygen that can be carried to the muscle, and the longer the athlete can exercise. Increased blood count and hemoglobin have significantly enhanced performance in laboratory endurance tests. Blood doping is the use of exogenous red blood cells—either one's own or another person's—to boost the oxygen-carrying capacity of the blood. The standard procedure has been to have blood withdrawn well before a competition, spin it down to concentrate it, freeze it, and then to thaw and reintroduce the blood just before the event. But it's now possible to accomplish the same goal through use of **erythropoietin,** a natural hormone produced by the kidney and the primary stimulus to development of red blood cells in the bone marrow.

Erythropoietin is given by injection subcutaneously or intravenously to stimulate the bone marrow to produce more red blood cells. Now produced synthetically, it is used to treat people who are anemic; it is particularly helpful for patients whose kidneys are failing. Cyclists, long-distance runners, Nordic skiers, speed skaters, and other endurance athletes sometimes use erythropoietin or blood doping to improve endurance. Because they increase the thickness of the blood, however, too many red cells in the bloodstream can easily lead to a heart attack or stroke—particularly if the athlete becomes dehydrated, thereby thickening the blood even more. Increased blood count is also associated with hypertension, which boosts the heart's workload and can lead to heart failure and leakage of fluid in the lungs. Athletes receiving legitimate medical treatment with these interventions should therefore be monitored very carefully.

Erythropoietin is particularly dangerous in that it is a very potent stimulator of red blood cell production. Researchers are currently investigating ways to detect blood doping and use of erythropoietin. Lab assays can detect erythropoietin, but there is no way at this time to determine if the excess blood levels are natural or caused by exogenous sources.

Another way to increase the production of red blood cells is to train at high altitude, where lower oxygen levels stimulate the kidneys to produce more erythropoietin and therefore more red blood cells. This practice is controversial but is not banned by any group, whereas blood doping and use of erythropoietin are generally prohibited.

RECREATIONAL DRUGS

Sports' governing bodies ban many of these substances not necessarily because they convey an unfair advantage but simply because they are harmful, or because they are illegal, or because taking them sets an inappropriate example. Athletes, in general, do not use recreational drugs any more frequently than nonathletes. Some of the drugs that are used recreationally are also used to enhance performance and can be considered ergogenic.

Stimulants

Virtually any drug that is considered a stimulant has the potential for enhancing performance. Because they are considered "uppers," these drugs also have the potential for recreational use. The stimulants below are those most commonly used and include amphetamines, cocaine, caffeine, and nicotine.

■ Amphetamines are potent stimulants as well as appetite suppressants. They probably can enhance performance in selected events, as they appear to decrease the sense of fatigue while boosting energy level, ability to concentrate, and feelings of self-confidence; many athletes also believe that amphetamines improve reaction time. Chronic use can lead to a decrease in body fat, because these drugs are potent appetite suppressants. Amphetamines produce a variety of adverse effects. They can make a person anxious, distractible, and agitated. Some users become quite paranoid, and a few experience hallucinations. The stimulant effect of these drugs can affect heart rhythm sufficiently to cause the heart to stop. Amphetamines make a person more likely to become hyperthermic as a result of constriction of the blood vessels in the skin. And they can be addicting. Fatigue and depression are common problems after people stop using them.

■ Cocaine is an old drug that has gained new popularity. It is used in medicine as an excellent local anesthetic for the nose and respiratory tract; it also prevents swelling and bleeding of these tissues because of its properties as a vasoconstrictor. It is a stimulant of the brain, heart, and lungs. It produces an intense euphoric feeling that leads to abuse and is thought to be one of the most addictive drugs known. People ingest it by sniffing the powder through the nose or by smoking it—or, after dissolving it in a liquid, injecting it into a vein. Even though an athlete might believe he can perform better under the influence of cocaine, it is more likely that performance will be impaired. Although it has some of the same effects as amphetamines, cocaine is very short-acting (20-30 min) and affects mental processing more than amphetamines. The user is likely to experience accelerated mental processes, euphoria, feelings of increased mental and physical power, and paranoia. Because the purity of cocaine on the street varies, overdoses are common, causing heart rhythm disturbances, coma, seizures, hyperthermia, and death. Cocaine causes the blood vessels to constrict (narrow); as a result it can cause a heart attack in a very young person. Chronic use of cocaine may result in tremulousness, agitation, restlessness, insomnia, and anxiety. A toxic psychosis associated with cocaine is characterized by hallucinations, paranoia, and delusions.

■ Caffeine can enhance performance in endurance events via two mechanisms: At the tissue level, it enhances utilization of fatty acids (a source of energy) during activity, thereby sparing muscle glycogen (the storage form of sugar); and it increases skeletal muscle contractility, thereby increasing endurance. Because caffeine is a mild stimulant, it decreases the perception of fatigue. Adverse effects include gastrointestinal upset, including vomiting or diarrhea. As a mild diuretic, caffeine can be a problem in distance events, resulting not only in more trips to the bathroom but also in dehydration. Caffeine also can cause heart rhythm problems and may raise blood pressure. Withdrawal from caffeine use can cause headache, drowsiness, irritability, lethargy, and nervousness.

■ Nicotine is a stimulant of the sympathetic and parasympathetic nervous systems. It increases heart rate, blood pressure, and intestinal muscular activity and leads to increased production of saliva, bronchial mucus, and sweat. Because it stimulates the satiety center in the brain, people who stop using nicotine often gain weight. *Despite their subjective feelings of being calmed or more relaxed, people who use nicotine are actually stimulating nearly every system in the body.* Research has not shown any improvement in performance with use of nicotine and occasionally shows diminished performance. Although most such studies have focused on smoking, more recent research on chewing tobacco has led to similar findings. The adverse effects of smoking are well known and include emphysema, lung cancer, and an increased risk of hardening of the arteries. Use of chewing tobacco is associated with mouth cancer and many dental problems. Nicotine overdose is associated with heart arrhythmias, convulsions, and death.

Depressants

Although athletes occasionally use depressants ("downers") to calm themselves before a competition, they more commonly use them to relax after an event. The two most important drugs in this category are alcohol and marijuana.

Alcohol

Alcohol remains the most abused drug in all age groups. Absorbed in both the stomach and small intestine, it exhibits peak blood levels about 45 min after ingestion. The liver metabolizes alcohol at a constant rate (about 10-15 ml/h), regardless of the amount ingested. Although low-level intoxication might improve self-confidence and relaxation for a sport-related task, these apparent benefits are usually far outweighed by adverse effects—for example, impaired reaction time, reduced hand-eye coordination, reduced accuracy of movements, and impaired balance. Even one alcoholic drink affects reaction time and fine-motor coordination. Because alcohol acts as a diuretic, it may lead to dehydration.

Chronic alcohol use is associated with a variety of problems including damage to heart muscle, hardening of the arteries, reduced sexual performance, damage to peripheral nerves, damage to various parts of the brain, increased risk of stomach ulcers, damage to the pancreas, and damage to the liver. In addition to these physical events, the social implications of alcohol abuse are extensive. Many studies point to the role alcohol plays in assaults, unwanted sexual contact, increased motor vehicle accidents, and accidental deaths. Athletes who are becoming dependent on alcohol (or any other drug) show a variety of symptoms, including decreased athletic performance. See *Symptoms of Emerging Drug Dependence* to get a good idea of what should alert you to the possibility that an athlete may be developing

Symptoms of Emerging Drug Dependence

- Sudden personality changes
- Severe mood swings
- Changing peer groups
- Dropping out of extracurricular activities
- Decreased interest in leisure activities
- Decrease in grades
- Less-responsible behavior
- Frequent depression
- Poor personal hygiene
- Changes in eating and sleeping habits
- Smell of alcohol or marijuana
- Weight loss or weight gain
- Lying
- Trouble with the law
- School truancy
- Job loss or frequent job changes
- Increased time spent alone
- Poor family relationships
- Hidden alcohol or other drugs
- Increased amount of negative behavior
- Signs of physical intoxication

a dependence on or addiction to alcohol, recreational drugs, or even some of the ergogenic aids discussed earlier. Some of these symptoms were apparent in the case-study athlete, who had developed a dependency on anabolic steroids.

A number of preliminary screening tools are available to identify people at risk for alcohol or other drug dependency. One of the most useful and easy to remember is the CAGE questionnaire, which includes the following questions that are specifically targeted at alcohol abuse:

- Have you ever felt you ought to **C**ut down on your drinking?
- Have people **A**nnoyed you by criticizing your drinking?
- Have you ever felt bad or **G**uilty about your drinking?
- Have you ever had a drink first thing in the morning to steady your nerves or to get rid of a hangover? (**E**ye-opener)

Athletes who answer positively to one or more questions should be referred to the team physician for a more thorough assessment.

Marijuana

Marijuana has been used as a muscle relaxant, analgesic, sedative/hypnotic, topical anesthetic, appetite stimulant, and bronchodilator. It was declared illegal in the United States in 1937. Its popularity increased in the drug culture in the 1960s, and it remains a popular drug of abuse among young people. The active ingredient, **tetrahydrocannabinol (THC),** is absorbed rapidly when smoked and produces a high that usually lasts about 30 min to 1 h but that can last longer with repeated exposure and with high concentrations of THC. The potential medical benefits include a decrease in pressure within the eyes (potentially useful for people with glaucoma), bronchodilation, increased appetite, and reduction of nausea following chemotherapy for cancer.

Some of the adverse side effects may last much longer than the euphoric effects. Although marijuana relieves anxiety, it can produce either sedation or excitement. It can adversely affect coordination and it decreases both blood pressure and the depth of breathing. There are numerous adverse affects on performance. It alters perception, resulting in a sense of slow motion; and it impairs depth perception, a problem in any sport that involves a ball. It immediately impairs short-term memory and occasionally causes an increase in suspiciousness and panic reactions—all of which can adversely affect athletic performance. Chronic use can produce amotivational syndrome: apathy, unwillingness to complete tasks, low threshold to frustration, unrealistic thinking, increased introversion, and total involvement in the present at the expense of future goals. Probably the greatest acute danger of marijuana use is its psychological and behavioral side effects on people who drive cars or operate machinery. Because THC is fat-soluble, it stays in the fat in the body for many days and may be detectable in the urine for at least a month after use.

OTHER SEDATIVES

Athletes use many other sedatives to relax, sleep, or escape from reality. Most are prescription drugs like the benzodiazepines (e.g., Valium®, Klonopin®) and barbiturates (e.g., Nembutal®, Amytal®), although myriad street drugs are versions of barbiturates.

Benzodiazepines are central nervous system (CNS) depressants and are addictive. Sudden withdrawal may cause seizures and sometimes withdrawal psychosis or even death.

Barbiturates are somewhat similar to alcohol in their effects on the body, but the combination of barbiturates and alcohol can be lethal. Moreover, antihistamines—

Dealing With the Athlete Who May Be in Trouble

Your most valuable efforts in dealing with drug abuse will probably be in educating athletes about the adverse affects on performance. It may also be helpful to discuss the moral issues involved, the dangers of side effects, and the consequences of being caught. It is important to provide the closest possible network of adults and peers so that anyone who is experimenting or having trouble with drugs will be intercepted as quickly as possible and directed to professionals who can help get the person back on the right track. It is important to know local alcohol and other drug abuse (AODA) counselors who can provide a good confidential assessment and provide treatment when it is needed. Usually these individuals can provide other resources such as local Alcoholics Anonymous and Narcotics Anonymous meetings when indicated.

Here are some Web resources for information on helping your athletes whom you suspect of having trouble with addictions:

- The National Council on Alcoholism and Drug Dependence is a group that works to fight the stigma and break stereotypes surrounding dependence.
  www.ncadd.org/programs/advocacy/policytest.html

- The Medline Plus National Library of Medicine Web site offers many resources and a great deal of information regarding alcoholism and drug dependence. This government-sponsored site provides information on research, screening, and treatment.
  www.nlm.nih.gov/medlineplus/alcoholism.html

- The National Clearinghouse for Alcohol and Drug Information (NCADI) is the information service of the Center for Substance Abuse Prevention of the Substance Abuse and Mental Health Services Administration in the U.S. Department of Health and Human Services. NCADI is the world's largest resource for current information and materials concerning substance abuse.
  www.health.org/about/aboutncadi.aspx

- The Center for Substance Abuse Prevention (CSAP) is a federal organization whose mission is to decrease substance use and abuse by bringing effective prevention to every community. CSAP is the sole federal organization with responsibility for improving accessibility and quality of substance abuse–prevention services.
  www.prevention.samhsa.gov/about/

found in many allergy and cold medicines—are also CNS depressants and in combination with barbiturates can cause respiratory arrest. Barbiturates are highly addictive. Peddlers of street drugs sometimes combine barbiturates with stimulants such as amphetamines or cocaine to soften the effects of coming down off the stimulant high, but this mixture is extremely dangerous in that it can increase heart rate and cause coronary arrest. Nearly one-third of all drug-related deaths (including suicides and accidental drug poisonings) stem from barbiturate overdoses. Moreover, withdrawing "cold turkey" from many barbiturates can also lead to death.

BETA-BLOCKERS

Adrenaline (more properly called epinephrine) speeds up the heart, raises blood pressure, and constricts blood vessels. Beta-adrenergic blockers (e.g., metoprolol, brand name Lopressor®) inhibit some of the effects of adrenaline; they slow the heart rate and reduce blood pressure but also reduce anxiety. They are very popular in medicine for treatment of high blood pressure, migraine headaches, heart arrhythmias, and even stage fright. The first beta-blocker discovered was propranolol (brand name Inderal®), which was used for angina (chest pain from coronary blood vessel constriction). Beta-blockers have an adverse effect on endurance athletic performance: The longer the event, the more profound the effect.

The principal class of athletes who might make unfair use of beta-blockers are competitive shooters and archers, who can use them to enhance performance by lowering the heart rate. Slowed pulse is an advantage in shooting in that shooters squeeze the trigger between heartbeats when the hands are steadiest, and slower heart rates provide a longer window during which to fire. Beta-blockers are banned in international competition in the shooting sports.

HERBAL SUPPLEMENTS

Recent increases in the availability and popularity of herbal supplements have created an environment of confusion and misinformation for both patients and health-care providers. With Americans spending billions of dollars annually on supplements, the need to distinguish fact from fiction is critical when educating patients regarding possible side effects, harmful drug interactions, and potential problems with drug testing. These issues are reviewed by Winterstein and Storrs (2001), and points from that article are summarized in *Herbal Supplements: Considerations for the Athletic Trainer*, page 220.

Recent high-profile deaths in college and professional football athletes have raised questions about the role that herbal supplements (in particular, ephedrine or ma huang) may have played in those deaths. The situation for health-care providers is further compounded by current laws that limit the ability of the Food and Drug Administration (FDA) to regulate any product labeled as a supplement.

Athletes wishing to learn more about such supplements often call upon the athletic trainer to serve as an educational resource. Herbal products are vigorously marketed to both competitive and recreational athletes with claims of performance enhancement and improved health and wellness. Care providers must be aware of the current regulations, potential risks, and known harmful effects of such products.

Regulation of Herbal Supplements

In the United States, the FDA is responsible for ensuring the public of the safety of drugs. Since the early 1960s the FDA has required that all drugs be evaluated for safety and efficacy. Herbal products have traditionally been listed as food supplements to avoid the burden of proof associated with research and testing. In addition, the FDA recognizes a list of approximately 250 herbs as "generally safe"; however, these are herbs used in food flavoring and not for medicinal purposes. More than 1,400 herbs are used worldwide for medicinal purposes. Manufacturers in the United States have had little incentive to seek FDA approval due to the costs associated with drug research. Such an environment has left the public with limited credible information about which products are both safe and effective.

In 1993 the FDA responded to reports of herb-related deaths with an advance notice of their intent to propose a rule to regulate dietary supplements. This is the FDA's method of indicating a desire for stricter regulation. The result was an unanticipated public and political backlash from manufacturers and consumers of specific supplements. This massive lobbying campaign led to the establishment of the 1994 Dietary Supplement and Health Education Act (DSHEA), a political compromise that has left the FDA with limited influence on herbal products. Under the current legislation, supplement makers do not have to prove that a product is safe; the FDA can take action only if a product is found to present a significant or unreasonable risk of illness or injury. The DSHEA does not allow manufacturers to make claims about an herb's ability to cure a disease, but they can make claims about the supplement's effect on the "structure" and "function" of the body. This nebulous language is confusing. For example, a manufacturer may not claim an herb cures arthritis but can claim it promotes healthy joints. When you consider

Herbal Supplements: Considerations for the Athletic Trainer

- The athletic trainer and other allied health professionals must be able to provide honest, unbiased information when educating physically active people about herbal supplements. Despite an increasing tendency to seek natural therapies, patients need to be aware that "natural" does not equal "safe."

- The Dietary Supplement and Health Education Act of 1994 allows herbal manufacturers to sell products without any testing for efficacy.

- Companies cannot make claims to cure a disease but can make claims to how a supplement affects "structure" and "function." For example, a manufacturer cannot claim to cure inflammation but can claim a product promotes "healthy joints" without a requirement to scientifically prove this statement. These products must be labeled with a disclaimer stating that the FDA has not reviewed the product.

- Many guidelines for the appropriate dosage of herbal products have been adopted from the international community (e.g., World Health Organization, German Commission E); these data rely on a significant amount of historical use information and only some clinical trials. A long history of use may allow for good safety information; however, it does not address efficacy.

- Multiple risk factors exist in the use of herbal supplements that can range from minor skin irritations to death. The FDA, herbal manufacturers, and herbal experts do not agree on how to interpret the wide range of evidence on various types of herbal remedies.

- Herbal products may have varied levels of concentration and purity. Many independent lab tests have shown products to contain widely varying amounts of active ingredients. Because physiologic responses are dictated by the amount of the active ingredient, this is of concern.

- Patients who wish to take an herbal supplement should use a standardized product that contains the scientific name and quantity of the botanical on the label. The name and address of the manufacturer, the lot number, and the expiration date should be provided.

- Product adulteration is a concern with herbal supplements, and multiple cases are presented in the literature. Contamination of Ayurvedic and Chinese herbs is common because of the multiple ingredients found in such preparations. Patients should avoid preparations that are not standardized and packaged as described above.

- Toxicity and adverse reactions are of particular concern. Numerous cases of toxicity have been linked to herbal products. Most notably are the concerns over the herb ma huang and all ephedrine alkaloids. These ingredients are frequently found in over-the-counter stimulants often marketed as weight-loss products, or thermogenic metabolism boosters. Adverse effects range from irritability to cardiac arrhythmia and death.

- Patients often fail to report their herbal supplement use when providing a medical history. Herbal products in combination with prescription medications may adversely mimic, magnify, or oppose the desired effect of a medication. Questions regarding herbal supplement use must be part of a complete history.

- Care providers must be aware that herbal use can be deeply rooted in folk medicine and is commonplace in certain cultures. An appropriate level of cultural sensitivity is necessary when discussing herbal use with patients. Being judgmental or dismissive can erode the patient's trust.

Adapted, by permission, from A.P. Winterstein and C.M. Storrs, 2001, "Herbal supplements: Considerations for the athletic trainer," *Journal of Athletic Training* 36(4): 425-432.

studies showing that consumers believe products sold in pill form have been reviewed for safety by the FDA, the landscape is fairly perplexing.

RISKS OF HERBAL SUPPLEMENTS

Although most herbal side effects are benign, some have been associated with a range of adverse reactions, including death. Concerns have been voiced about the purity and concentration of herbal products. Even though manufacturing practices and standardization of product content have improved, several purity issues have been documented. Several independent consumer groups have conducted laboratory tests on herbal products and have found significant variations in the concentration of the herbal contents. For example, *Consumer Reports* tested 10 brands of ginseng and found substantial differences in concentration among them ("Herbal roulette" 1995). An herb's ability to elicit a desired physiologic response (or promote a potentially dangerous response) is based on the amount of the purported active ingredient. Variability of active ingredients is of particular concern because of the profound risks of toxicity and drug-herb interactions. Drug-herb interactions may be problematic because of the patient's reluctance to divulge his use of herbal supplements. The known effects of using prescription medication and herbs in combination are that herbs may mimic, magnify, or oppose the desired effect of the drug. Care providers must form a trusting relationship with patients and ask about possible use of herbal products in a nonthreatening manner. Table 14.3 outlines some possible drug-herb interactions.

Toxicity and Adverse Reactions

Numerous cases of toxicity have been linked to herbal products. Most notably are the concerns over the herb ma huang and all ephedrine alkaloids. These ingredients are frequently found in over-the-counter stimulants often marketed as weight-loss products, or thermogenic metabolism boosters. These are examples of herbs commonly ingested by athletes looking to enhance performance. Though ma huang and ephedra are the most common names, these stimulants may be found under as many as 25 names, including Chinese joint fir, bitter orange, country mallow, and Brigham's tea. This is significant in that even an informed consumer may mistakenly ingest these herbs by not recognizing the name. High-profile cases involving professional and collegiate athletes who died while training or practicing have raised questions about the role supplements containing ephedrine may have played in these deaths. Northwestern University has sued the manufacturer of a supplement that contains ephedrine after toxicology reports found that football player Rashidi Wallace had ephedrine in his system when he died. The suit alleges negligence in the labeling and selling of the product.

A *New England Journal of Medicine* report from December 2000 by Haller and Benowitz reviewed 140 reports of adverse effects linked to use of ephedra alkaloids. Ten of the 140 cases resulted in death, with 13 producing a permanent disability. The most serious of the side effects impact the central nervous system and the cardiovascular system (table 14.4). Ephedra, like all stimulants, increases a user's risk for heat-related illnesses. Given the risks of toxicity and potential drug interaction, athletic trainers and medical staff must ask questions regarding supplement use as part of the medical history for any exam.

In 1996 the FDA issued a warning to consumers about the use of ephedrine alkaloid products and encouraged consumers to avoid products containing more than 8 mg per serving, and eliminate products containing combinations of ephedrine and caffeine. The FDA received over 14,000 public comments about the warning, and the FDA's Center for Drug Evaluation has evaluated hundreds of reports from consumers who have experienced adverse effects, including reports of deaths associated with use of the product. To date, despite the volume of information, the FDA has yet to change the rules concerning ephedrine alkaloid regulation and continues to meet resistance and political pressure from herbal manufacturers. In August 2002 the Justice Department announced it was seeking a criminal investigation into whether the company Metabolife (Metabolife International Inc., San

Table 14.3 Possible Herbal-Drug Interactions

Drug name	Common use	Herbal name	Common use	Known interactions
Anti-inflammatories				
Aspirin	Anti-inflammatory Analgesic Antipyretic Antirheumatic	Ginko biloba	Increases circulation, increases short-term memory	Spontaneous hyphema
Hydrocortisone	Anti-inflammatory	Licorice	Expectorant, antiulcer	Glycyrrhetinic acid (an acid in topical anti-inflammatories) potentiates cutaneous vasoconstrictor response
Oral and topical corticosteroids	Anti-inflammatory	Licorice	Expectorant, antiulcer	Potentiates corticosteroids
Oral contraceptives				
Combined oral contraceptive	Birth control	St. John's wort	Alleviates depression and anxiety	Breakthrough bleeding
Oral contraceptives	Birth control	Licorice	Expectorant, antiulcer	Hypertension, edema, hypokalemia
Antidepressants				
Antidepressants	Antidepressant	Panax ginseng	Stimulant	Induces mania in depressed patients
Lithium	Manic depression	Psyllium	Reduces cholesterol	Decreases lithium concentrations
Paroxetine	Antidepressant	St. John's wort	Alleviates depression and anxiety	Lethargy, incoherence
Phenelzine	Monoamine oxidase inhibitor, antidepressant	Ginseng	Stimulant	Headache, tremor, mania
Serotonin-reuptake inhibitors	Antidepressant	St. John's wort	Alleviates depression and anxiety	Mild serotonin syndrome, decreased bioavailability of digoxin, theophylline, cyclosporin, phenprocoumon
Trazodone, sertraline, and mefazodone	Antidepressant, obsessive/compulsive disorders	St. John's wort	Alleviates depression and anxiety	Mild serotonin syndrome
Bronchodilator				
Theophylline	Bronchodilator	St. John's wort	Alleviates depression and anxiety	Decreased theophylline concentration

Reprinted, by permission, from A.P. Winterstein and C.M. Storrs, 2001, "Herbal supplements: Considerations for the athletic trainer," *Journal of Athletic Training* 36(4): 425-432.

Diego, CA) misled the public as to the safety of its product. Metabolife is a leading seller of a weight loss/metabolic stimulant that contains ephedra.

Athletes seeking an edge in performance or an energy boost for practice or competition, or those concerned about weight loss, may be tempted to consume these

Case Study

On an August afternoon, a 19-yr-old college soccer player becomes light-headed and nauseated during her second practice of the day; she is pale and has heart palpitations. She has eaten both breakfast and lunch and has never had a similar reaction. She is on no medications. Because she does not improve with rest, you have an ambulance take her to the emergency room.

In the emergency room, her electrocardiogram reveals a normal but fast heart rhythm; her blood pressure is slightly elevated at 140/85. She is pale but coherent and talkative during the entire evaluation. She remains slightly nauseated but does not vomit. Upon further questioning, she reveals that she has begun a new supplement to try to lose weight. She also admits that, although the instructions on the bottle recommended that a person take one or two capsules per day, she has taken six capsules today. After her roommate retrieves the bottle, you learn that the active ingredients in the supplement are ephedrine and caffeine. The athlete is quite embarrassed to learn the cause of her illness. Fortunately, after about 2 h in the emergency room, she begins to feel better and is discharged.

Table 14.4 Side Effects Associated With Ephedra Use

Central nervous system	Cardiovascular	Behavioral
Tremors	↑Heart rate	Mood changes
Headaches	↑Blood pressure	Memory
Dizziness	Irregular heart rhythm	Vigilance
Syncope	Myocardial infarction	Euphoria
Insomnia	Stroke	Anorexia
Seizures		↓Sexual function
Psychomotor function changes		Dependency
Stroke		

supplements. Problematic with all supplement use is the misguided notion that if the recommended dose is good, more will be better. In addition to the aforementioned adverse effects, the possibility that a person may fail a drug test following prolonged supplement use is a possibility. These substances have been banned by the NCAA, IOC, and National Football League. Both competitive and recreational athletes must be educated about the risks of these products.

SUMMARY

1. *Identify various drugs and supplements as performance-enhancing (ergogenic), restorative, or recreational.*

Drugs that are used to potentially improve athletic performance are called performance-enhancing, or ergogenic, drugs. Whereas anabolic-androgenic steroids are probably the most publicized performance-enhancing drugs, a long list of other substances potentially fit into that category. Restorative drugs are used to treat injuries or illnesses and are not very controversial. They are called restorative because they are intended to restore sick athletes to a healthier state. Recreational drugs alter moods and are usually used to provide a high or euphoria. This group includes alcohol,

For Further Information

Print Resources

American College of Sports Medicine Position Stand on the Use of Blood Doping as an Ergogenic Aid. 1996. *Medicine and Science in Sports and Exercise* 28(3): i-viii. Available at www.acsm-msse.org

Bahrke, M., and C. Yesalis, eds. 2002. *Performance-enhancing substances in sport and exercise.* Champaign, IL: Human Kinetics.

Hutchins, G.M., S.J. Traub, W. Hoyek, R.S. Hoffman, C.A. Haller, and N.L. Benowitz. 2001. Dietary supplements containing ephedra alkaloids. *New England Journal of Medicine* 344: 1095-97.

National Institute on Drug Abuse. 2000. *NIDA Research Report—Steroid abuse and addiction* (revised). NIH Publication no. 00-3721, revised April.

Ray, R., and D. Wiese-Bjornstal, eds. 1999. *Counseling in sports medicine.* Champaign, IL: Human Kinetics.

Yesalis, C.E. 2000. *Anabolic steroids in sport and exercise,* 2d ed. Champaign, IL: Human Kinetics.

Web Resources

National Library of Medicine and National Institutes of Health
www.nlm.nih.gov/medlineplus/anabolicsteroids.html
A Web site maintained by the National Library of Medicine and National Institutes of Health, with public information on anabolic steroids, current research, and links to up-to-date articles and information.

National Collegiate Athletic Association
www.ncaa.org/sports_sciences/drugtesting/banned_list.html
A list of the substances currently banned by the NCAA, along with details of its rules about drug use.

U.S. Anti-Doping Agency (USADA)
www.usantidoping.org/prohibited_sub/list.asp
USADA manages testing and adjudication for athletes involved in U.S. Olympic, Pan American, and Paralympic competitions. This Web site has the most up-to-date information on substances banned by the International Olympic Committee.

marijuana, amphetamines, cocaine, hallucinogens, and many others. Athletes appear to use recreational drugs at about the same frequency as the general population.

2. *Access current U.S. Olympic Committee and National Collegiate Athletic Association (NCAA) information on which drugs and substances are banned.*

A list of the substances currently banned by the NCAA, along with details of its rules about drug use, is available from the NCAA and is posted on the World Wide Web. The U.S. Anti-Doping Agency (USADA) manages testing and adjudication for athletes involved in U.S. Olympic, Pan American, and Paralympic competitions. The most up-to-date information on substances banned by the International Olympic Committee is updated regularly and can be found on the World Wide Web.

3. *Recognize the side effects and potential dangers of using anabolic steroids and human growth hormone.*

Although steroids can increase an athlete's lean body mass as well as strength, anabolic steroids also have both physiological and psychological adverse effects. They can produce unacceptable levels of aggressiveness, both on and off the playing field. They can be toxic to the liver and are associated with a variety of liver tumors, including cancer. Anabolic steroids are associated with permanent pattern baldness both in men and in women; can greatly worsen acne; and can increase hair growth, especially in females. In adolescents they can cause premature cessation of bone growth. During use, anabolic steroids cause fluid retention that can create swelling (edema) of the skin and soft tissue, especially in the face. Males who take anabolic steroids experience shrinkage of their testicles and are temporarily sterile because of a low sperm count. These compounds stimulate the prostate gland, which becomes enlarged; sometimes the enlargement obstructs the urinary tract, causing difficulty urinating. Anabolic steroids are associated with cancer of the prostate and (rarely) of the kidney. In some males, the estrogenic metabolites of anabolic steroids produce breast tissue (a condition called gynecomastia) that does not subside with disuse. When withdrawing from use of anabolic steroids, some males become impotent. In females, the permanent side effects can be quite dramatic. Females who use anabolic steroids can be masculinized—they develop a deep voice, body hair, and an enlarged clitoris.

Human growth hormone affects all the organs in the body and therefore can have significant adverse affects. When taken in excess, it produces all of the signs of gigantism, including acromegaly (enlargement of the nose, jaw, fingers, and toes). Exogenous growth hormone is associated with damage to the heart muscle and can cause enlargement of several organs, including the liver and spleen. Human growth hormone can cause osteoporosis and is associated with sexual dysfunction. Prolonged use of growth hormone may lead to the development of diabetes mellitus.

4. *Identify the signs of drug dependence and the risks associated with alcohol abuse.*

Alcohol remains the most abused drug in all age groups. Chronic alcohol use is associated with a variety of problems including damage to heart muscle, hardening of the arteries, reduced sexual performance, damage to peripheral nerves, damage to various parts of the brain, increased risk of stomach ulcers, damage to the pancreas, and damage to the liver. In addition to these physical events, the social implications of alcohol abuse are extensive. Many studies point to the role alcohol plays in assaults, unwanted sexual contact, increased motor vehicle accidents, and accidental deaths. Athletes who are becoming dependent on alcohol (or any other drug) show a variety of symptoms, including decreased athletic performance.

The athletic trainer and personnel who interact with athletes on a daily basis are in a good position to notice behavioral changes. Some signs of drug dependence can include personality changes, mood swings, changing peer groups, decreased interest in leisure activities, poor academic performance, irresponsible behavior, depression, changes in eating and sleeping patterns, weight loss or gain, legal troubles, truancy, poor family relationships, smells of alcohol or marijuana, and physical signs of intoxication.

5. *Explain current regulatory issues surrounding herbal supplements.*

The 1994 Dietary Supplement and Health Education Act (DSHEA) is the legal standard for the herbal supplement industry. Unfortunately, this legislation has left the U.S. Food and Drug Administration (FDA) with limited influence on herbal products. Under the current legislation, supplement makers do not have to prove a product is safe; the FDA can take action only if a product is found to present a significant or unreasonable risk of illness or injury. The DSHEA does not allow manufacturers to make claims on an herb's ability to cure a disease, but they may make claims about the supplement's effect on "structure" and "function" of the body. This language associated with herbal supplements is confusing for consumers and health-care providers alike.

6. *Recognize the potential dangers of using herbal supplements.*

Although most herbal side effects are benign, some have been associated with a range of adverse reactions, including death. Concerns have been voiced over the purity and concentration of herbal products. Even though manufacturing practices and standardization of product content has improved, several purity issues have been documented. Laboratory tests on herbal products have found significant variations in the concentration of the herbal contents. Variability of active ingredients is of particular concern because of the profound risks of toxicity and drug-herb interactions. Drug-herb interactions may be problematic due to patients' reluctance to divulge their use of herbal supplements. The known effects of using prescription medications and herbs in combination are that herbs may mimic, magnify, or oppose the desired effect of the drug. Care providers must form a trusting relationship with patients and ask about possible use of herbal products in a nonthreatening manner.

CHAPTER 15

Drug Testing in the Athletic Setting

OBJECTIVES

Upon completion of this chapter the reader will be able to do the following:

1. Identify the origin of drug-screening programs for athletic competition

2. Explain the components of a drug-screening program, including methods of drug screening and common confirmatory tests

3. Discuss the issue of false positives and false negatives and their impact on screening programs for athletes

4. Appreciate the legal and ethical issues that surround drug-screening programs

Testing for performance-enhancing (ergogenic) drugs in athletes is a fairly recent phenomenon. Moreover, the media have given increasing attention to athletes' use of alcohol and other drugs (those that are anything but performance enhancing)—especially when high-profile athletes are involved. After several deaths in the 1960s due to amphetamine abuse, and with the recognition that many athletes were using anabolic steroids, Olympic organizers asked chemists to come up with ways to identify users of these compounds. The International Olympic Committee (IOC) conducted preliminary testing for the 1968 Olympic Games, but comprehensive testing did not take place until the 1972 Summer Games in Munich. Athletes at many levels—from Olympic to college and sometimes even high school—are subject to drug testing, so allied health professionals need to be knowledgeable about the processes and issues related to drug testing.

Health providers are often asked to perform drug tests on athletes simply because the athletes are having problems. The most critical part of this process is not the testing itself but rather identifying athletes who truly need to be tested. If you work with athletes, especially at the college level or higher, you may become involved, whether you like it or not, with drug screening. To best serve the athletes with whom you work, you need to keep apprised of the substances that are banned by your sport's governing organization (chapter 14) and of the protocols required for drug testing. Athletic trainers and other health-care personnel should develop a sensitivity to athletes' personalities and performance abilities so that, as early as possible, they can identify individuals who may be using drugs (page 218).

Case Study

A basketball coach sends a 16-yr-old player to see the team physician for a drug test. The coach says the player is not performing well and believes that the youth is using drugs. The athlete asks the athletic trainer if he is required to undergo the test and asks why the coach is picking on him.

Further history from the coach, teammates, and teachers reveals that the coach is not the only one worried about this athlete. His grades have dropped from As and Bs to Cs and Ds. He is hanging out with a different group of friends, some of whom are known drug users. He recently broke up with a girlfriend of 8 months and has not been dating anyone else in that time.

The athlete reluctantly meets with the team physician. He is angry and can't believe the coach has required a drug test. The physician informs the athlete that the entire meeting is confidential and that the results of a drug test can also be confidential between the athlete and the physician (there is no drug-testing program at their school). The athlete then admits that he has been distraught over the breakup with his girlfriend and that he has had difficulty sleeping. He says that a drug test for marijuana would be positive because he used last weekend. He also binge drinks on some weekends but prefers to use pot. He says he has not experimented with any other drugs. His family history is negative for alcoholism and drug abuse.

He reluctantly agrees to see a psychologist and agrees not to use marijuana until he meets again with the team physician in a week. The physician and the athlete agree to tell the coach that this player is in trouble and also agrees to get help. The young man sees the psychologist weekly, and eventually the team physician runs a drug test for marijuana when the athlete states he has not used for 4 weeks. The test comes back negative. His grades begin to improve, and his performance on the court improves, too.

Terms and Definitions

anabolic-androgenic steroid (AAS)—Name for synthetic derivative of the male sex hormone testosterone that stimulates the biosynthesis of tissue and causes masculine sex characteristics.

gas chromatography (GC)—A process used to identify chemical compounds from a mixture using an inert gas that is run through a column. The individual components separate along the column in a certain order based on their chemical composition.

mass spectrophotometry (MS)—A sophisticated analytical tool used to identify chemicals based on how chemicals break down atomically when bombarded with electrical energy. Every chemical has a unique mass spectrophotometric fingerprint.

metabolite—A chemical that is a breakdown product of a larger chemical usually produced by an enzyme in the body.

pH—A measure of acidity; because urine is normally slightly acidic (pH < 7.0), alkaline urine (pH > 7.0) indicates possible tampering with the sample.

specific gravity—The ratio of the density of a sample to the density of water. If urine has a specific gravity <1.015, the person may have ingested large amounts of liquid to dilute drug residues in the urine.

T/E ratio—The ratio of testosterone to epitestosterone in the urine. A ratio greater than 6.0 usually implies that the person has taken exogenous testosterone.

tetrahydrocannabinol (THC)—The primary active ingredient in marijuana.

venipuncture—The puncture of a vein with a needle to obtain a blood sample.

OVERVIEW OF DRUG SCREENING

Most drug-screening programs are designed to detect drug use, enforce a banned list, and punish offenders of the ban. Table 15.1 gives examples of some of the policies, banned lists, and penalties. Although the IOC and the National Collegiate Athletic Association (NCAA) primarily test for ergogenic drugs, other governing bodies screen for illicit drugs as well to identify athletes who need treatment for dependency. At the professional sports level, screening is largely a business decision: Team owners do not want the performance of multimillion-dollar players hampered by drugs. At the professional level, players' unions closely scrutinize drug-testing programs and often influence the content of banned lists as well as the penalties for positive tests. Any drug-screening program is a potential deterrent to use.

Drug use is a significant problem at the international level. Table 15.2 summarizes the results of drug screening in past Olympic Games. It has become quite clear that when tests are announced ahead of time, athletes have learned how to avoid testing positive for those tests.

Drug-screening sessions may be scheduled publicly, such as during a championship event; they also may be unannounced and random, such as the NCAA's **anabolic-androgenic steroid (AAS)** drug-screening program that gives athletes at a college less than 24 h notice of a screening session; or there may be scheduled tests of randomly selected athletes, such as those conducted weekly by each National Football League team. Drug tests are also performed ad hoc on individuals who show behavior suggestive of alcohol and other drug abuse. Positive findings at the international level occur most often after unannounced, random tests.

Identifying Athletes Who Use Banned Substances

Epidemiologists define *screening* as the *presumptive* identification of an unrecognized disease or defect by procedures that can be administered rapidly. In other

Table 15.1   Examples of Drug Policies, Banned Lists, and Penalties From Various Sporting Organizations

Organization	Policy	Banned list	Penalties
U.S. Olympic Committee (USOC)	Tests at Olympic and Pan American trials, USOC-sponsored competitions	Stimulants, narcotics, AAS,* diuretics, and others (see text)	Decongestant or codeine: first positive: 3-month suspension, second positive: 2 yr, third positive: life ban AAS, amphetamines, diuretics, etc.: first positive: 2-yr suspension, second positive: life ban
National Collegiate Athletic Association (NCAA)	Tests at NCAA championships and football bowl games; random during school year for football and track	Stimulants, diuretics, AAS, and others, plus "street drugs": marijuana, heroin	First positive: loss of a minimum one season + postseason until negative test; second positive: loss of all eligibility in all sports (for street drugs, second positive: ineligible for 1 yr)
Major League Baseball (MLB)	Regular and random	Any illegal drug	No penalty for first positive if in treatment, second positive results in discipline, severity depends on individual
National Basketball Association (NBA)	Based on cause for veterans; random for rookies	Cocaine, heroin	Veterans: disqualification from NBA, can be reinstated in 2 yr; rookies: at least 1-yr suspension
National Football League (NFL)	Regular and random, plus reasonable cause	Cocaine, AAS, amphetamines, opiates	First positive: outpatient or inpatient counseling, second positive: 6-game suspension, third positive: banned from NFL for 12 mo

*AAS = anabolic-androgenic steroids.

Data from Gall et al. 1988, 155-61.

areas of medicine, screening tests *are not meant to be diagnostic*: Patients who test positive for a screening test usually undergo further evaluation to pin down the diagnosis. Although drug testing does indicate whether a person has used one or more drugs, it documents use only at a particular time. It makes no diagnosis but rather identifies a user who may be at risk of drug dependency. Screening for alcohol is usually done by blood or breath test, though it can also be done by urinalysis. Peptide hormones such as human growth hormone and the blood booster erythropoietin are not excreted in urine and therefore cannot be detected through urine tests. Researchers are working on ways to detect use of these compounds using blood testing. Testing for other drugs usually uses urine samples, with two types of procedures:

- a laboratory screening test, and, if that test is positive,
- a confirmatory test.

As in other areas of medicine, screening tests should have a high sensitivity (few or no false negative results), whereas confirmatory tests should have a high specificity (few or no false positive results).

Table 15.2 Results of Drug Screening in Past Olympic Games			
Location	**Year**	**Athletes tested**	**Positive test results (AAS*)**
Grenoble	1968	86	0
Mexico City	1968	668	1 (0)
Sapporo	1972	211	1 (0)
Munich	1972	2,079	7 (0)
Montreal	1976	2,061	11 (8)
Lake Placid	1980	NA	0
Moscow	1980	2,200	0
Sarajevo	1984	408	1 (1)
Los Angeles	1984	1,520	11 (10)
Calgary	1988	428	11 (1)

*AAS = anabolic-androgenic steroids.

Adapted from *The team physician's handbook*, M.B. Mellion, W. Walsh, and G.L. Shelton, p. 112, © 1999, with permission from Elsevier.

Most laboratories use screening tests that are highly sensitive, fast, and as inexpensive as possible. For confirmatory tests, a somewhat elaborate system has been developed using analytical tools called **gas chromatography (GC)** and **mass spectrophotometry (MS),** which together can provide unambiguous identification of a given substance. GC has the added benefit of measuring precisely how much of a particular substance is present. This methodology is the gold standard for confirmatory tests. The rigorous standards set up by the GC/MS system delayed effective testing for anabolic-androgenic steroids because the **metabolites** of all such compounds had not yet been well documented using MS. Not until 1976, in the Montreal Olympic Games, were anabolic-androgenic steroids tested. (Note: Employers do not always spend the money required to conduct confirmatory tests. As a result, employees should not assume that workplace drug testing is as vigorous or as accurate as the testing used for athletes. Laboratories employ a variety of screening methods, some more accurate and quantitative than others. Athletes undergoing drug screening through an employer should learn as much about the program as possible before consenting to undergo testing.)

An accreditation system exists for laboratory testing of Olympic athletes. The NCAA has developed a similar accreditation system. Because the protocols are very stringent and require testing for anabolic steroids, only a handful of laboratories in the United States meet these accreditation standards. Every step in the process is critical and must follow rigorous protocols in both collecting samples and analyzing them.

Collecting Samples

Urine is almost always the preferred body fluid used in drug tests. Not only are large specimen volumes easily obtained, but in addition most banned drugs are concentrated more highly in urine than in blood. And, of course, collecting urine is much less invasive than collecting blood. In the past, both athletes and athletic federations have argued that obtaining blood by **venipuncture** is too invasive—that it is unnecessarily traumatic, has potential for transmitting disease, and requires good technique on the part of the venipuncturist. Today coaches, federation officials, and even athletes are beginning to reconsider blood testing favorably, particularly to detect evidence of doping with polypeptides such as erythropoietin and growth hormone. The question is still open.

Regardless of the policy for scheduling, it is imperative that *everyone* involved in the testing process follow security measures to guarantee that the urine specimen tested is from the person identified on the specimen container. Testing officials must follow strict chain-of-custody procedures that document every person who handles the specimen—procedures similar to those followed in forensic cases. When a specimen is not in the possession of a person, it must be locked in a secure area to prevent tampering or administrative errors.

Collection of urine at drug-screening stations must follow a strict protocol. The Olympic program and NCAA protocols are almost identical and follow those set up originally by the U.S. Olympic Committee (USOC). Before an Olympic competition, a courier notifies an athlete that she has been selected for drug screening and has 1 h to report to the drug-screening station. *USOC Protocols for Collecting Specimens for Drug Testing* summarizes how the USOC specifies that urine be collected. For random testing sessions outside of competition, such as those that occur at the collegiate level, a student athlete selected for drug screening is notified approximately 24 h before the test. The notification must make clear, of course, the exact time and place of the drug-screening session.

USOC Protocols for Collecting Specimens for Drug Testing

After a doping control official (DCO) positively establishes your identify, proceed as follows under constant DCO observation:

1. Select a sealed container from a group of at least three; using your collection center's specified procedure, verify that it is empty and clean and is labeled as yours.
2. With a same-sex DCO, go to the toilet area and provide the urine sample with your shirt to mid-torso, sleeves above your elbows, and pants to mid-thigh.
3. After leaving the toilet area, choose a sample kit from a group of at least three; confirm that it is undamaged, properly numbered, and empty and clean.
4. Pour a specified amount of the sample into each of the two bottles in the kit and secure them. The DCO will confirm that the bottles will not leak.
5. Observe the DCO testing the urine left in the original collection container for pH and specific gravity.
6. Sign a statement that all procedures were followed properly. If they were not, any variations must be recorded on an official form before you leave.

Adapted from USADA, 2003. Available: www.usantidoping.org.

Upon arrival at the testing location, athletes begin by verifying their identity. They sign a log sheet with their time of arrival and choose their own specimen container, which has been sealed in plastic. Athletes are assigned a same-gender observer who follows the entire process. An athlete proceeds to a bathroom and, with the observer in the same room, produces a minimum of 85 ml of urine. Still under direct observation, the athlete carries the specimen to a processing station, where she chooses a sealed transport container. The athlete pours about half the specimen into one bottle and half into another, leaving a small amount of urine at the bottom of the specimen container for testing of specific gravity and acidity (see *Testing Urine for Specific Gravity and pH* on page 233). After pouring urine into the containers, the athlete is assisted in sealing each container and signs paperwork documenting that the numbers on the paperwork are indeed the same as those on the bottles that contain her urine. The athlete is then given a copy of this form with the specimen number. Providing that the pH is less than 7.0 and the specific grav-

Testing Urine for Specific Gravity and pH

Specific gravity is a measure of the concentration of the urine. Whereas water has a specific gravity of 1.000, most fluid in cells has a specific gravity of 1.010 to 1.015. Because urine is usually concentrated with the body's waste products, it should measure 1.015 or higher.

Acidity is measured with a **pH** test. A pH of 7.0 is neutral, meaning it is neither acidic nor alkaline. Because the body's waste products are acidic, urine should be acidic. If it is alkaline (pH > 7.0), something may have been added to the urine.

ity is greater than 1.015, the athlete may proceed to the checkout station to sign the log sheet and indicate the time of departure.

The athlete must be observed urinating. Although this is probably the most humiliating aspect of this procedure (for both the athlete and the observer), lack of direct observation invites tampering with the samples. At one major university, a dramatic increase in the number of positive tests accompanied a change from unobserved to observed collections.

False Positives

Many tests indicate a positive only if a substance is above a threshold level; below that level, the test is called negative even though the substance may be present. At an extremely low threshold level, for example, a test might be positive for metabolites of **tetrahydrocannabinol** (**THC**, the principal active ingredient in marijuana) for a person who had simply been in a room where marijuana was smoked. Some laboratories call a test positive for marijuana if the concentration of THC metabolites in urine exceeds 50 ng/ml. The NCAA calls positive a level over 15 ng/ml. In either case, a positive reflects relatively recent use of marijuana by the individual, not merely passive exposure to smoke or use by the individual many months before the test.

Because drug screening in the athletic arena is punitive, the tolerance for false positives is low and the tolerance for false negatives is high. The assumption is that it is better not to detect a user than to falsely accuse a nonuser—an approach quite different from that followed in drug-rehabilitation centers or in prisons. There are essentially three possible sources of error in drug screening, any one of which can produce false positives or false negatives:

1. *Clerical error* may occur because of a human or computer error in record keeping.
2. *Technical factors* may cause either human or instrument error in the laboratory (these errors are most common in laboratories that do not perform confirmatory tests).
3. A *break in the chain of custody* during collection or transport of samples can mean that a specimen does not correspond to the person who produced it.

Drug testing does not determine why a person uses a drug but simply addresses its presence or absence. Sometimes athletes ingest banned substances inadvertently. One of the biggest problems at the Olympic level is the use of pseudoephedrine found in many cough and cold preparations. More recently, nutritional supplements that contain ephedrine and similar compounds have also led to positive drug tests. Unfortunately, almost all athletes who test positive claim publicly that there must be an error, and many claim that their positive drug test is from an inadvertent ingestion. It is rare for athletes to admit they were caught cheating.

Some types of tea contain chemical relatives of ephedrine, which is banned by both the IOC and the NCAA. It is important for participants in the Olympics to be aware of this problem. The naturally occurring herb ma huang (Chinese ephedra) is a constituent of many common teas, including Bishop's tea, Brigham Tea, Chi Powder, Energy Rise, Ephedra, Excel, Joint Fir, Mexican Tea, Popotillo, Squaw Tea, Super Charge, and Teamster's Tea.

Poppy seeds may contain significant amounts of morphine that are excreted in amounts indistinguishable from those excreted by drug users as reported by Landry et al. in 1994. Poppy seeds grown in the United States have negligible amounts of opiates, but many foods have foreign poppy seeds that may have a high morphine content as well as lesser amounts of codeine. Confirmatory tests can usually determine whether the opiates are due to ingested poppy seeds as opposed to drug use. In the workplace, however, employees subject to drug testing for opiates will do well to avoid eating poppy seeds.

Theoretical Ways to Avoid Detection

Although a variety of ways exist to avoid detection during drug screening, most do not work if the athlete is under constant observation. Athletes have tried to use other drugs to mask use, but these drugs are also banned by the IOC and the NCAA; for example, diuretics will dilute the urine and reduce the concentration of drugs in the urine, but the IOC and the NCAA now ban all diuretics.

If drug testing is performed infrequently and with prior announcement, athletes can avoid detection if they know the retention times of drugs they take (table 15.3). Retention times for anabolic-androgenic steroids are quite variable, from a few days for oral preparations and water-soluble injectable preparations to months for oil-based injectables. Knowledge of retention times is probably the primary means of avoiding detection.

To make it more difficult for tests to detect use of anabolic steroids, by the 1976 Olympics most athletes had switched from synthetic steroids to natural testosterone. Since that time, tests have been developed to measure metabolites of testosterone: In the body, testosterone (T) is broken down to epitestosterone (E). Because the body breaks down its own testosterone at a relatively constant rate relative to the rate at which it is produced, there should never be an overabundance of testosterone compared to the amount of its metabolite, epitestosterone. Although a **T/E ratio** greater than 6.0 has long been considered evidence of exogenous testosterone use, this benchmark is not foolproof; occasionally a person naturally has a ratio greater than 6.0. But if that is the case, repeated testing can exonerate the athlete, whose T/E ratio should remain stable if he is not taking exogenous testosterone. The T/E ratios of anyone using exogenous testosterone will vary from test to test.

Because drug users frequently complain of "shy bladders" (inability to produce urine when someone is watching), it is important to be firm about production of urine at a drug-screening station. It is true that some people with elevated anxiety experience shy bladders when asked to void under observation. An adequate amount of time along with insisting that athletes drink fluids at the drug-screening sites ultimately will lead to successful voiding for a drug-screening specimen.

Table 15.3 Approximate Retention Times for Illicit Drugs

Drug	Approximate duration of detectability
Amphetamines	1-3 d
Barbiturates	
Short-acting	24 h
Intermediate-acting	48-72 h
Long-acting	>7 d
Cocaine metabolites	2-4 d
Codeine, morphine	48 h
Cannabinoids	
Single use	4 d
4 ×/week	5-7 d
Daily use	>28 d
Anabolic-androgenic steroids	
Water-soluble injectable or oral preparations	7-14 d
Fat-soluble injectable	1-12 months

Reprinted, by permission, from Council on Scientific Affairs, 1987, "Scientific issues in drug testing," *Journal of the American Medical Association* 257(22): 3112.

Table 15.4 Some Adulterants Used to Produce Deceptive Results in Drug-Screening Tests

Adulterant	pH	Relative density	Appearance
Unadulterated urine	5-7	1.005-1.030	
NaCl			
25-75 gm/L	5.5	1.035	
Liquid Drano®			
12-23 ml/L	6-7	1.018-1.019	
42-125 ml/L	8-11	1.020-1.028	
Liquid hand soap			
12-42 ml/L	6-7	1.018-1.021	Cloudy to turbid
107 ml/L	8	1.033	Cloudy to turbid
Visine®			
107-125 ml/L	7	1.016-1.018	
Vinegar			
125 ml/L	4	1.018	
Golden Seal tea			
15-30 gm/L	6	1.022-1.024	Brown
Water		<1.005	
Temperature			
°C	32.5-37.5		
°F	90.5-99.8		

Reprinted, by permission, from S.L. Mikkelsen and K.O. Ash, 1988, "Adulterants causing false negatives in illicit drug testing," *Clinical Chemistry* 34(11): 2333-2336.

Table 15.4 describes some of the adulterants used to produce deceptive results in drug-screening procedures. Adulterants are popular in the business sector, where direct observation is less common than in sports. Any source of water that dilutes the urine increases the chance that the test results will fall below the testing threshold. Because many individuals use toilet water for this purpose, federal officials recommend that bathrooms involved with drug testing have blue toilet water and that federal employees avoid medications containing methylene blue, the dye used in toilet bowl preparations. Most drug-screening procedures examine the specific gravity or concentration of urine to prevent deception by diluted urine. Because amphetamine excretion is decreased by ingestion of sodium bicarbonate, most screening sessions test urine's pH (see *Testing Urine for Specific Gravity and pH* on page 233). Some legitimate medications can lead to alkaline urine, however, as can some urinary tract infections. An athlete who has recurrent vomiting may also have alkaline urine.

NOTIFICATION OF RESULTS

Athletic organizations' policies vary in how they notify athletes of test results. Unfortunately, with the high stakes in the sports community, drug-testing results are often leaked to the press. Health providers involved in drug testing should clarify to athletes, *before* they begin a test, who will have access to the results. Every drug-testing program should clearly and publicly outline its policies in this respect.

The most important person to notify concerning positive test results is the athlete. Once a person has been identified as a drug user, that person's coach, physician, and athletic trainer have the choice of viewing the data as an opportunity to halt a trend that can prove quite destructive for the athlete, or they can adopt a purely punitive attitude and exile the athlete to his own devices. A drug-screening program ideally is a means to a beneficent end, not a weapon to weed out supposed ne'er-do-wells. The physical and mental health of athletes is far more important than any win-loss record. It is critical that all athletes identified with a problem have access to professionals who can assess and treat them for alcohol or other drug abuse. Providing such professional help is a much more complex issue than merely screening urine for chemicals, and it requires much greater investment of time and financial resources. But the net results are far more beneficial to a school or business—not to mention the people who have problems with substance abuse—than simple policies of punishing offenders. They are worth the investment many times over.

EFFECTIVENESS AND COST OF DRUG SCREENING

Despite wide use of drug screening, no one has clearly studied its effectiveness in preventing drug use. Athletes generally like the idea of providing a level playing field without ergogenic drugs, especially if they can be guaranteed that users will be caught—a result that unfortunately is difficult to attain. Drug-testing programs provide one clear benefit: They give athletes a good reason not to use drugs. Peers who want their athletic friends to use drugs seem more understanding and less likely to apply pressure when they know the athlete faces penalties if caught using drugs.

Some argue that because there are so few positive tests at the Olympic and NCAA level, drug screening must be working. Yet it is equally possible that athletes are simply getting better at avoiding positive tests. By tallying self-reports from anonymous surveys since 1989, the NCAA has documented a decrease in use of anabolic-androgenic steroids. Although similar surveys have not been done on Olympic athletes, anecdotal evidence suggests that banned drug use is very common because athletes have learned how to use drugs without getting caught.

Drug screening can be very expensive and time-consuming. Costs vary from laboratory to laboratory and are even more expensive if personnel must be provided to assist with the collection procedure. As discussed by Kammerer (2000), in 1999 testing one urine sample for anabolic steroids in the United States was performed at a cost of approximately $100 or more. Tests for a specific drug or for a small battery of drugs not including anabolic steroids are considerably less costly. The high cost of urinary drug screening precludes the use of such tests in all but a minority of high school athletic programs. Note that the total cost represents not only the dollars spent and the labor of personnel who do the collecting; drug screening also takes time away from athletes' studies or workouts, and health providers involved in collecting samples have that much less time to treat athletes for illnesses and injuries.

LEGAL AND ETHICAL QUESTIONS

The legality of screening athletes for drugs is still controversial in the United States. There are many different kinds of drug-screening programs, and many issues have yet to be tested in court. Drug screening in the workplace has been examined more carefully and has generally been upheld. It is clear that drug screening is legal when substance abuse endangers or infringes on the rights of others. Drug screening is usually examined by state courts, and drug-screening programs in the athletic setting have been challenged infrequently. Courts have provided inconsistent rulings, because almost every drug-screening program has different rules.

Some aspects of drug-screening programs can be problematic for health providers. To preserve the rapport they have built in their confidential relationships with athletes, athletic trainers and physicians should not be asked to participate in the selection process for drug screening (i.e., deciding who will be tested). They also should not be involved in communicating test results to anyone but the athlete unless doing so is explicitly stated in the drug-testing policy. As in any other situation, all medical information obtained from an athlete should be considered

For Further Information

Print Resources

Fuentes, R.J., and J.M. Rosenberg. 1999. *Athletic drug reference '99.* Research Triangle Park, NC: Glaxo Wellcome.

Ray, R. 2000. *Management strategies in athletic training,* 2d ed. Champaign, IL: Human Kinetics.

Voy, R., and K. Deeter. 1991. *Drugs, sport and politics.* Champaign, IL: Human Kinetics.

Web Resources

National Collegiate Athletic Association
www1.ncaa.org/membership/ed_outreach/health-safety/drug_testing/index.html
Includes NCAA drug-testing program information from the NCAA Committee on Competitive Safeguards and Medical Aspects of Sports.

World Anti-Doping Agency
www.wada-ama.org
An autonomous agency that coordinates antidoping efforts for all Olympic events. Its mission is to promote and coordinate, at the international level, the fight against doping in all its forms.

strictly confidential unless the athlete has previously authorized its release to a third party. The NCAA Drug-Screening Program (www1.ncaa.org/membership/ed_outreach/health-safety/drug_testing/index.html) clearly delineates this principle for collegiate athletes.

SUMMARY

1. *Identify the origin of drug-screening programs for athletic competition.*

Testing for performance-enhancing (ergogenic) drugs in athletes is a fairly recent phenomenon. After several deaths in the 1960s caused by amphetamine abuse, and with the recognition that many athletes were using anabolic steroids, Olympic organizers asked chemists to come up with ways to identify users of these compounds. The International Olympic Committee (IOC) conducted preliminary testing for the 1968 Olympic Games, with comprehensive testing beginning during the 1972 Summer Games in Munich. Athletic organizations including the IOC, the National Collegiate Athletic Association (NCAA), and individual institutions (including some high schools) sponsor drug-testing programs.

2. *Explain the components of a drug-screening program, including methods of drug screening and common confirmatory tests.*

Strict protocols exist for obtaining urine samples from athletes and for guaranteeing that laboratory results are correctly attributed to a specific athlete. Athletic trainers need to be knowledgeable about these procedures to legitimately identify athletes who are using drugs and to protect those who may be falsely accused of using them. Health-care providers must also be aware of the methods athletes use to produce deceptive results on the drug tests. A key component of the screening process is security. Measures must be followed to guarantee that the urine specimen that is tested is from the person identified on the specimen container. Testing officials must follow strict chain-of-custody procedures that document every person who handles the specimen. These procedures are similar to those followed in forensic cases. Urine samples must meet criteria for pH and specific gravity. A usable sample must have a pH <7.0 and specific gravity >1.015.

Most laboratories use screening tests that are highly sensitive, fast, and as inexpensive as possible. For confirmatory tests, a somewhat elaborate system has been developed using analytical tools called gas chromatography (GC) and mass spectrophotometry (MS), which together can provide unambiguous identification of a given substance. GC has the added benefit of measuring precisely how much of a particular substance is present. This methodology is the gold standard for confirmatory tests.

  3. *Discuss the issue of false positives and false negatives and their impact on screening programs for athletes.*

A test may be indicated as positive only if a substance is above a threshold level; below that level, the test is called negative even though the substance may be present. Drug screening in the athletic arena is punitive; the tolerance for false positives is low and the tolerance for false negatives is high. The assumption is that it is better not to detect a user than to falsely accuse a nonuser. There are essentially three possible sources of error in drug screening, any one of which can produce false positives or false negatives:

- Clerical error may occur because of a human or computer error in record keeping.

- Technical factors may cause either human or instrument error in the laboratory (these errors are most common in laboratories that do not perform confirmatory tests).

- A break in the chain of custody during collection or transport of samples can mean that a specimen does not correspond to the individual who produced it.

  4. *Appreciate the legal and ethical issues that surround drug-screening programs.*

Drug screening remains a controversial yet important part of both the national and international sports cultures, and numerous legal issues remain to be decided in the United States. Some evidence exists that drug-testing programs are effective at deterring drug use in athletes, but this has not been well studied. Drug testing is complex and costly—too costly for most high school programs to implement. There are many different kinds of drug-screening programs, and many issues have yet to be tested in court. State courts usually examine drug screening, and drug-screening programs in the athletic setting have been challenged infrequently. Court rulings have been inconsistent, because almost every drug-screening program has different rules.

Aspects of drug-screening programs can be problematic for health providers. Health providers must be able to preserve professional relationships and maintain medical confidentiality. Athletic trainers and physicians should not be asked to participate in the selection process for drug screening (i.e., deciding who will be tested). They also should not be involved in communicating test results to anyone but the athlete unless doing so is explicitly stated in the drug-testing policy.

It is important to follow through with athletes who are caught using illegal substances and not simply banish them from your team. See to it that they become actively engaged with professional counselors who can help them stop their potentially destructive behavior.

PART IV

SPECIAL ISSUES

CHAPTER 16

Environmental Concerns

OBJECTIVES

Upon completion of this chapter the reader will be able to do the following:

1. Explain the metabolic and environmental factors that contribute to heat loss and heat gain

2. Recognize the spectrum of heat- and cold-related injury and illnesses

3. Describe appropriate prevention strategies to avoid heat- and cold-related conditions

4. List the factors that make up an appropriate lightning-safety plan

5. Identify the potential problems associated with exercise at altitude

Athletes who exercise in extremes of high or low temperature, or at high altitude, are subject to a variety of afflictions—from those that merely annoy to those that kill. You should know how to recognize when athletes are in trouble and, even more important, should know how to help athletes avoid problems. Environmental stress can be tricky. Athletes can become hypothermic at temperatures that might seem quite comfortable (e.g., 70° F, or 21.1° C); or they can suffer dangerous heat illness in somewhat mild temperatures if they fail to ingest enough electrolytes or enough water, or in some cases if they drink *too much* water. This chapter provides basic information about environmental stresses you and your athletes are likely to encounter.

Case Study

You are working with a high school football team during a summer practice session. You are concerned about the heat, because the temperature has risen to 86° F (30° C) and the humidity is 55%. The coaches have been very good about providing frequent water breaks during the afternoon practice, and for the first hour of practice everything has gone well. During one of the drills, however, one of the players drops to his knees and refuses to stand up. He reports that he is dizzy and nauseated, and he is breathing rather hard. You remove him from the sun and get him into the shade. He still reports that he is dizzy and nauseated. His skin is flushed and he is sweating profusely. You ask him to drink some water, but he is very hesitant to do so because of his nausea. After just a few sips, he says he cannot drink any more. At that time he begins to develop cramps in his calves. Despite ice and stretching, the cramps persist. He remains alert, oriented, and responsive. Your best guess is that he has sodium depletion heat exhaustion.

You call the team physician for advice. Because the athlete refuses to take fluid orally, the physician says he will give fluids intravenously. The physician is not available to come to the practice site, so he asks you to transport the athlete to his office, where he gives the athlete 2 L of normal saline solution. The athlete reports that both nausea and cramps have disappeared. The team physician asks to monitor the athlete's weight carefully and holds him out from practice the next day. The physician will see him again before he is to return to practice.

HEAT-RELATED ILLNESSES

Illnesses attributed to heat may be a direct result of high temperatures or may be more directly related to dehydration or to electrolyte imbalance. These conditions place additional stress on the thermoregulatory systems of the body. Most heat-related illnesses result from combinations of these factors. These conditions combined with the stress of exercise can lead to catastrophic consequences.

Physiology

Muscles can generate over 20 times as much energy during maximal exercise as they can at rest. At maximal exercise, the human body's work efficiency is approximately 25%—which means roughly 75% of the muscle energy consumption is converted to heat rather than work. Early in exercise, heat production exceeds heat loss, thereby increasing core body temperature. Exercising muscles lose heat in four ways: *evaporation, radiation, convection,* and *conduction.* Evaporation is the

Terms and Definitions

acute mountain sickness (AMS)—An illness that can affect anybody who ascends too rapidly to high altitude.

alkalotic—Having abnormally high pH (alkalinity) in the blood and tissues.

anticholinergic—Side effects of blocking action of neurotransmitter (acetylcholine) that results in constipation, dry mouth, and decreased sweating.

erythropoietin—Hormone that stimulates the bone marrow to make more red blood cells; high-altitude exercise leads to greater synthesis of erythropoietin in the kidneys.

gangrene—Death of tissues caused by insufficient blood supply, with complete breakdown of tissue; it is often followed by bacterial infection and cell death.

hyponatremia—Abnormally low blood levels of sodium.

hyponatremic collapse—Low sodium content related to overhydration with water resulting in myriad symptoms, from confusion to death (also called *exercise-induced hyponatremia*).

hypovolemia—Abnormally low volume of blood plasma in the body.

nonshivering thermogenesis—Hormone-regulated production of heat.

syncope—Loss of consciousness caused by inadequate blood flow to the brain; fainting.

conversion of a liquid into a vapor. Radiation is the transmission of heat energy from a surface. Convection is the transmission of heat in a fluid by circulation of the fluid's heated molecules. Conduction is the transfer of heat from one substance to an adjacent substance. Heat from muscle is conducted to the adjacent blood vessels and carried by convection to the heart and out into the arteries into the small vessels in the skin. The heat is conducted to the surface of the skin, where it is radiated into the air. Heat is also lost by evaporation via sweat and via the moisture in exhaled gases. Radiation and convection dissipate most of the heat from the body when the ambient temperature is less than 68° F (20° C). In warm environments, evaporation is the most physiologically important means of heat loss in human beings. During heavy exercise, evaporation can account for up to 85% of the heat loss. A 154-lb (70-kg) athlete sweats at a rate of 1 to 2 L/h during intense exercise in the heat. Larger athletes may sweat at a considerably higher rate. Above 95° F (32.2° C), convection and radiation do not contribute to heat loss. After the heat-dissipating mechanisms are working during exercise, the core body temperature reaches a plateau until the athlete reduces the intensity of the exercise. In some athletes, the core temperature may increase as much as 1° to 4° F (0.6-2.2° C) with no diminution in performance. Temperature elevation of 1° to 4° F by itself is not dangerous, but if the heat-dissipating mechanisms fail to keep up with heat production, the core temperature may rise to dangerous levels.

Over time, the human body acclimates to exercising in heat. In adults, four to seven daily sessions of exercise in the heat, consisting of 1 to 4 h per session, will facilitate acclimation. Children take slightly longer to acclimate. During acclimation, basal plasma volume (fluid in the heart and blood vessels) increases and electrolyte concentration in sweat diminishes; sweating begins to be initiated earlier in the exercise bout, with an increased rate of sweating; and there is increased production of the hormone aldosterone, which helps the body save electrolytes.

Heat-Related Illnesses

The spectrum of heat illness ranges from very mild symptoms to heatstroke and death.

Heat edema is a transitory swelling of the hands and feet that occurs when an unacclimated person is exposed to heat. It is usually just a nuisance that typically resolves over the first few days of heat exposure. Patients with heat edema should take note to remove rings and other jewelry from the hands and feet that may cause discomfort or interfere with circulation.

Heat syncope is a transient episode of **hypovolemia** that causes the affected person to faint from low fluid in the bloodstream. It most often occurs at the end of a running race, when athletes are maximally vasodilated to get blood and oxygen to the muscles and heat to the skin. When they stop their vigorous activity, much of the blood volume pools in the lower extremities. This is one of the reasons that athletes should cool down, or continue to walk or jog, immediately after a running competition. Treatment, which involves simply getting more blood volume to the trunk and head, requires that athletes lie down and slightly elevate their legs (preferably in a cool place). They also should drink some fluids.

Heat cramps, which can be quite painful, are muscle spasms that occur during or after intense prolonged exercise in the heat. Usually the lower-extremity muscles are affected, but virtually any muscles can be involved. Heat cramps are more likely to occur in people who are not acclimated to the heat, and in athletes who have a high sweat volume or high sweat sodium and who have not replaced the lost sodium. Treatment consists of rest and cooling down the athlete. Massage of the cramping muscles is sometimes helpful. It is important for the athlete to replace both fluids and electrolytes. If the athlete is unable to take oral fluids, intravenous fluids may be necessary, as in the case history at the beginning of this chapter.

Heat exhaustion occurs when the body temperature is significantly elevated but usually by less than 1° to 3° F (0.6-1.7° C); the athlete is dizzy and weak but is still quite responsive and thinking clearly. It is a serious, acute disorder, with hyperthermia caused by dehydration, **hyponatremia,** or both. It may progress to become a form of **syncope.** Usually the athlete is still sweating, but dehydration may reduce the level of sweating. Depletion of sodium and depletion of water lead to slightly different syndromes. *Sodium-depletion heat exhaustion* occurs in unacclimated athletes who replace sweat loss only with water that contains no electrolytes. It is usually caused by inadequate dietary sodium intake. The symptoms are fatigue, profound weakness, light-headedness, sweating, muscle cramps, and occasionally flulike symptoms. *Water-depletion heat exhaustion* results from exercising in the heat with inadequate water intake (see *Strategies for Preventing Heat Illness* on page 249, which provides guidelines for fluid intake before, during, and after exercise). Symptoms are thirst, headache, mild anxiety, muscle weakness, generalized fatigue, and poor neuromuscular coordination; symptoms may also include high fever, tachycardia (elevated heart rate), decreased skin tone (more elasticity or stretchiness), mental confusion, and sometimes emotional agitation. These athletes sweat but with reduced volume. *The difference between heat exhaustion and heatstroke lies in the changes of mental status.* Any time you observe a sudden change in an athlete's mental status, you should consider the possibility of heatstroke. Figure 16.1 compares the signs and symptoms of heat exhaustion and heatstroke.

Treatment of heat exhaustion involves rest and rapid cooling. It is very important to provide fluid and electrolyte replacement in the form of hypotonic (i.e., containing only a small amount of electrolytes) oral fluids or half-normal (0.45%) saline intravenously. (Normal saline has the same concentration of sodium chloride as blood, which is 0.9%.) A body temperature reading should be obtained to ensure the patient's temperature is not significantly elevated (see *Measuring Body Temperature*). The team physician may request lab work to measure serum sodium for an indication of precisely how much sodium is needed.

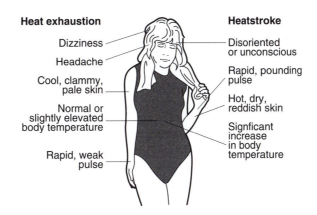

■ **Figure 16.1**   Signs and symptoms: Heat exhaustion versus heatstroke.
Adapted, by permission, from S. Hillman, 2000, *Introduction to athletic training* (Champaign, IL: Human Kinetics), 216.

Heatstroke is the most severe form of heat illness and is a medical emergency. Heatstroke occurs when the elevation in body temperature is greater than 5° F (2.8° C). Athletes with heatstroke appear confused, disoriented, and agitated; when heatstroke is severe, athletes may exhibit hysterical behavior, be delirious, have seizures, or collapse. *The hallmark of heatstroke is profound central nervous system dysfunction such as confusion, disorientation, and agitation.* In traditional heatstroke the patient is hot, flushed, and dry with no sweating; this form of heatstroke occurs in the elderly and is not related to exercise. Athletes and physically active individuals who suffer heatstroke will most often experience exertional heatstroke. These patients will exhibit the red, hot skin associated with traditional heatstroke. Unlike traditional heatstroke patients, however, their skin will most likely appear wet from the profuse sweating that took place during exertion before their collapse. Whether the skin is wet or dry, this is a medical emergency, and you need to activate an emergency action plan.

Heatstroke is not spontaneously reversible or self-limited and requires immediate cooling. If left untreated, heatstroke causes all the major organ systems to stop functioning. The most serious problems are brain dysfunction, kidney failure, and liver failure. An athlete with symptoms of heatstroke should be transported to an emergency facility as soon as possible. While waiting for the transport, immediately begin to cool the athlete. One good way to do this is to wet him with a cool

Measuring Body Temperature

Common methods of measuring body temperature—such as oral (a thermometer in the mouth), axillary (a thermometer in the armpit), or aural (measured in the ear canal)—generally underestimate the true *core body temperature.* In the laboratory or in the hospital, temperature probes are used to measure the temperature in the esophagus or a large blood vessel. In the field, the most accurate and practical way to measure core temperature is by use of a rectal thermometer. The sicker the patient, the less likely the oral temperature will be accurate.

If you believe an athlete's symptoms may suggest serious illness, such as heatstroke or severe hypothermia, your first priority should be to get the athlete to an emergency room, not to worry about the accuracy of the temperature measurement. If for any reason you need highly accurate temperature measurement in the field (i.e., if such knowledge might alter your method of treatment), use a rectal thermometer. This can be done more easily than most people realize. Even in a busy first aid tent at the end of a road race, for example, a large towel to cover the athlete allows enough privacy for a rectal temperature measurement.

spray and expose him to a large fan to speed evaporation. Remove the athlete's clothing and apply ice, especially to the armpits, neck, and groin. The priority should be cooling the patient. Immersion in ice water provides the most rapid cooling, so sports medicine personnel monitoring events where the possibility of heat-related illness exists should prepare by having ample adequate supplies of ice water to rapidly cool a patient in the event of an emergency such as heatstroke.

A syndrome defined only recently, **hyponatremic collapse** (also called *exercise-induced hyponatremia*) occurs when ultraendurance athletes (and sometimes marathon runners) drink excessive amounts of water without replenishing the electrolytes they have lost through sweating. Symptoms can range from mild confusion, weakness, and apathy to nausea, headache, and cramps, and in severe cases to pulmonary edema, seizures, coma, and death. Replenishing electrolytes too quickly can cause seizures and other serious complications of the central nervous system. Whenever possible, therefore, a physician should measure serum sodium before giving intravenous fluids to correct hyponatremia; but if there is no way to measure sodium levels, the attending medical professional should go ahead and give saline intravenously—to be safe, many physicians prefer to use half-normal saline when the serum sodium is unknown. A nonsymptomatic athlete should be rehydrated at a rate not exceeding 0.5 meq of sodium/kg body weight/h. For symptomatic individuals, the rate should not exceed 1.0 meq/kg/h. This is information you may want to tuck away in your brain for future reference, because on occasion a medical professional unfamiliar with treatment for hyponatremic collapse may be tempted to introduce sodium at too fast a rate during rehydration. Note that for hyperthermic ultraendurance athletes, cooling is still the treatment priority.

Risk Factors for Heat Illness

A number of factors predispose individuals to heat-related disorders. Athletes can control some factors, whereas others are out of their sway. Keep a close watch on the following people who are at risk for heat illness:

- Healthy individuals who are poorly acclimatized or poorly conditioned, or who are inexperienced competitors
- Anyone who is depleted of either salt or water
- Athletes who have large muscle mass or who are obese
- Children (because, relative to their body mass, they sweat more than adults)
- The elderly (people as young as age 50 may have reduced physiological response to heat)
- Any person who has had a previous heat injury
- Anyone who is sleep-deprived
- Any individual who has an acute illness—especially one that produces fever, or one whose gastrointestinal symptoms increase loss of water or electrolytes
- People with certain chronic illnesses such as any cardiac disease (which causes poor circulation and a decrease in conduction of heat to the skin), cystic fibrosis (increased sodium in the sweat), poorly controlled diabetes (poor circulation), any kind of eating disorder (fluid losses and dehydration), or uncontrolled hypertension
- Anyone who has recently drunk alcohol or abused illegal drugs
- Anyone who is taking medication that may affect sweating—especially a drug that has an **anticholinergic** effect (e.g., common antihistamines)

It is clear, then, that simply guzzling lots of water during an ultralong event can be quite dangerous. Encourage ultraendurance athletes to ingest small amounts of fluid frequently, always being sure to include some sodium along with their fluids. Remind them that, in an ultraendurance or marathon event under hot conditions, they can lose up to a liter of water an hour. Because that liter includes 2 to 3 g of electrolytes, it is common to replace these electrolytes by means other than sport drinks. During ultraendurance competitions, the use of gels, fruit, and bland snack foods as a mechanism to elevate carbohydrates and electrolytes is common. Remember, these suggestions are for ultraendurance athletes only. For most athletic situations, a balanced diet and judicious use of water and sports drinks will be enough to maintain electrolyte balance. For non-ultraendurance athletes, drinks, snacks, and gels with greater than 8% carbohydrate will slow the rate of fluid and electrolyte absorption.

Preventing Heat-Related Illnesses

The best way to prevent heat illness is to identify at-risk athletes (see *Risk Factors for Heat Illness,* page 246), encourage proper acclimatization, and make certain that athletes are well hydrated during the event. You might want to require at-risk athletes to reduce their workout time or to exercise during a cooler part of the day. For outdoor sports or indoor sports without air-conditioning, weather conditions play an important role in heat illness. Whenever possible, use objective measures of environmental conditions rather than relying on weather forecasts. *Always take humidity into consideration when estimating the dangers of heat stress.* The higher the humidity, the less effective evaporation is at cooling the body and the higher the heat stress. Although there are several ways to measure relative humidity, it is typically done on the athletic field using a sling psychrometer that measures dry bulb and wet bulb temperatures; relative humidity is then determined from a chart supplied with the instrument (figure 16.2). The heat stress index (table 16.1) evaluates the relative degree of heat stress; the resultant temperature on the chart is the heat sensation felt for a given humidity and temperature. Recommendations can be made based on the findings. The 1996 Olympic Marathon race in Atlanta was moved to an early-morning start time to avoid heat-related stress. Officials reached this decision following close monitoring of the weather conditions over a 24-h period. Table 16.1 shows the heat stress when you compare the relative humidity to air temperature.

Adjust athletes' workout schedules for hot and humid days, rescheduling them when possible to a cooler time of the day. Workouts can have a shorter duration, decreased intensity, more frequent breaks, or any combination of these. If there is any way to reduce the amount of clothing athletes wear on days with high heat stress, doing so will help reduce risk of heat illness by facilitating evaporation. Monitoring body weight will help you assess the degree of dehydration in that all acute weight loss is caused by water loss. Recording pre- and postpractice body weights will assist in determining the amount of fluid lost during a single practice session. In addition, it

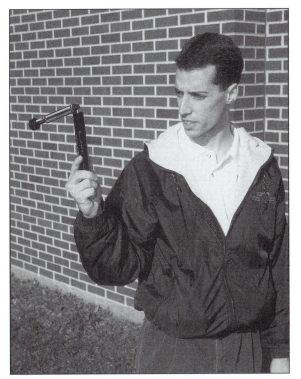

■ **Figure 16.2**   Sling psychrometer.

Reprinted, by permission, from S. Hillman, 2000, *Introduction to athletic training* (Champaign, IL: Human Kinetics), 218.

Table 16.1   Heat Stress Index

	Air temperature (°F)									
	70°	**75°**	**80°**	**85°**	**90°**	**95°**	**100°**	**105°**	**110°**	**115°**
	Heat sensation									
0%	64°	69°	73°	78°	83°	87°	91°	95°	99°	107°
10%	65°	70°	75°	80°	85°	90°	95°	100°	105°	111°
20%	66°	72°	77°	82°	87°	93°	99°	105°	112°	120°
30%	67°	73°	78°	84°	90°	96°	104°	113°	123°	135°
40%	68°	74°	79°	86°	93°	101°	110°	123°	137°	151°
50%	69°	76°	81°	88°	96°	107°	120°	135°	150°	
60%	70°	76°	82°	90°	100°	114°	132°	149°		
70%	71°	77°	85°	93°	106°	124°	144°			
80%	72°	78°	86°	97°	113°	136°				
90%	73°	79°	88°	102°	122°					

Reprinted, by permission, from W.D. McArdle, F.I. Katch, and V.L. Katch, 2000, *Essentials of exercise physiology,* 2nd ed. (Philadelphia, PA: Lippincott, Williams, and Wilkins).

Table 16.2   Practice and Competition Recommendations

Temperature	Recommendation
Heat sensation below 90° F	No adjustments needed
Heat sensation 91-104° F	Increase rest breaks, increase fluid intake, monitor for signs of heat illness
Heat sensations 105-129° F	Adjust practice time or activity. Decrease intensity unless acclimated. Monitor for heat illness. Change wet clothing during breaks.
Heat sensation 130° F and above	Consider suspending activity or changing time of day. Extreme caution must be taken. Risk for heat illness is high.

Adapted, by permission, from S. Hillman, 2000, *Introduction to athletic training* (Champaign, IL: Human Kinetics), 220.

will allow the athletic trainer the opportunity to monitor hypohydration states for athletes who are not replacing lost fluids. Athletes who lose 5% or more of their body weight over several days should be evaluated by a physician and their activity restricted until they are rehydrated. Do not permit athletes to work out if they are more than 3% dehydrated in 1 d (i.e., they have lost more than 3% of the body weight they had at the beginning of the day). Monitoring weight is especially important when there is more than one workout per day. Provide frequent water breaks during workouts in hot weather. Table 16.2 provides practice and competition recommendations based on the temperature and relative humidity.

In addition to identifying at-risk athletes and providing proper fluids to ensure hydration, the other factor that appears to have the greatest impact on preventing heat-related illnesses is acclimatization. People must acclimatize themselves to the heat. Heat acclimatization refers to the physiological adaptations that improve heat tolerance. Several physiological adaptations take place as acclimatization improves. These include the following:

Strategies for Preventing Heat Illness

Obtain a complete medical history. Athletes with a history of heat-related illness must be identified. Previous episodes of heat illness are risk factors for future events.

Acclimatize gradually. Gradual exposure to warm environments combined with good aerobic fitness is an essential prevention strategy. A period of 7 to 10 d is needed to achieve acclimatization.

Wear proper clothing and uniforms. Lightweight, lightly colored clothing that helps transfer sweat away from the body is desirable. Avoid dark colors that absorb solar radiation. If sweating is significant, rest periods that allow for changing from wet to dry clothing are advised. Athletes participating in activities that require lots of protective equipment (e.g., football) should slowly acclimate to the full required equipment. Rubberized clothing that does not transfer sweat away from the body should *never* be used.

Monitor environmental conditions. The air temperature and relative humidity must be measured. Wet-bulb, dry-bulb, and globe temperatures can be taken to assess the impact of the humidity, temperature, and solar radiation.

Fluid replacement. Water must be available to athletes as needed. Make sure athletes follow these guidelines:

Before Exercise

Drink 17 to 20 oz of water or a sports drink 2 to 3 h before exercise.

Ten to 20 min before exercise drink another 7 to 10 oz of water or a sports drink.

During Exercise

Drink early. Even minimal dehydration compromises performance.

In general, every 10 to 20 min drink at least 7 to 10 oz of water or a sports drink.

To maintain hydration, remember to drink beyond your thirst. Optimally, drink fluids based on amount of sweat and urine loss.

After Exercise

Within 2 h drink enough to replace any weight loss from exercise.

Drink approximately 20 to 24 oz of a sports drink per pound of weight loss.

Avoid diuretics. Substances that act as stimulants may increase your risk of heat illness. In addition, diuretics cause increases in fluid loss and can contribute to poor hydration states. Caffeine and ephedra are stimulants commonly found in over-the-counter nutritional supplements.

Use weight charts. Recording pre- and postpractice body weights will assist in determining the amount of fluid lost during a single practice session. In addition, it will allow the athletic trainer the opportunity to monitor hypohydration states for athletes who are not replacing lost fluids.

Identify athletes at risk. History of heat illness, poor acclimatization, poor fitness, increased body fat, athletes who are febrile (have a fever), poorly hydrated athletes, and those with a history of pushing themselves to capacity are at increased risk and should be monitored appropriately.

Educate. Participants, coaches, and support personnel must all be aware of the signs and symptoms of heat-related illness. The responsibility for a safe environment is shared; it is not the sole domain of the athletic trainer.

Adapted, by permission, from NCAA Committee on Competitive Safeguards and Medical Aspects of Sports, 2002, *2001-2002 NCAA Sports Medicine Handbook* (Indianapolis: NCAA), 22-24.

- Improved peripheral blood flow
- Earlier onset of sweating
- Greater volume of sweat

All of these adaptations will assist with improved heat dissipation. The acclimatized person must be properly hydrated to keep these systems functioning at an optimal level. Gradual exposure to the heat will improve the capacity for exercise with less discomfort during elevated temperatures. A period of 7 to 10 d is needed to achieve acclimatization. Exercise must begin for short periods and increase gradually. Unfortunately the major physiological benefits of acclimatization will dissipate 2 to 3 weeks after temperatures return to a temperate level.

COLD-RELATED INJURIES

When exposed to cold, the body adapts to keep the heart, lungs, and central nervous system warm. The body produces extra heat in three ways: (1) by increasing basal metabolism; (2) by increasing muscle activity (which may include shivering, exercise, or both); and (3) through **nonshivering thermogenesis,** a metabolic adaptation involving thyroid hormone and epinephrine (adrenaline). Symptoms of hypothermia begin when the body can no longer keep up with heat loss.

Hypothermia

Hypothermia is defined as a core temperature that falls below 95° F (32.2° C). Between a core temperature of about 95° and 98° F (35.0-36.7° C), a person feels cold and begins shivering. There is numbness in the skin and slight motor impairment. With a core body temperature from about 93° to 95° F (33.9-35.0° C), there is a profound feeling of deep cold and numbness, violent shivering, more-severe problems with muscular coordination, difficulty speaking, mental confusion, and memory loss; the skin becomes pale and cold. Below about 91° F (32.8° C), a person stops shivering and becomes incoherent and irrational; muscles become rigid, and the individual generally can neither walk nor stand. If the core temperature drops below 86° F (30.0° C), coma ensues and the heart may go into fibrillation. Below about 80° F (26.7° C), there is respiratory failure and the heart stops. Keep in mind, of course, that a person's descent into these various stages is gradual and that individual differences exist in the manifestation of symptoms and in the temperatures at which they are evident.

Anyone who is shivering probably has a core temperature greater than 90° F, with mild hypothermia. This level of hypothermia can almost always be treated in the field. First, get the athlete out of the cold and wind and into a tent or other shelter to prevent further heat loss. Replace wet clothing with dry. Cover the head (a great deal of heat is lost from the head), and have her lie down. Do not let her sit, stand, or walk until she is rewarmed. Whenever possible, get the person to a hospital. Any warming device can help with mild hypothermia. Have the athlete drink warm or hot beverages (but not alcohol). Warm her with a sleeping bag, hot water bottle, or heating pad. Hot tubs are useful if available. Be careful, of course, that none of these devices are so hot that they cause burns.

Someone with very dull mental reactions who is not shivering probably has a core temperature of 90° F (32.2° C) or lower, with moderate to severe hypothermia. The highest priority in this case is to prevent further heat loss. *Make no attempt to rewarm such an athlete in the field, since serious—even fatal—electrolyte and metabolic changes can occur that are impossible to diagnose or treat in the field.* Follow the usual procedures of basic life support, except that cardiopulmonary resuscitation should not be given unless ventricular fibrillation is likely. In severe hypothermia, the chest may be rigid and incompressible. Transport the athlete to an emergency facility as soon as possible. Remember that a person is not dead until he is warm and dead. The pulse of an extremely cold person can be so slow that it is difficult to assess, and people who were taken for dead have been successfully resuscitated. At low temperatures, the brain and vital organs have some protection from damage.

Frostbite

Frostbite is cold injury to the extremities. *Superficial frostbite* involves the outer layers of the skin. The mildest form of this is called *frostnip*, whose symptoms include a burning feeling followed by numbness, and a grayish or pale area of skin, usually on the face or extremities; deeper tissues are soft and pliable. After thawing, the area becomes red, sensitive, and swollen to varying degrees. In more severe cases, a few small blisters may appear. A few days later, the skin is shed by flaking or peeling.

Superficial frostbite can be thawed on the spot by direct body heat—for example, placing a warm hand on a frozen cheek or holding a frozen finger under the armpit inside a jacket. In some cases, you may have to add protective layers of clothing to athletes with superficial frostbite or take them to a shelter where the entire body can be warmed.

Deep frostbite is less common and much more damaging. It occurs most often in the ears, nose, fingers, toes, and extremities. The affected part typically becomes painfully cold; then it stops hurting, becomes numb, and feels like a block of wood. The affected body part appears cold, firm, rigid, pale, or waxy, resembling a piece of chicken meat removed from the freezer. After the area thaws, blisters develop within hours to days.

It is best to rewarm deep frostbite under controlled conditions in a hospital—warming the body part too quickly can increase tissue damage. Refreezing is especially dangerous to the tissue. If there is deep-tissue damage and blood circulation does not return, **gangrene** may develop and the damaged tissue must be removed surgically, usually by amputating that part of the extremity. Loss of fingers and toes is a common complication of prolonged exposure to the cold.

Prevention of Hypothermia and Frostbite

There are two fairly obvious ways by which people can prevent hypothermia and frostbite. First, they can *increase heat production.* Eating regularly to keep glycogen and fat stores replenished is helpful, especially for athletes who will be working out or competing in the cold. Voluntary muscular activity produces heat much more effectively than the involuntary activity of shivering.

Second, they can *decrease heat loss* by wearing adequate clothing and by covering vulnerable body parts (figure 16.3). Instruct athletes to wear enough to stay warm and dry. Clothing insulates more effectively when worn in layers; tight garments interfere with the insulating effect. Dress in layers and make every effort to stay dry. Wear a base layer that will not stay wet. Base layers should *wick* or move the perspiration away from your skin. The best fabrics for covering the body are polypropylene, treated polyesters such as Capilene®, and hollow-core polyesters such as Thermastat®. Cotton is a poor base layer because it holds moisture.

The head should be covered to prevent excess heat loss; jackets should have hoods. The outside layer of a garment should provide wind protection and ideally should be water repellent (e.g., Gore-Tex®). When the temperature is below freezing, consider one layer of protective clothing for every 5 mph of wind. Remember to dress in base layers to wick moisture, middle layers for warmth, and outer layers to stop wind. Cotton is a poor insulator and is even worse when wet. Pile garments such as down, Dacron®, Hollofil®, and Thinsulate™ are too thick for many activities. Fleece is a good second layer for trapping warmth.

In very cold environments, athletes should cover the face, extremities, head, eyes, hands, and feet. Covering the face requires use of a face mask or neck gaiter. Fingers and toes need extra protection even during intense exercise. The best gloves are made with polypropylene or wool; wool or pile mittens with a windproof shell are best in extreme conditions. Shoes should be large enough to

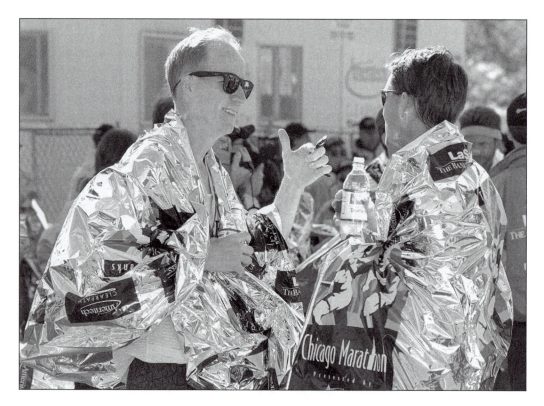

■ **Figure 16.3**   Athletes warming up after a race with aluminum foil wraps.

accommodate several layers of socks. For running, there should be at least one inner pair of polypropylene socks and at least one outer layer of heavy wool socks. Instruct male athletes to pay special attention to their genitalia and nipples if they are exercising in conditions of extreme cold. Insulated, windproof front panels for running shorts are helpful in protecting the genitalia. Women should wear insulated bras to protect their nipples from cold injury. Runners are at higher risk for hypothermia due to constant exposure and the energy demands of exercising in the cold (Sallis and Chassay 1999). Keeping the trunk warm also helps extremities, especially areas of high blood flow such as the groin, armpits, and neck. A good ski cap works well for the head; because of the high blood flow to the head, an uncovered head can account for 25% to 50% of an individual's heat loss.

It is extremely important to remain dry. People can develop hypothermia even at 70° F (21.1° C) if they are wet and exposed to the wind. (A woman we know who moved from Wisconsin to Houston said that Houston was the coldest place she had ever been, because she was so often exposed to drizzle when she exercised outdoors—even though winter temperatures were rarely below 40° F [4.4° C].) Instruct athletes to remove wet clothing as soon as possible and replace it with dry clothing. If you can postpone a workout to avoid cold rain or wet snow, do so. It is always best for athletes to exercise when they can remain dry.

HIGH ALTITUDE

High altitude stresses the human body in several ways. The most significant stressor is the decreased amount of oxygen available to the lungs. Greater levels of ultraviolet light also increase the risk of sunburn (and eventually of skin cancer). The air is drier and colder at altitude, with temperature decreasing on average about 11.7° F (6.5° C) every 1,000 m (3,281 ft). Dealing with athletes exposed to

Altitude Definitions

Health professionals use the following generally accepted definitions when referring to altitude above sea level:

Extremely high altitude	Above 5,000 m (16,405 ft)
High altitude	3,000-4,999 meters (9,843-16,404 ft)
Moderately high altitude	2,000-2,999 m (6,562-9,842 ft)
Low altitude	1,000-1,999 m (3,281-6,561 ft)
Sea level	0-999 meters (0-3,280 ft)

extreme altitude is not a common occurrence for most sports medicine professionals. However, those who work with teams that travel to high altitude may find an understanding of the physiology associated with high altitude helpful.

The reduction in available oxygen at higher altitudes dramatically reduces the body's ability to work. Any exercise that requires aerobic metabolism is more difficult to perform at altitude, but short sprints or track events such as jumping or throwing, which depend primarily on anaerobic metabolism (glycolysis) rather than aerobic processes, are generally no more difficult.

Acclimatization

Chronic exposure to altitude induces physiological adaptations that improve the body's ability to do work. The most immediate adaptation is an increase in ventilation that enhances oxygen delivery to blood vessels in the lungs. (Unfortunately, the hyperventilation expels so much excess carbon dioxide that it makes the blood **alkalotic**—that is, less acidic, with pH > 7.45. This alkalosis reduces the efficiency of the body's enzymes; over time it also causes loss of minerals that may be excreted in the urine. Although alkalosis is dangerous, healthy kidneys correct it by excreting bicarbonate in the urine over the first 5 to 7 d of exposure to high altitude.) The heart rate increases, and the heart pumps harder to increase oxygen delivery to muscle and other tissues. Oxygen-carrying capacity increases in 1 to 2 d from an increase in hemoglobin (the oxygen-carrying molecule) concentration and an increase in hematocrit (the percentage of blood volume that is composed of red blood cells)—both caused by a small decrease in blood plasma because the kidneys are excreting more water. Over weeks and months at high altitude, the lower amount of oxygen delivered to the kidneys increases their production of **erythropoietin,** a hormone that stimulates the bone marrow to make more red blood cells. Athletes must have adequate dietary intake of iron at higher altitudes, because the bone marrow cannot respond if the body has inadequate iron stores.

For competitions at even moderately high altitude, athletes from lower altitudes should try to provide time for acclimatization. Although a minimum of 1 week is required, some athletes need about 2 weeks to adjust to lower oxygen levels. When acclimatization is not possible, anecdotal experience suggests that competing immediately upon arrival may optimize performance. Athletes in endurance events have attempted to take advantage of the physiological changes at altitude to improve their performance at sea level. Research has shown that living at altitude and training at altitude do not seem to improve performance at sea level because it is so difficult to train intensely at altitude (Fulco et al. 2000). Living at altitude (e.g., at 2,500 m [8,202 ft]) and training close to sea level (e.g., 1,200 m [3,937 ft]), however, do seem to improve performance at sea level. That way an athlete can train hard yet still get the physiological benefit of altitude. Those athletes who live and train at altitude year-round and compete at sea level may have an advantage over those who live and train at sea level.

High-Altitude Illness

Failure of the body to acclimate can lead to **acute mountain sickness (AMS),** the symptoms of which include headache, nausea, loss of appetite, fatigue, and difficulty sleeping. AMS rarely occurs below about 7,000 ft (2,130 m); it can strike people of any age or health status. The chances of experiencing severe symptoms tend to be proportional to altitude and to the rapidity of ascent; though it is not practical in most cases, once people are above 7,000 to 8,000 ft (approx. 2,132 to 2,440 m), they ideally should ascend only about 1,000 additional feet (305 m) per day to avoid AMS.

Usually the symptoms of AMS are mild and self-limiting. Sleep can exacerbate AMS, because breathing is shallower during sleep. Because sedatives (including alcohol) produce the same effect as sleep, they should be avoided (although analgesics such as aspirin or ibuprofen are OK for treating the pain of headaches). If possible, people with AMS should not sleep at high altitudes until their symptoms have cleared. If they must remain at high altitudes, however, they should *rest* (not sleep) as much as possible, preferably with feet elevated above the head. Because dehydration is a partial cause of AMS, they should remain well hydrated and

For Further Information

Print Resources

American College of Sports Medicine. 1996. Position stand on exercise and fluid replacement. *Medicine and Science in Sports and Exercise* 28: i-vii. Available at www.acsm-msse.org

American College of Sports Medicine. 1996. Position stand on heat and cold illnesses during distance running. *Medicine and Science in Sports and Exercise* 28: 12. Available at www.acsm-msse.org

Bellis, F. 2002. Acute mountain sickness: An unexpected management problem. *British Journal of Sports Medicine* 36(2): 147.

Bouvhama, A., and Knochel, J.P. 2002. Heat stroke. *New England Journal of Medicine* 346(25): 1978-88.

Moran, D.S. 2001. Potential applications of heat and cold stress indices to sporting events. *Sports Medicine* 31(13): 909-17.

Web Resources

National Athletic Trainers' Association
www.nata.org
Copies of position statements regarding fluid replacement and exercise in the heat, and lightning safety can be found at the NATA Web site.

National Collegiate Athletic Association
www1.ncaa.org/membership/ed_outreach/health-safety/index.html
Links to NCAA Sports Sciences page provide copies of position papers, NCAA-sponsored research, and links to the sports medicine handbook. The Sports Sciences section is under the guidance of the NCAA Committee on Competitive Safeguards and Medical Aspects of Sports.

National Lightning Safety Institute
www.lightningsafety.com
The National Lightning Safety Institute (NLSI) is an independent, nonprofit consulting, education, and research organization that advocates a proactive risk-management approach to lightning safety.

should avoid caffeine and other diuretics. If rest, water, and treatment with analgesics do not ameliorate the symptoms (and they usually do), descent to a lower altitude will provide relief. Medical treatments that may help include acetazolamide (brand name Diamox®) and the anti-inflammatory dexamethasone (brand names Decadron®, Dexon®), which also are sometimes used to help prevent AMS. Because acetazolamide is a diuretic, it is particularly important for people receiving this drug to replenish their fluids. How these medications work to relieve and prevent altitude sickness is not clear.

LIGHTNING

The final environmental issue we will discuss is lightning. Of all weather-related hazards, lightning is the one that most consistently can affect athletic events. The

Lightning Safety Recommendations

A comprehensive lightning-safety policy should include the following:

- A designated chain of command that establishes who should make the call to remove participants and spectators from the athletic activity.
- A designated weather watcher. This person will actively look for signs of threatening weather and notify the chain of command if conditions warrant.
- A method for monitoring local weather forecasts and warnings.
- Knowing where the closest safe structures or locations are located near the athletic fields or playing areas.
- The primary choice for a safe location from the lightning hazard is any building normally occupied or frequently used by people. Buildings with plumbing or electrical wiring can act to electronically ground the structure. Avoid using showers for safe shelter, and do not use the shower of plumbing facilities during a thunderstorm.
- If a building is unavailable, any vehicle with a hard metal roof can serve as protection. The roof can dissipate the lightning strike. *DO NOT TOUCH THE SIDES OF THE VEHICLE.*
- Educating participants as to how to minimize the body's surface area to help avoid a ground strike.
- If a safe structure cannot be found, try to find a thick grove of small trees surrounded by taller trees or a dry ditch. Assume a crouched position with only the balls of your feet touching the ground, wrap your arms around your knees, and lower your head. *MINIMIZE YOUR BODY'S SURFACE AREA, AND MINIMIZE CONTACT WITH THE GROUND! DO NOT LIE FLAT!*
- Avoid tall objects, metal objects, standing water, and individual trees. Never take shelter under a single tall tree.
- Be aware of how close the lightning is occurring. Use appropriate lightning-detection technology or the strike-to-bang method (see *Strike-to-Bang Method*).
- Established criteria for suspension and resumption of activities.

Adapted, by permission, from NCAA Committee on Competitive Safeguards and Medical Aspects of Sports, 2002, *2001-2002 NCAA Sports Medicine Handbook* (Indianapolis: NCAA), 12-14.

Strike-to-Bang Method

- The observer begins counting when a lightning flash is sighted.
- Counting is stopped when the associated bang (thunder) is heard.
- Divide this count by 5 to determine the distance to the lightning flash (in miles).

Walsh et al. 2000.

National Severe Storms Laboratory (NSSL) estimates that 100 fatalities and 400 to 500 injuries requiring medical treatment occur from lightning strikes annually. Lightning strikes occur most often in the summer between late morning and early evening. These are times of year and times of day when athletic and outdoor activities frequently take place. Athletic facilities are often open spaces surrounded by tall backstops and metal poles that make them targets for lightning strikes. Direct strikes are only one mechanism of lightning injury. Injury can occur from indirect mechanisms such as touching an object that is struck, being next to an object that has been stuck, the ground itself, or being thrown by the force of a strike.

The key to lightning safety is prevention and education. Institutions must develop a lightning-safety policy that can provide written guidelines for safety during lightning storms. Walsh et al. (2000) found that 92% of National Collegiate Athletic Association (NCAA) Division I athletic departments responding to a survey did not have a formal, written lightning-safety policy. The National Athletic Trainers Association (NATA) has established a position statement on lightning safety for athletics and recreation. See *Lightning Safety Recommendations* on page 255 for a summary of recommendations for lightning safety.

SUMMARY

1. *Explain the metabolic and environmental factors that contribute to heat loss and heat gain.*

Muscles may generate over 20 times as much energy during maximal exercise as they do at rest. At maximal exercise, the human body's work efficiency is approximately 25%—which means roughly 75% of the muscle energy consumption is converted to heat rather than work. Early in exercise, heat production exceeds heat loss, thereby increasing core body temperature. Exercising muscles lose heat in four ways: evaporation, radiation, convection, and conduction. Evaporation is the conversion of a liquid into a vapor. Radiation is the transmission of heat energy from a surface. Convection is transmission of heat in a fluid by circulation of the fluid's heated molecules. Conduction is the transfer of heat from one substance to an adjacent substance. Heat from muscle is conducted to the adjacent blood vessels and carried by convection to the heart and out into the arteries into the small vessels in the skin. The heat is conducted to the surface of the skin, where it is radiated into the air. Heat is also lost by evaporation via sweat and via the moisture in exhaled gases. Radiation and convection dissipate most of the heat from the body when the ambient temperature is <68° F (20° C). In warm environments, evaporation is the most physiologically important means of heat loss in human beings. During heavy exercise, evaporation can account for up to 85% of the heat loss.

2. *Recognize the spectrum of heat- and cold-related injury and illnesses.*

The spectrum of heat illness ranges from very mild symptoms to heatstroke and death. The most serious of the heat illnesses is heatstroke, which is a medical emergency. Heatstroke occurs when the elevation in body temperature is >5° F (2.8° C). Athletes with heatstroke appear confused, disoriented, and agitated; when heatstroke is severe, they may exhibit hysterical behavior, be delirious, have seizures, or collapse. The hallmark of heatstroke is profound central nervous system dysfunction such as confusion, disorientation, and agitation. In traditional heatstroke the patient is hot, flushed, and dry with no sweating; this form of heatstroke usually occurs in the elderly and is not related to exercise. Athletes and physically active individuals who suffer heatstroke will most often experience exertional heatstroke. These patients will exhibit the signs and symptoms of traditional heatstroke; their skin, however, may appear wet from the profuse sweating that took place before their collapse.

Cold injuries may run the spectrum from skin and tissue injury associated with exposure to hypothermia. Symptoms of hypothermia begin when the body can no longer keep up with heat loss. Prolonged exposure with significant drops in core temperature can lead to system failures and ultimately death.

3. *Describe appropriate prevention strategies to avoid heat- and cold-related conditions.*

With proper planning and attention to prevention strategies, athletes can avoid most problems associated with environmental stresses. Mild symptoms of heat illness are common, and most are preventable with adequate fluid intake, adequate electrolyte intake, proper use of cool-downs after major workouts or competitions, and judicious scheduling of events for cooler times of day. Athletes can prevent cold injuries by wearing adequate clothing, remaining dry, maintaining appropriate dietary intakes, and postponing workouts or competitions until the weather is less dangerous.

4. *List the factors that make up an appropriate lightning-safety plan.*

The key to lightning safety is prevention and education. Institutions must educate participants and supervisors about strategies to minimize the risk of a lightning-strike injury. In addition, institutions should develop a lightning-safety policy that can provide written guidelines for safety during lightning storms. Such a policy should include a designated chain of command, a designated weather watcher, a method for monitoring local weather forecasts and warnings, identification of the closest safe structures or locations near the athletic fields or playing areas, and criteria for suspension and resumption of activities.

5. *Identify the potential problems associated with exercise at altitude.*

Failure of the body to acclimate can lead to acute mountain sickness (AMS), the symptoms of which include headache, nausea, loss of appetite, fatigue, and difficulty sleeping. Athletes who will compete at altitude will benefit from a gradual acclimatization. Although AMS is usually self-limiting, active people should avoid rapid ascents (particularly those above 7,000 ft) when possible.

CHAPTER 17

Psychological Aspects of Sport and Rehabilitation

OBJECTIVES

Upon completion of this chapter the reader will be able to do the following:

1. Identify psychological issues related to injury and rehabilitation

2. Describe common mental health issues, including mood and anxiety disorders

3. Explain specific mental-imaging techniques to assist athletes in preparing for competition

Tiger Woods, Boris Becker, Eric Heiden, Bonnie Blair, Wayne Gretzky, Mary Lou Retton, and Michael Jordan are all superstar athletes who have excelled in their sports at least in part because of a psychological mastery over their competitors. In these instances the mind affects performance during competition. Great athletes also may exhibit psychological strength on the sidelines—having an easier time recovering from difficult practice sessions, for example, or finding it relatively easy to deal with injury, illness, or rehabilitation. The purpose of this chapter is to help you recognize the normal and abnormal emotions of athletes, and to help you understand the psychological factors that affect sport performance.

Case Study

A basketball player has recently been diagnosed with a tear in her anterior cruciate ligament. She expresses frustration and is visibly angry that her season is over. Her teammates report that she is withdrawn, she socially isolates herself, and she seems to have rapidly changing emotions. A history of depression runs in her family. Because of her family history and singularly negative response to her injury, you do two things:

- You refer her to a sport psychologist for counseling.
- In consultation with the physician who is treating her torn ligament, you devise a rehabilitation protocol that permits her to perform workouts *in the presence of the team* so that she can be building up those muscles that are not affected by her injury while maintaining her aerobic fitness with an eye toward next year's season.

PERSONALITY TRAITS OF ATHLETES

Data from a number of researchers indicate that on average, athletes have psychological and behavioral profiles somewhat different from those of nonathletes. Morgan and colleagues reported that compared to nonathletes, athletes exhibited higher levels of vigor and extroversion—and lower levels of tension, depression, anger, fatigue, neuroticism, and confusion (Morgan et al. 1987; Raglin et al. 1991). On the other hand, athletes studied by Nattiv and Puffer (1991) on average consumed more alcohol per sitting than nonathletes, were more likely to drive while intoxicated, were less likely to wear seat belts or motorcycle helmets, and were more likely to engage in a variety of risky sexual behaviors. Studies within genders have shown similar differences: Compared to male nonathletic counterparts, male athletes were more likely to ride with a driver under the influence, fight, use snuff, and engage in thrill-seeking behavior. Women athletes, however, were less likely than female nonathletes to use alcohol, cigarettes, or marijuana (Kokotailo et al. 1996).

Not only do athletes tend to differ from nonathletes, but male athletes tend to have different personality traits than female athletes. In a study by Pedersen (1997), male athletes tended to be more active, aggressive, competitive, dominating, and controlling; females were more goal oriented, organized, and governed by rules.

Teams can even exhibit personality traits, which often are characterized by a culture—the combination of underlying beliefs, values, and behaviors shared in common by the team. Try to become sensitive to personality differences among both individuals and teams, because these traits can affect a team's overall health, response to success or failure, and rate of injury.

PSYCHOLOGY OF INJURY AND REHABILITATION

Psychosocial factors strongly influence the risk of injury (figure 17.1). Psychosocial stress, overtraining syndrome (burnout), risk taking, coping mechanisms, and

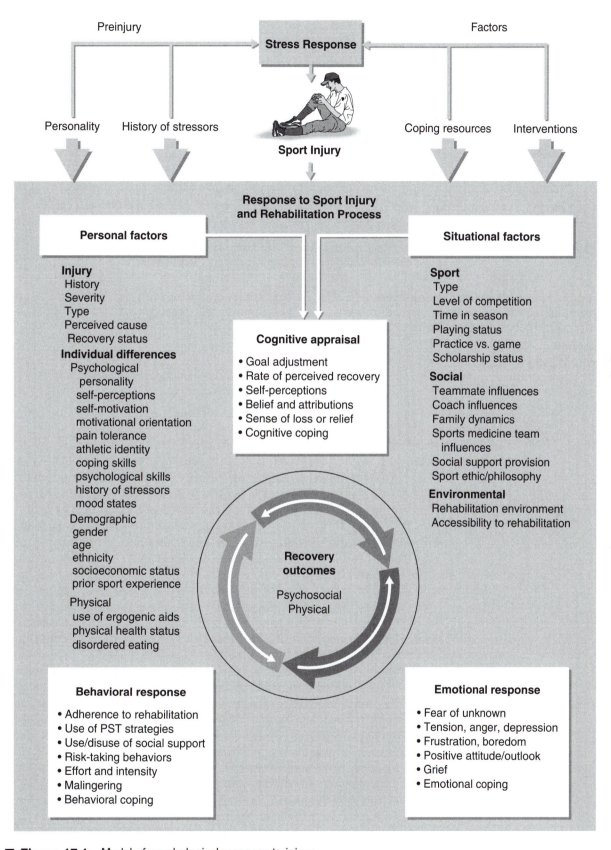

Preinjury

Stress Response

Factors

Personality   History of stressors   Coping resources   Interventions

Sport Injury

**Response to Sport Injury
and Rehabilitation Process**

Personal factors

Situational factors

Injury
History
Severity
Type
Perceived cause
Recovery status

Individual differences
Psychological
  personality
  self-perceptions
  self-motivation
  motivational orientation
  pain tolerance
  athletic identity
  coping skills
  psychological skills
  history of stressors
  mood states
Demographic
  gender
  age
  ethnicity
  socioeconomic status
  prior sport experience

Physical
  use of ergogenic aids
  physical health status
  disordered eating

Cognitive appraisal

• Goal adjustment
• Rate of perceived recovery
• Self-perceptions
• Belief and attributions
• Sense of loss or relief
• Cognitive coping

Sport
Type
Level of competition
Time in season
Playing status
Practice vs. game
Scholarship status

Social
Teammate influences
Coach influences
Family dynamics
Sports medicine team
  influences
Social support provision
Sport ethic/philosophy

Environmental
Rehabilitation environment
Accessibility to rehabilitation

**Recovery
outcomes**

Psychosocial
Physical

Behavioral response

• Adherence to rehabilitation
• Use of PST strategies
• Use/disuse of social support
• Risk-taking behaviors
• Effort and intensity
• Malingering
• Behavioral coping

Emotional response

• Fear of unknown
• Tension, anger, depression
• Frustration, boredom
• Positive attitude/outlook
• Grief
• Emotional coping

■ **Figure 17.1** Model of psychological response to injury.

Terms and Definitions

malingering—In athletes, intentionally pretending to have symptoms of mental or physical illness to avoid returning to play. Usually involves a conscious decision to intentionally deceive sports medicine professionals about their injury.

obsessive-compulsive disorder (OCD)—Recurrent obsessions or compulsions that are severe enough to be time consuming or cause marked distress or significant impairment.

paresthesia—Tingling or prickly sensation in the skin.

psychiatrist—A medical doctor who treats individuals with behavioral or mental disorders; main function is to prescribe drugs that can ameliorate symptoms of disorders.

psychologist—A professional with clinical training (usually a PhD) who treats behavioral or mental disorders through psychotherapy and does not prescribe drugs.

secondary gain—An unconscious advantage a patient may receive from physical illness or other complaints. Athletes who unconsciously perceive advantages to negative events such as injuries, defeats, and the like may not do their best to overcome their compromised situation.

selective serotonin reuptake inhibitor (SSRI)—A medication that blocks the reuptake of the neurotransmitter serotonin into neurons and has only weak effects on the reuptake of other neurotransmitters such as norepinephrine and dopamine.

tricyclic antidepressant (TCAD)—A medication that is composed of three chemical rings and is used to treat depression.

psychosocial support all can affect both the risk of injury and recovery from injury (Ahern and Lohr 1997).

A study at the Mayo Clinic showed that injured athletes, regardless of gender or age, often experience frustration, anger, and depression after the initial assessment of an injury. When injuries are relatively mild, the mood disturbance usually subsides within 2 weeks after the injury as the athlete returns to active participation in sport. For athletes with a more severe injury, emotional symptoms tend not to abate until about 4 weeks after the injury (Smith et al. 1990). Some athletes have a prolonged emotional response and may require psychotherapy to cope with the stress of imposed rest, rehabilitation, and the pressure to return to sport.

Ideally, people derive their sense of self-worth from a broad scope of individuals, events, and experiences. For some athletes, however, a great deal of their self-worth derives from their sport and their daily exercise routine. Most of the time, this is not a problem—but injury or illness can remove a large component of their self-identity, leading to problems with self-esteem, isolation, feelings of helplessness, and anxiety. These negative feelings increase athletes' difficulties in overcoming an injury, completing the rehabilitation process, and returning to their sport in a timely manner. Although a few athletes may use their injury as an excuse to quit their sport because of burnout or some other reason, most athletes want to continue to participate and are extremely frustrated when they are away from their sport and team. *Do all within your power to keep injured athletes involved in sport, even on a limited basis, to help them maintain their athletic identity.* One useful approach is to have athletes perform their rehabilitation in the physical presence of the team; another is to work on specific techniques that may improve the athletes' overall performance after rehabilitation. Your goal is to help athletes focus their obsessive traits, determination, goal setting, and physical abilities on the rehabilitation process to make it a more positive experience.

Athletes who continue to have difficulty with the rehabilitation process may be developing **secondary gain**—an unconscious indulgence in the benefits of adversity. The increased attention a player receives after an injury, for example, can lead him to unconsciously extend the rehabilitation period as long as possible. Do your best to read between the lines in dealing with injured athletes so that you can learn to recognize secondary gain when it occurs. You then need to explore the issue with the athlete: In some cases if you simply bring up the possibility that the individual is unconsciously benefiting from his injury and explore the ramifications in a completely nonthreatening and nonaccusing manner, that may be enough to motivate the athlete to move forward in the rehabilitation process. If the athlete continues to have difficulty, you may need to refer him to a psychologist.

The other possible reason for extremely prolonged rehabilitation may involve **malingering**—a conscious decision the athlete makes, because of fears, attention, liability issues, or perhaps to gain a year of eligibility at the collegiate level, to fake symptoms or pain. Other causes of malingering may include loss of starting position on the team, lack of desire to continue to play the sport but fear of disappointing a parent or coach, and failure to live up to others' expectations as the level of competition increases. Maintaining a trusting, caring, empathetic relationship with the athlete is essential to help you recognize these psychological factors so that you can offer psychological support and the athlete can move past these obstacles of rehabilitation if possible.

Compliance with the rehabilitation plan is another area where you may have to employ psychological tools to assess whether an athlete is doing too much or too little. *One trick for improved compliance is to convince athletes to view rehab as an inherent part of their athletic performance.* This approach can lead athletes not only to develop other areas of their bodies that their sport-specific training may be neglecting, but also to remain focused on the same rituals of setting goals, practicing, and achieving goals that they use when they are healthy.

The psychological effects of an injury also involve cognitive components. Athletes continually think about the perceived cause of their injury and their perceived recovery status. They may worry about changes to their role on the team; collegiate and professional athletes may worry about losing their scholarships and incomes, respectively. How an athlete copes with all of these perceptions and worries will greatly influence his recovery and compliance with therapy. Social support from teammates, friends, family, coaches, and medical professionals can greatly influence the athlete's coping ability.

Case Study

A 20-yr-old female field hockey player comes to you with fatigue. She has been playing elite-level field hockey for the last 5 yr and has not taken a break from her sport for the last 2 yr until a recent knee injury forced her to take a 2-month layoff. Now that she has returned, she does not seem connected with the team. You take her history and determine that her diet has not changed, her weight is stable, and she is not suffering from any other symptoms such as fever, chills, sweats, hair loss, gastrointestinal symptoms, sore throat, swollen joints, or any other illness she can identify. She denies any possibility of pregnancy. Ruling out almost any medical problem, you turn your attention to possible psychiatric disorders. You notice her affect (mood) is extremely flat and she has no energy. On further questioning, she reports a recent breakup with a significant other, problems relating to teammates, overwhelming fatigue, spontaneous crying without reason, and difficulty getting out of bed in the morning. When questioned about self-harm, she relates occasional suicidal thoughts but no mechanism of how she would follow through on them. At your suggestion she agrees to meet with a psychologist and would also like to consider medication, as this has helped her mother.

ATHLETES AND MENTAL ILLNESS

Athletes suffer from mental illnesses just as often as nonathletes do. Overidentification as an athlete can contribute to some of these disorders, although other factors are certainly important, such as family history, death, divorce, injury, or illness. Major life events that affect an athlete's practice schedule, performance, or interpersonal relationships may contribute to the development of mental illness—especially in people genetically predisposed to mental health problems. Because you work with athletes on a regular basis, *you may be the first person to recognize a problem;* therefore you must have a practical understanding of the signs and symptoms of common psychiatric disorders so that you can refer athletes to appropriate professionals at appropriate times.

Mood Disorders

Mood disorders (which are fairly common among athletes and nonathletes alike) include major depression, dysthymia, and bipolar disorders. Affected athletes demonstrate impairments in psychosocial, academic, and athletic functioning. Note that athletes with mood disorders sometimes *do not* overtly display changes in mood, exhibiting instead decreased energy, poor performance, or dissatisfaction with their sport.

Depressive disorders include major depression and dysthymia. Diagnosis with major depression requires that an individual have a disturbance of mood (sadness, irritability) that affects feelings and behavior nearly every day for most of the day; or there must be loss of interest or pleasure in most activities nearly every day for most of the day. In addition, five of seven other associated symptoms must be present (see *Symptoms of Major Depression*). Major depression can be episodic, with full recovery between episodes.

Dysthymia denotes a chronically depressed mood that is less intense than major depression but has no prolonged well states—that is, it is less episodic. By definition, the depressed mood must be evident to self or others for at least 1 yr in children and adolescents, and for at least 2 yr in adults. Associated symptoms include at least two of the following: poor appetite, sleep disorder (either hypersomnia or insomnia), low energy, low self-esteem, poor concentration, and feelings of hopelessness.

Symptoms of Major Depression

Major depression is diagnosed if five or more of the following symptoms have been present during the same 2-week period *and* when they represent a change from previous functioning. At least one of the symptoms must be (1) depressed mood or (2) diminished interest or pleasure in most activities.

1. Depressed mood
2. Diminished interest or pleasure in most activities
3. Significant weight loss or weight gain, or change in appetite
4. Insomnia or hypersomnia
5. Psychomotor agitation or retardation (feelings of agitation, restlessness, or being slowed down)
6. Fatigue
7. Feelings of worthlessness or excessive guilt
8. Diminished ability to think or concentrate
9. Recurrent thoughts of death or suicide

Adapted from American Psychiatric Association 1994.

If you suspect that an athlete suffers from a mood disorder, refer the individual to his or her primary care physician (or caregiver) or to a **psychologist** or **psychiatrist** for further evaluation. Medical causes of depression must be considered in the initial evaluation of an athlete with suspected depression. These disorders include mononucleosis and other infections, hypothyroidism, medications (beta-blockers, corticosteroids, anabolic steroids), lupus, and renal insufficiency. More often, however, no identifiable cause is evident, and the assumption is that the depression stems from unknown neurohormonal, biochemical, or genetic causes.

Treatment of persistent, disabling depressive disorders ideally involves psychotherapy and medications. *Encourage athletes to resume all daily routines including exercise, as this can help stabilize their mood.* In fact, studies have shown that regular aerobic exercise by itself often can significantly mitigate (but not completely cure) the symptoms of depression (Martinsen et al. 1985; Doyne et al. 1987).

Medications routinely used to treat depression include the traditional **tricyclic antidepressants (TCADs)** and the newer **selective serotonin reuptake inhibitors (SSRIs)**. Because SSRIs are well tolerated, have fewer side effects than TCADs, and require less monitoring of drug levels, most caregivers prefer them for initial treatment of depression. Common side effects for SSRIs are gastrointestinal distress and either drowsiness or insomnia.

Bipolar disorder is characterized by sequential periods of major depression and manic episodes, the latter involving an abnormally and persistently elevated expansive and irritable mood that lasts for at least 1 week or requires hospitalization. Associated symptoms include inflated self-esteem, decreased need for sleep, unusual loquaciousness, racing thoughts or flights of ideas, distractibility, and excessive involvement in pleasurable activities that have high potential for painful consequences (promiscuity, binge drinking, shopping sprees).

A person with suspected bipolar disorder requires a thorough medical and psychological evaluation. Although bipolar disorder is usually of unknown etiology, medical causes include prescription psychostimulants (e.g., Ritalin® [methylphenidate] or Dexedrine® [dextroamphetamine]), cocaine, corticosteroids, anabolic steroids, hyperthyroidism, head trauma, and seizures. Management involves both treatment of the manic phase and maintenance treatment. Lithium is the standard treatment for most people suffering from mania, although the tricyclic drugs or carbamazepine may be used as well (see table 17.1). Noncompliance with mood-stabilizing agents is a major problem in people with bipolar disorder. If you identify a relapse resulting from noncompliance, do your best to help the athlete obtain appropriate evaluation from the psychological professionals responsible for her care.

Anxiety Disorders

Anxiety disorders come in many forms, including post-traumatic stress disorder and different types of social phobias. Our focus in this section is on generalized anxiety disorder, panic attacks, obsessive-compulsive disorder (OCD), and conversion reactions, as these are the disorders you are most likely to see.

Generalized anxiety disorder is characterized by excessive worry that occurs in multiple settings, often creating difficulty in social or academic functioning. As with mood disorders, there are usually periods of worsening and remission. Associated but variable symptoms include fatigue, difficulty concentrating, and sleep disturbance. All athletes experience anxiety or nervousness about their athletic performance. But when these worries overtake a person's day-to-day functioning, affect athletic performance, or result in academic problems or sleep disorders, you should refer the individual for a more thorough evaluation. Treatment for anxiety

Table 17.1   Common Prescribed Psychotropic Drugs

Drug name	Typical dose	Indications	Possible side-effects	
Citalopram (Celexa®)	20-40 mg daily	Depression	Nausea, dry mouth, sweating, somnolence, ejaculation disorder	SSRI
Fluoxetine hydrochloride (Prozac)	20 mg daily; 90 mg weekly 60 mg daily 20-120 mg daily 20 mg daily	Depression Bulimia OCD PMS	Anorexia and weight loss anxiety, sweating, insomnia, asthenia, tremor, headache, GI complaints	SSRI
Paroxetine hydrochloride (Paxil®)	20-50 mg daily 40-60 mg daily 40-60 mg daily 20 mg daily	Depression OCD Panic attacks Social anxiety disorder, post-traumatic disorder	Headache, sedation, dry mouth, insomnia, dizziness, nausea, constipation, tremor, sweating, asthenia, sexual dysfunction	SSRI
Bupropion hydrochloride (Wellbutrin®)	100 mg BID 100 mg TID MAX 450 mg daily	Depression	N/V, seizures/ tremors, agitation, insomnia, hypersensitivity reaction (arthralgia, myalgia, fever, rash), hypertension, anorexia, dry mouth, headache/ migraine, constipation, dizziness	Not SSRI or TCAD Also can be used for smoking cessation
Sertraline hydrochloride (Zoloft®)	50-200 mg daily	Depression, panic attacks, anxiety, OCD	GI complaints, tremor, headache, insomnia, male sexual dysfunction	SSRI
Venlafaxine hydrochloride (Effexor®)	75-225 mg BID	Depression, anxiety	Nausea, anorexia, sedation, dizziness, dry mouth, insomnia	Phenethylamine bicyclic antidepressant

SSRI = selective serotonin reuptake inhibitor; OCD = obsessive-compulsive disorder; PMS = premenstrual syndrome; GI = gastrointestinal; N/V = nausea/vomiting; TCAD = tricyclic antidepressant; BID = twice daily; TID = three times daily.

initially involves psychotherapy that focuses on adaptive coping strategies. When medical treatment is needed, SSRIs or benzodiazepines are the most effective drugs at present.

A panic attack consists of a period of intense fear, discomfort, or terror accompanied by thoughts of impending doom or loss of control. Systemic symptoms can include tachycardia, sweating, shortness of breath, chest pain, choking, nausea, abdominal distress, fear of dying, fear of losing control, paresthesias, chills, or hot flashes. Panic disorder is defined by recurrent episodes of unexpected panic attacks followed by persistent worries about future attacks and their consequences.

As with anxiety disorder, treatment usually involves psychotherapy and medications such as SSRIs or benzodiazepines.

Obsessive-compulsive disorder (OCD) is marked by recurrent obsessions (ruminating thoughts) or compulsions (ritualistic behavior) that can be time-consuming or cause significant impairment. The disorder is often episodic, with stress exacerbating the symptoms. OCD may manifest itself as obsessive thoughts about a person's own sport, success, or failure. The most at-risk athletes are those who identify themselves only through their sport. Most people with true OCD require long-term medical treatment and should be referred to a physician for treatment. Pharmacotherapy with SSRIs appears effective for both children and adolescents with OCD. Cognitive behavioral therapy in conjunction with pharmacotherapy is often effective in treating this disorder.

Conversion reactions are characterized by a loss or change in bodily functioning that results from psychological conflict. Medical disorders and pathophysiological processes are unable to explain the dysfunction or symptoms. Individuals are not aware of the psychological basis for their symptoms. Typical manifestations include paralysis, blindness, aphonia (loss of voice, as with laryngitis), coordination deficits, and **paresthesias.**

Serious medical illness, school problems, previous conversion reactions, and preexisting psychopathology are all risk factors for developing a conversion reaction. Classically, the affected person demonstrates *la belle indifference,* a term that refers to an inappropriately casual attitude toward a serious symptom. An example in our experience was a teenage athlete with newly diagnosed insulin-dependent diabetes who attempted to control his diabetes through obsessive exercise. When the endocrinologist discussed the ramifications of this behavior, the athlete became increasingly frustrated; within months, both hands were paralyzed in a clenched position. A few months after this first episode resolved, the athlete exhibited an acute onset of aphonia, which because of the previous episode was immediately identified as a conversion reaction.

The most important step in managing those with conversion reaction is a prompt and firm diagnosis. The physical exam is often atypical and inconsistent, and the affected person may demonstrate either overly dramatic concern or indifference to the problem.

Supportive interventions incorporating a strong element of suggestion sometimes result in prompt elimination of the symptom. If you point out to the athlete the seriousness of the problem, demonstrate the lack of a medical explanation, and suggest a possible need for psychological evaluation, these actions in themselves may open the door to a resolution of the problem. It is also important to prevent secondary gain, which only reinforces the problem. If these initial steps are not helpful in alleviating symptoms, refer the athlete to a psychologist (Dvonch et al. 1991).

PERFORMANCE ENHANCEMENT

Anxiety surrounding performance may stem from fear of failure, self-imposed or outside expectations, poor mental or physical preparation, fear of injury, or unforeseen events. Inordinate anxiety about an athletic event impairs performance. Athletes who are not able to control their anxiety may benefit from referral to a sport psychologist, who can help them prepare mentally for their events. You can help by scheduling fixed preperformance routines before the event—such as meals, relaxation times, warm-ups, and even visualization exercises (figure 17.2). Pre-enactment of possible scenarios athletes may experience during an upcoming game or event can also be helpful.

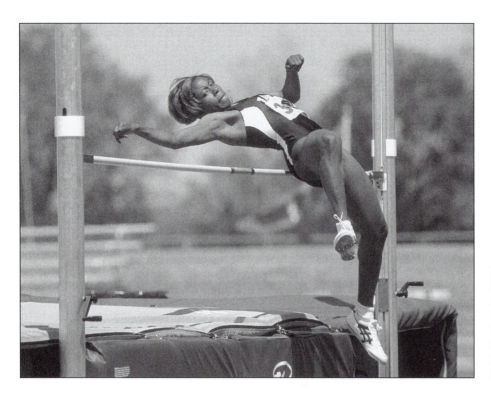

■ **Figure 17.2** Athletic trainers who can skillfully apply principles of sport psychology to improve performance can make major contributions to the success of their athletes.

Note that too little anxiety can also reduce the level of performance. *Optimal performance occurs when anxiety occurs within a narrow precompetition range—in other words, some level of anxiety is healthy and desirable.* Psychologists often use *imaging, positive self-talk,* and *relaxation* to help athletes prepare for important competitions.

Imaging

Active imaging is particularly useful just before and after practice; before and after competition; during breaks in the action of a competition; and during recovery from an injury, when physical workouts are impossible. The essential nature of imaging is that athletes first close their eyes and relax as much as possible; then imagine a particular event or series of events *in real time;* and in so doing, imagine they are reacting or performing *perfectly.*

The purpose of imaging can be simply to rehearse a particular action—such as going through an entire slalom course perfectly or making the perfect dive. Or an athlete might visualize a game in which she experiences every possible difficult tennis shot from her opponent, and she "practices" in her imagination with the appropriate responses. Or the aim might be to practice appropriate emotional responses: If a wide receiver has problems with inordinate anger when he is tackled roughly, he first imagines violent tackles (remember, imaging must be in real time) and then mentally practices a cool, reasoned response ("Man, you sure got me that time. That hurt! Good tackle!"). Or an athlete who is bedridden due to a serious injury can greatly benefit by going through winning scenarios over and over in her head.

Imaging works. It is used by 90% of Olympic athletes. Encourage your athletes to use imaging as much as possible. Remind them that they will get much better at the imaging process as they practice (it's a learned skill) and that it can significantly improve their performance (Weinberg and Gould 1999).

For Further Information

Printed Resources

Parmalee, Dean X., ed. 1996. *Child and adolescent psychiatry.* Neurology Psychiatry Access Series. St. Louis: Mosby.

Ray, R., and D. Wiese-Bjornstal, eds. 1999. *Counseling in sports medicine.* Champaign, IL: Human Kinetics. Reference for sports medicine professionals. Discusses the special psychological needs of athletes and demonstrates the role sports medicine professionals play in counseling.

Web Resources

Association for the Advancement of Applied Sport Psychology
www.aaasponline.org/index2.html
Association for the Advancement of Applied Sport Psychology provides a forum for people who are interested in research and theory development and in the application of psychological principles in sport and exercise.

National Library of Medicine
www.medlineplus.gov
A division of the National Institutes of Health, Medlineplus provides a searchable Web resource with information available on mood disorders, anxiety disorders, and mental health treatment.

National Institute of Mental Health
www.nimh.nih.gov
An extensive Web resource with information for both patients and practitioners. The site provides considerable information about government-sponsored research on a variety of topics.

Self-Talk

Self-talk is simple and can be quite effective. The basic idea is that athletes repeatedly say aloud what would be the ideal case, *using present tense.* Statements that begin with "I'm going to" or "I will" or "I should" are less helpful. Rather, the athlete repeats over and over to himself what he perceives to be the ideal scenario: "I always keep my eye on the ball"; "I am completely cool and confident"; "The rest of the team supports me completely"; "I *love it* when the other team outweighs us by 20 pounds per team member"; "I always follow through completely on my swing"; "I always feel a surge of energy during the last 100 meters of the 800-meter run," and so on. Athletes should decide on appropriate phrases, and repeat them over and over to themselves many times a day (preferably when they are alone)—including right before (and even during, when that's feasible) the time they need to succeed in the skill in question.

The theory behind this practice is to "convince" the brain that these things are true so that in the appropriate circumstances, the brain will provide the maximum possible neurological and physiological boosts to performance. It is common knowledge that "attitude"—loosely, what happens in the brain—strongly affects physical performance, whether in a negative or a positive way. Self-talk is simply a tool to prime the brain to be on its best behavior.

Needless to say, an important aspect of self-talk is to eliminate negative comments. Encourage athletes to avoid saying negative things about themselves after they miss a shot ("I'm terrible!") or make a mistake ("I always do that!"). The more positive the talk, the more an athlete's performance will be enhanced (Gill 2000).

Relaxation

There are two general kinds of relaxation techniques: physical and emotional/mental. Physical relaxation is relatively simple and can be learned with little difficulty. An athlete sits quietly, then in turn tenses and relaxes each part of her body: left toes, left foot, right toes, right foot, and so on, progressing through the lower leg, thighs, buttocks, back, abdomen, hands, arms, shoulders, neck, jaw, tongue, and face. After a good bit of practice, a person can learn to relax any part of the body at will. One benefit of this skill arises when an athlete realizes a particular part of his body is tense—a tennis player whose serving arm is tense, for example, or a javelin thrower with a tight shoulder. Athletes who have learned the skill of consciously relaxing any part of the body can quickly eliminate the tightness that otherwise would undermine their performance.

Much more complex and time-consuming are meditative techniques that can, after months of practice, enable athletes to focus much more effectively on their game or event without being distracted, and to relax their minds and emotions no matter how stressful the circumstances during a competition. These techniques usually employ periods of deep, slow breathing and are quite similar to Eastern meditation (but can be done without the religious trappings). It is not possible in this short space to describe these techniques in detail—Weinberg and Gould (1999) provide a comprehensive summary.

SUMMARY

1. *Identify psychological issues related to injury and rehabilitation.*

Studies show that injured athletes, regardless of gender or age, often experience frustration, anger, and depression after the initial assessment of an injury. When injuries are relatively mild, the mood disturbance usually subsides within 2 weeks postinjury as the athlete returns to active participation in sport. Athletes with more severe injury will experience emotional symptoms longer postinjury (about 4 weeks). Some athletes have a prolonged emotional response and may require psychotherapy to cope with the stress of imposed rest, rehabilitation, and the pressure to return to sport. For some athletes, however, a great deal of their self-worth derives from their sport and their daily exercise routine. Most of the time, this is not a problem—but injury or illness can remove a large component of the athlete's self-identity, leading to problems with self-esteem, isolation, feelings of helplessness, and anxiety. For some, these negative feelings increase their difficulties in overcoming an injury, completing the rehabilitation process, and returning to their sport in a timely manner.

Patient compliance is always a concern when an athlete must complete an extended rehabilitation program. Developing challenging rehabilitation programs that the athlete views as an extension of her preparation for performance and maintaining a connection to the team will assist in compliance.

2. *Describe common mental health issues, including mood and anxiety disorders.*

Your frequent contact with athletes may make you the first person to note symptoms of mental illness. As is true with the nonathletic population, the mental disorders that occur most often in young athletes are mood disorders (major depression, bipolar disorder, and dysthymia) and anxiety disorders (generalized anxiety disorder, panic attacks, obsessive-compulsive disorder, conversion reactions). Practitioners should be aware of the symptoms of these disorders so that they will know when to refer athletes to mental health professionals. Athletes with mood disorders may demonstrate impairments in psychosocial, academic, and athletic functioning. An athlete with a mood disorder may not overtly display changes in mood, exhibiting instead decreased energy, poor performance, or dissatisfaction with her sport. Generalized anxiety disorder is characterized by excessive worry that occurs in multiple settings, often creating difficulty in social or academic functioning. Symptoms are variable and may include fatigue, difficulty concentrating, and sleep disturbance. All athletes experience anxiety or nervousness about their athletic performance. However, when these worries overtake a person's day-to-day functioning, affect athletic performance, or result in academic problems or sleep disorders, proper referral for an evaluation is indicated. The athletic trainer can also play an important part in the treatment process, by working hand in hand with the mental health professionals.

3. *Explain specific mental-imaging techniques to assist athletes in preparing for competition.*

Anxiety surrounding performance may stem from fear of failure, self-imposed or outside expectations, poor mental or physical preparation, fear of injury, or unforeseen events. Inordinate anxiety about an athletic event impairs performance. Athletes who are not able to control their anxiety may benefit from referral to a sports psychologist, who can help them prepare mentally for their events. Too little anxiety can also reduce the level of performance. Optimal performance occurs when anxiety occurs within a narrow precompetition range—that is, some level of anxiety is healthy and desirable. The most successful athletes tend to use a variety of mental or behavioral "tricks" to enhance their performance. Such techniques as imaging, self-talk, and relaxation exercises not only can boost athletes' performance but they can also help the athletes excel in other activities of their daily lives.

CHAPTER 18

Growth and Maturation During Adolescence

OBJECTIVES

Upon completion of this chapter the reader will be able to do the following:

1. Define adolescence and appreciate the wide range of physical and emotional development possible among athletes in this age group

2. Discuss the differences in physical development common in boys and girls

3. Classify the Tanner stages of development and identify specific events related to puberty

4. Describe injuries common to growing bone and the potential complications

5. Discuss the psychological development of the adolescent

Dealing with issues of growth and maturation in high school or even college athletes requires skills and understanding that may appear unrelated to sports. Adolescents' bodies are not merely slightly smaller versions of those of adults; they are quite different anatomically, physiologically, and developmentally. In addition, adolescents' psyches are passing through an extremely difficult time of change, in which a young person's brain chemistry, hormonal development, and neurological functioning can whipsaw emotions, motivations, and rationality of thought—and even strongly affect physical performance or the nature of physical injuries.

Coaches and athletic trainers who are unaware of what is natural or unnatural in adolescent development may miss clues to underlying pathologies or may take too seriously supposedly "aberrant" behavior that is in fact quite normal and should be met with graciousness rather than unyielding adherence to rules.

Adolescence is the period of life beginning with the appearance of secondary sex characteristics and ending with cessation of somatic growth—roughly ages 11 to 19. This chapter provides an overview of the adolescent's physical and psychological development and discusses how these matters pertain to your interactions with young athletes. Please keep in mind that we are dealing with trends and averages (i.e., normal curves); young people can be quite some distance from the average in all kinds of physical or psychological characteristics and still be considered normal. Although you may occasionally see abnormal (i.e., pathological) states of physical or emotional development, your most frequent challenge will be to determine where on the normal continuum an individual lies—because the way you treat a broken leg or a broken heart may depend significantly on whether the injured athlete is in early or late adolescence. And that status does *not necessarily* correlate with biological age.

Case Study

As an athletic trainer at the local high school you have suddenly been fielding lots of questions from the girls on the freshman volleyball team. The one you hear most frequently is "How much more should I expect to grow?" You are at a loss as to how to answer. One of your athletes, a 14-yr-old who plays volleyball and basketball, has been coming to you for 2 yr with intermittent knee pain. You refer her to a physician, who has taken X rays of her knee. He tells her that the images reveal no bony abnormalities and show normal physes that are beginning to close. Her discomfort is likely due to some patellar tendinitis. She asks the physician what physes are, and after hearing his explanation, she asks how much taller she will get. The physician informs her that although there is no foolproof way to predict her adult height, he can give her a decent estimate if she will answer a few questions for him. He learns that she is currently 5 ft 6 in. (167 cm), her mother is 5 ft 8 in. (172 cm), and her father is 6 ft 3 in. (190 cm) tall. She has not experienced menarche, and she developed breast buds at about 11.5 yr. The physician tells her that she is probably not finished growing, since she is premenarcheal. Then he uses this calculation, based on her parents' heights (in inches): (68 + 75) − 5 = 138; 138/2 = 69. Her predicted height is 69 in., or 5 ft 9 in. (175 cm). The team physician promises to follow up with you to report on her X-ray result, discuss her course of treatment, and share the height-estimate formula with you so that you can satisfy her curious teammates.

PHYSICAL DEVELOPMENT

Tremendous variability exists among adolescents in their rate of physical growth and development. A person's rate of development in one area may significantly

---

Terms and Definitions

apophyseal growth plate—**Physis** that causes an outgrowth or bump on the bone; also called *traction physis or apophysis.* Occurs where large tendons insert into bones.

epiphyseal growth plate—**Physis** at the end of a long bone; also called *pressure physis.*

menarche—The beginning of menstrual functioning.

physis—Area of bone that is continuing to grow; also called *epiphyseal growth plate.*

spermarche—The first ejaculation.

---

trail the rate in another area, making it a challenge for you to estimate where someone is, not only in terms of physical growth but also in development of secondary sexual characteristics and internal anatomical development (e.g., the ossification of bone structures).

Stature and Body Composition

The major growth period in the teen years is usually closely linked with the onset of puberty. Because children tend to follow the growth pattern of one of their biological parents, they may gain insight into their potential growth pattern by asking biological parents (when available) how and when they grew. Though most parents will probably recall a definite growth spurt early in their high school years, with no growth late in high school, a few will report having additional growth after the high school years.

Although there are several ways to predict adult height, the most common estimate of the child's genetic growth potential uses the biological parents' height to determine an average predicted measurement based on the child's gender. This measurement is called the *midparental height.* For boys, add paternal height to maternal height in inches, add 5 in., and divide by 2 (or add parental heights in centimeters, add 12.7 cm, and divide by 2). For girls, subtract 5 in. (12.7 cm) from the parental sum and divide by 2. This rough estimate of an adolescent's adult height is accurate within a standard deviation of about 2 in. (5.08 cm).

Not only do girls have an earlier onset of puberty than boys, but they get their growth spurt earlier in puberty as well. A girl's growth spurt tends to occur around age 11 to 12. For males, the peak growth rate occurs around 14 to 15 yr.

The timing of puberty can influence success in athletics. Early-maturing boys and girls have an advantage in many sports that require strength, height, and (sometimes) agility, such as football, basketball, soccer, rugby, and volleyball. In some sports, however, late maturity conveys a strong advantage—with the most

Case Study

Roger is a high school sophomore who is 5 ft (152 cm) tall and weighs 105 lb (47 kg). He is a three-sport athlete and loves football. He is frustrated that all the other boys are taller than he is. He discusses this with the athletic trainer who recognizes the wide variety of "normals" among developing boys but refers to the boy's pediatrician for reassurance. His pediatrician notes that Roger is starting puberty and explains that he appears shorter than all the other boys because he is starting puberty a little later than they are. The pediatrician assures Roger that he likely will be of average height since his parents are both of average height. The pediatrician also learns that Roger's father had his major growth spurt late in high school.

obvious example being girls' gymnastics. Not all pubertal growth is lean body mass (muscle and bone): Whereas boys average about 4.3% body fat before puberty, young adult males average 11.2%. For girls the average is 15.7% before puberty and 26.7% for young adult females. The greater increase in body fat for females is a disadvantage for early-maturing girls in some sports that require thinness or speed, such as distance running.

Secondary Sexual Characteristics

The events of puberty follow a fairly clear pattern as discussed by Slap (1986). Knowing these patterns will help you understand what may be happening, both physically and emotionally, with individual athletes. The causes of depression, for example, in a rapidly growing 14-yr-old girl may be quite different from those in a short 17-yr-old boy. In addition, specific orthopedic injuries may also differ based on these differences in development.

The onset of puberty is signaled by physical changes in both sexes. Girls tend to develop before boys, with the onset of breast buds tending to occur around age 10. Boys tend to start puberty at about 12 yr, with early manifestations being enlargement of the testes and development of pubic hair (figure 18.1).

The most common description of physical sexual development defines five stages, often called *Tanner stages,* after the pediatrician who first described them (Tanner 1962; Marshall and Tanner 1969, 1970). Maturity ratings have been described for breast development, pubic hair, and genital development. These stages are important to know so that you are able to spot potential problems. But don't take them too seriously; genetic variability can play havoc with generalizations.

- Stage 1 of sexual maturity in both genders designates no signs of puberty and the body build and constitution of a young child.
- Stage 2 for female breast development is a raised breast bud under the nipple and areola; sparse growth of hair on the labia indicates stage 2 development for pubic hair. Stage 2 for male genital development is when the testes become larger and scrotal skin becomes redder and coarsens; pubic hair grows sparsely, mostly on the base of the penis.
- Stage 3 for female breast development shows more raising of the nipple and areola, with tissue extending beyond the diameter of the areola; pubic hair shows pigmentation, coarsening, and curling, with an increase in the amount of hair. Stage 3 for male genital development is a continuation of stage 2, with enlargement of the penis; pubic hair shows pigmentation, coarsening, and curling, with an increase in the amount of hair.
- Stage 4 for female breast development shows that the contour of the areola is raised, with breast tissue extending beyond its diameter; an adult pubic hair pattern develops but is limited to the labia and the area over the pubic bone. Stage 4 for male genital development is when the penis becomes longer with pigmentation of the scrotal skin; an adult pubic hair pattern develops but is limited to the area over the pubic bone.
- Stage 5 for female breast development is an adult breast with the areola at the same contour as the rest of the breast; stage 5 female pubic hair development shows adult hair with a horizontal upper border and hair usually extending to the thighs. Stage 5 for male genital development designates adult genitalia; stage 5 male pubic hair development shows adult hair with a horizontal upper border and hair usually extending to the thighs.

But here we see the problem of genetic variability—because breasts and genitals are related to overall body size, there is some subjectivity to the ratings. Thus, it is

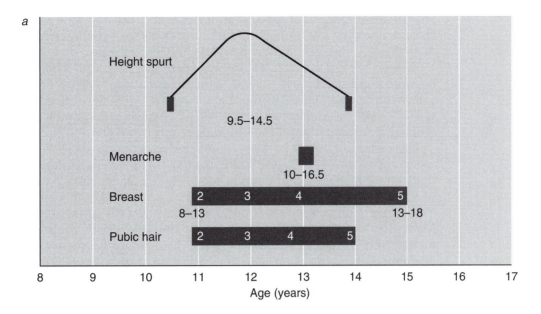

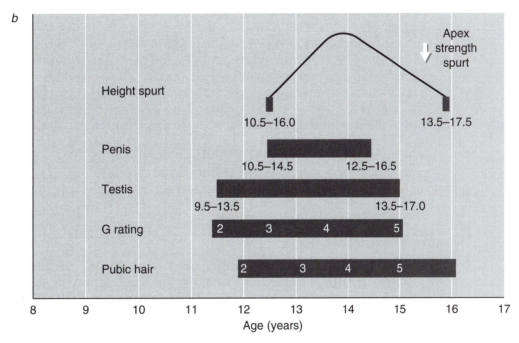

■ **Figure 18.1** Physical changes that signal the onset of puberty: *(a)* females, *(b)* males.

Adapted, by permission, from J.M. Tanner, 1962, *Growth at adolescence*, 2nd ed. (Oxford: Blackwell Scientific Publications).

not unusual for an adult woman to have stage 3 breasts or an adult man to have stage 3 penis and testes.

Though it is not appropriate for you to keep close tabs on sexual development in your athletes, you should be aware of the maturity stages and note if an adolescent appears not to be progressing through them. An interruption in progression may indicate a medical condition that disturbs the hormones responsible for growth. For example, an adolescent with hypothyroidism may experience an interruption in the progression of puberty, and progression will not resume until the thyroid deficiency is corrected; or, in addition to being anemic and having trouble gaining weight, an athlete with inflammatory bowel disease (e.g., Crohn's disease) may stall in one stage of puberty. Thus, if superficial observation (such as delayed growth) indicates to you that an athlete may be stalled in one stage, you should refer him or her to a physician to be sure that there is no underlying problem. It may be more appropriate to raise your concern about this sensitive topic with a parent rather than the athlete. Another benefit of knowing the Tanner stages is that you will often see them referred to in physicians' notes, and familiarity with the stages will help you understand the full import of those notes.

The two most important events related to puberty are the growth spurt and menarche (females) or spermarche (males). Figure 18.1 shows the average onset of these events along with the range of normal for some of the events. The numbers on the bar correspond to the Tanner stage as depicted in figure 18.1. Girls tend to experience a growth spurt about 6 months after the appearance of breast buds. Most girls and their mothers are appropriately concerned about when to expect **menarche** (the first menstrual period). On average this occurs about 24 months after breast buds develop. For males, the growth spurt tends to occur later in puberty—about 2 yr after onset of puberty. Not included in the bar graph is **spermarche,** which is the first ejaculation. Spermarche tends to occur at about the same time as the growth spurt. Whether it occurs in a wet dream or as a result of self-stimulation, boys sometimes need reassurance that this event is normal and simply means that all their "plumbing" is working the way it should.

Intense athleticism may delay the onset of puberty or lengthen the time during which all puberty events take place. The intensity and duration of physical stress are important factors in this respect, along with the individual athlete's body composition. Participation in sports that require thinness or that demand extraordinary physical effort (e.g., gymnastics, long-distance running, ballet, diving, figure skating) tends to delay puberty and growth. Though the delay does not appear to affect adult height in most cases, this matter is still under study. If you deal with adolescent girls' gymnastics, always be on the lookout for unhealthy dieting practices. A recent study found that the *majority* of adolescent female gymnasts are dieting in unhealthy ways that can affect not only their pubertal development but also their overall health.

Growth of Bone

Injuries to growing bones can differ from injuries to mature bones because of the presence of growth plates, also called *physes,* in the growing bones. Bones do not elongate along their entire length—rather, they grow only at the **physes,** which contain cartilaginous cells and collagen and exhibit rapid cell turnover. There are two types of physes: *Pressure physes* at the ends of long bones are responsible for longitudinal growth of long bones, and *traction physes* are present where large tendons insert into bones. Traction physes tend to cause an outgrowth or bump on the bone and are called **apophyseal growth plates,** or *apophyses.* The pressure growth plates are also called **epiphyseal growth plates** (figure 18.2). (Unfortunately, sometimes physicians mistakenly call them "epiphyses"—but that term should be reserved for the ends of long bones.)

Injuries to pressure physes can disturb the growth of long bones, and because a physeal fracture can stop long bone growth in its entirety or in only part of the growth plate, it can result in discrepancies of limb length or in limb deformities. Several people have devised classification systems to rate the probability that a fracture of a pressure growth plate will cause growth disturbance. The best known is the Salter Harris classification system shown in figure 18.3. A Salter Harris type I fracture has a low likelihood of causing growth disturbance, whereas a type V fracture (a crush-type injury) has a very high likelihood of doing so.

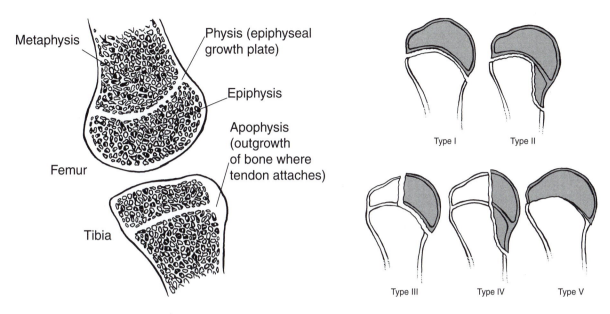

■ **Figure 18.2**   Epiphyseal growth plates.

■ **Figure 18.3**   Salter Harris classification system.

Because traction apophyses are formed from the insertion of large tendons, it is essential with developing athletes to pay close attention to muscle injuries in these regions. A severe hamstring injury, for example, can result in a fracture to the apophysis of the ischial tuberosity. If the avulsion fracture is incomplete, the injury may be mistaken for a severe muscle strain. Severe hamstring injuries with pain at the origin warrant a radiograph to determine the integrity of the apophysis. Apophyseal injuries can also be seen at the iliac crest and the tibial tuberosity.

Figure 18.4 shows the pressure growth plates and their usual time of closure during a person's development. Of note are the two latest physes to close. Because the iliac crest apophysis does not close until about age 18, a high school or collegiate runner with hip pain may have fractured this apophysis; and because the proximal end of the clavicle does not close until about age 20, an apparent sprain of the sternoclavicular joint may actually represent a fracture.

PSYCHOLOGICAL DEVELOPMENT OF THE ADOLESCENT

As you interact with ill or injured adolescents, try to remain aware of their psychological development; remember that their chronological ages may not correlate with their emotional or cognitive ages. In dealing with high school students, you may meet a 14-yr-old mind in a 17-yr-old body, or vice versa. Adolescents are undergoing a multitude of developmental challenges, and you need to be aware of these. They are trying to emancipate themselves from their families and may perceive you as a surrogate parent—which in this case may mean rebelling against you as they do against their own parents. They are also developing their sexual self-concepts, which can be manifested at different times by crushes on adults or on peers, or by outbursts of anger toward various people. Finally, they may be experiencing roller-coaster changes in their self-images, leading (you hope) in the end to a realistic and positive self-image. One athlete may exude self-confidence and superiority, whereas another may feel like a total loser. Or the same person may exhibit both feelings within a matter of days. Remember that for athletes, positive self-image can be closely related to athletic achievement. Condemning athletes for failure is often quite counterproductive, whereas applauding even slight

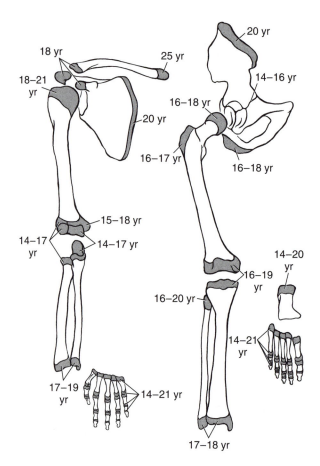

■ **Figure 18.4**   Pressure growth plates and time of closure.

achievements—as long as the praise is genuine and not affected—can improve both self-image and athletic performance. It is helpful to understand the three stages of cognitive development in adolescence as discussed in Schubert and Famolare (1998) and summarized in table 18.1.

In early adolescence (usually defined as <14 yr), athletes may experience wide mood swings and have low impulse control. There may be very intense feelings and crushes on idealized adults. Peers are very important in early adolescence. Young adolescents tend to use concrete thinking and literal interpretation and have limited ability to anticipate results of current actions or to project themselves into the future. Sometimes they have difficulty separating feelings from reality— for example, the high school freshman who, after spraining his ankle, has trouble comprehending why he cannot play in the game the next day, or the softball player with a sore shoulder who refuses to even think about long-term damage to her shoulder, insisting that she still be permitted to pitch.

Middle adolescents (approximate ages 15-17) tend to have a sense of invincibility and omnipotence and are trying to get more distance from their families. Their language skills have improved, and now they can understand metaphors and double entendres. The middle adolescent is beginning to be less self-centered—for example, the high school junior with a serious quad contusion who is more concerned about letting his teammates down than about how the injury will affect his future.

The late adolescent (>18 yr) has an increasing sense of vulnerability and may engage in less risk-taking behavior. (In some sports, however, the risk taking never diminishes.) The mature athlete uses formal operational thought and abstract thinking; she can compromise and set limits and understand others' thoughts and feelings—for example, the high school senior football player with a bad shoulder sprain who realizes that, by sitting out the next game against a lesser opponent, he will have a good chance of being stronger and more effective for the homecoming game 10 d later.

If you are not sure of an injured or sick athlete's level of maturity, it is usually best to err on the low side—assume that he needs concrete instructions for treatment and is probably fairly self-centered. You probably can avoid lengthy explanations about the whys and whats of your treatment of the illness or injury; instead, concentrate on the here and now of the treatment, explaining what you are doing and what the athlete needs to do until you see him again the next day. Let the athletes ask about the future. If they respond with questions about details

For Further Information

Print Resources

Ehrman, W.G., and S.C. Matson. 1998. Approach to assessing adolescent on serious issues. *Pediatric Clinics of North America* 45(1): 189-204.

Greynadeus, D.E., and D.R. Patel. 2000. The female athlete: Before and beyond puberty. *Pediatric Clinics of North America* 49(3): 553-80.

Neinstein, L.S. 2002. *Adolescent health care*, 4th ed. Baltimore: Lippincott Williams & Wilkins.

Ogden, J.A. 1990. *Skeletal injury in the child.* Philadelphia: W.B. Saunders.

Purcell, J.S., A.C. Hergenroeder, C. Kozinetz, E.O. Smith, and R.B. Hill. 1997. Interviewing techniques with adolescents in primary care. *Journal of Adolescent Health* 4: 300-5.

Slap, G.B. 1986. Normal physiological and psychosocial growth in the adolescent. *Journal of Adolescent Health Care* 7: 13S-23S.

Steiner, H., I.D. Yalom, and N. Steiner. 1996. *Treating adolescents.* San Francisco: Jossey-Bass.

Web Resources

National Institute of Child Health and Human Development: Endocrinology, Nutrition and Growth Branch
www.nichd.nih.gov/crmc/eng/eng.htm
Investigations supported by this branch are directed toward developing a better understanding of the roles nutritional and hormonal factors play in human growth and development.

National Institute of Arthritis and Musculoskeletal and Skin Diseases
www.niams.nih.gov/hi/topics/growth_plate/growth.htm
Excellent information about growth plate injuries in a question-and-answer format from this government-sponsored site.

U.S. Department of Health and Human Services
www.hhs.gov/kids/
Web resources pertaining to children and adolescents. Targeted to educators and children themselves; presents a variety of information and links to current government prevention programs.

National Library of Medicine/National Institutes of Health
www.nlm.nih.gov/medlineplus/anabolicsteroids.html
A Web site maintained by the National Library of Medicine and National Institutes of Health with public information on issues common to growth and development, current research, and links to up-to-date articles and information. Search feature using "adolescent" as a key word yields extensive listing of available information.

Table 18.1   A Review of Adolescent Development

Early (<14 yr)	Middle (15-17 yr)	Late (18+ yr)
Physical		
Experiences puberty changes 8-13 years for girls 9-14 years for boys Wonders, "Am I normal?" Seeks reassurance and respect	Experiences end to puberty changes Has better body acceptance except Girls concerned about fat Boys concerned about muscle	Has sense of responsibility for own health Feels, "I'm in control, not my hormones" Initiates teen preventive care
Emotional		
Experiences wide mood swings Has low impulse control Experiences intense feelings Wonders, "Who am I?" Tries different roles Daydreams Has "crushes" on idealized adults	Has sense of invincibility, omnipotence, and omniscience, which allows increased distance from the protection of the family	Has increasing sense of vulnerability Engages less in risk-taking behavior Can suppress needs of self and consider other's needs
Cognitive		
Uses concrete thinking and literal interpretation (e.g., illness exists if there is pain) Has limited ability to project and anticipate Believes that "Others think about me the way I do" Mind reader (they think they know what others are thinking) Has difficulty separating feelings from reality Has poor ability to project self into the future Tends to overthink situations, with actions denoting hidden attitudes (e.g., "Why is s/he asking me that?")	Has improved language skills Understands metaphor, double entendre Can conceptualize the ideal (e.g., justice, love, truth) and ideal family Has rise of interest in the spiritual Realizes that "People aren't always thinking about me"	Uses formal operational thought, abstract thinking (e.g., time), mental manipulation Can compromise and set limits Can understand others' thoughts and feelings Has increasing sense of how he or she fits into the world Can understand cynicism
Family		
Has need for privacy (stress confidentiality) Experiences periods of estrangement Tests to "See what I can get away with" Needs approval and a stable base	Rejects parental values Experiences peak of parental conflicts Has difficulty communicating with parents	Reaccepts parental values Has improved communication with parents
Peers		
Finds peers increasingly important Experiences intense same-sex relationships May experiment in sexual behaviors (same/opposite) May become sexually active	Arrives at peak of peer conformity Experiences rise of opposite-sex relationships Engages in serial monogamy Wonders, "Am I lovable?"	Finds peers less important Spends more time in mutually supportive, intimate relationships

(continued)

Table 18.1 *(continued)*

Early (<14 yr)	Middle (15-17 yr)	Late (18+ yr)
School		
Is "youngest" as enters junior high	Is "youngest" again as enters senior high	If enters college, may experience increased dependence on parents for certain needs (e.g., car, money)
Experiences class and teacher changes	Concerned about career and/or college	Exposed to new people, ideas, independence
Experiences rearranged peer groups	Experiences more peer pressure	Usually makes no major lifestyle changes during first 1-2 months
Has performance now evaluated on productivity, not effort	Experiences more sexual pressure	Faces issues of risk-taking behaviors in new setting
Engages in self-teaching		
Has long-term assignments		
Sees subtle but increased importance of reading ability (e.g., ADD/LD may become apparent)		
Work		
Views as something to do	Views as way to make money, but usually legally limited to 15 h per week	Will likely have 3-4 careers per lifetime

Reprinted, by permission, from P.S. Shubert and N.E. Fumolare, 1998, "Teaching and communication strategies: Working with the hospitalized adolescent with PID," *Pediatric Nursing* 24(1): 19.

of their diagnosis or treatment, by all means answer them with as much detail as the questions call for.

SUMMARY

1. *Define adolescence and appreciate the wide range of physical and emotional development possible among athletes in this age group.*

Adolescence is the period of life beginning with the appearance of secondary sex characteristics and ending with cessation of somatic growth—roughly ages 11 to 19. Adolescents' bodies are not merely slightly smaller versions of those of adults; they are quite different anatomically, physiologically, and emotionally. Adolescents' psyches are passing through an extremely difficult time of change, in which a young person's brain chemistry, hormonal development, and neurological functioning can affect emotions, motivations, and rationality of thought—and even strongly affect physical performance or the nature of physical injuries. Coaches and athletic trainers must be aware of what is natural or unnatural in adolescent development, or they may miss clues to underlying pathologies or may take too seriously supposedly "aberrant" behavior that is, in fact, quite normal.

2. *Discuss the differences in physical development common in boys and girls.*

Tremendous variability exists among adolescents in their rate of physical growth and development. A person's rate of development in one area may significantly trail the rate in another area, making it a challenge for estimating where someone is, not only in terms of physical growth but also in development of secondary sexual characteristics and internal anatomical development (e.g., the ossification of bone structures). The onset of puberty is signaled by physical changes in both sexes. Girls tend to develop before boys, with the onset of breast buds tending to occur around age 10. Boys tend to start puberty at about 12 yr, with early manifestations being enlargement of the testes and development of pubic hair.

3. *Classify the Tanner stages of development and identify specific events related to puberty.*

The most common description of physical sexual development defines five stages, often called Tanner stages, after the pediatrician who first described them. Maturity ratings have been described for breast development, pubic hair, and genital development. These stages are important to know so that you are able to spot potential problems. But don't take them too seriously; genetic variability can play havoc with generalizations. The most important reason for you to know the maturity stages is so that you can observe whether an adolescent is in fact *progressing* through the stages. An interruption in progression may indicate a medical condition that disturbs the hormones responsible for growth. For example, an adolescent with hypothyroidism may experience an interruption in the progression of puberty, and progression will not resume until the thyroid deficiency is corrected; or, in addition to being anemic and having trouble gaining weight, an athlete with inflammatory bowel disease (e.g., Crohn's disease) may stall in one stage of puberty.

The two most important events related to puberty are the growth spurt and menarche (females) or spermarche (males). Most girls and their mothers are appropriately concerned about when to expect menarche (the first menstrual period). On average this occurs about 24 months after breast buds develop. For males, spermarche, which is the first ejaculation, tends to occur at about the same time as the growth spurt. Intense athleticism may delay the onset of puberty or lengthen the time during which all puberty events take place. Participation in sports that require thinness or that demand extraordinary physical effort (e.g., gymnastics, long-distance running, ballet, diving, figure skating) tends to delay puberty and growth. Though the delay does not appear to affect adult height in most cases, this matter is still under study.

4. *Describe injuries common to growing bone and the potential complications.*

Injuries to growing bones can differ from injuries to mature bones because of the presence of growth plates, also called physes. There are two types of physes: Pressure physes at the ends of long bones are responsible for longitudinal growth of long bones, and traction physes are present where large tendons insert into bones. Traction physes tend to cause an outgrowth or bump on the bone and are called apophyseal growth plates or apophyses. The pressure growth plates are also called epiphyseal growth plates.

Injuries to pressure physes can disturb the growth of long bones, and because a physeal fracture can stop long bone growth in its entirety or in only part of the growth plate, it can result in discrepancies of limb length or in limb deformities. Several people have devised classification systems to rate the probability that a fracture of a pressure growth plate will cause growth disturbance; the best known is the Salter Harris classification system. Given the potential complications involved with epiphyseal fractures and apophyseal avulsions, fractures and soft-tissue injuries in adolescents must be evaluated with care to determine involvement of growing bone.

5. *Discuss the psychological development of the adolescent.*

The psychological development of adolescents has important implications for you as an athletic trainer. Remember that psychological development may not correlate with physical development or chronological age. Adolescents are undergoing a multitude of developmental challenges, and you need to be aware of these. They are trying to emancipate themselves from their families and may perceive an athletic trainer as a surrogate parent—which in this case may mean rebelling against you as they do against their own parents. They are also developing their sexual self-concepts, which can be manifested at different times by crushes on adults or on peers, or by outbursts of anger toward various people. Finally, they may be experiencing roller-coaster changes in their self-images, ideally leading to a realistic and positive self-image.

CHAPTER 19

Preparticipation Physical Examination

OBJECTIVES

Upon completion of this chapter the reader will be able to do the following:

1. Discuss the different types of examinations and identify advantages and disadvantages of each type of preparticipation physical exam (PPPE)

2. Explain the limitations of the PPPE and be able to educate athletes and their families about these limitations

3. Recognize the importance of the medical history in assessing the athlete's health, risk factors, and playability; make sure a comprehensive history form is used that can document assessment for key aspects of this screening tool

4. Identify the components of the physical exam portion of the PPPE

Every year, millions of middle school, high school, and collegiate student athletes complete a preparticipation physical examination (PPPE) during the months leading up to the sport season. For many young athletes, this exam is their only encounter with the health-care system—and for nearly one-third of the athletes, this single encounter involves a somewhat impersonal school-based screening exam rather than an in-depth appointment with a private physician (Krowchuk et al. 1995). Such "drive-through" exams often provide young people with signed waivers that do not represent adequate examination. It is a mistake to assume, based merely on a signed waiver, that an athlete is in good health. Always be certain that each athlete has undergone a complete, thorough annual history and physical examination before the first practice of the season. Minimum requirements in terms of how frequently these examinations must be completed vary by region at the high school level and are done at matriculation at the collegiate level. Incomplete exams, on very rare occasions, fail to reveal underlying problems that lead to serious injury or even sudden cardiac death—or that result in long-term damage to an athlete's health. On the other hand, even complete physical examinations may not uncover serious medical problems, usually cardiac, that could have profound implications for an athlete's ability to compete and could possibly result in sudden death. Athletes, parents, coaches, athletic trainers, primary care physicians, and other primary caregivers must be aware of the limitations of this type of examination.

Case Study

You are asked to organize a preparticipation physical exam for Harry Potter and all the Quidditch athletes at the Hogwart's Wizard Academy. Is organizing a station-based exam in the best interest of the athletes, or does it merely fulfill the legal requirements for the academy? Does the traditional office-based exam offer an advantage by permitting anticipatory guidance and providing time to explore Harry's troubled past? How might each kind of exam affect Harry's self-esteem, academic performance, and the like? What potentially serious injuries related to the game of Quidditch might be prevented by proper education during this examination?

REASONS FOR PERFORMING THE PREPARTICIPATION PHYSICAL EXAMINATION

The most important reason for performing PPPEs is to guarantee athletes' safety. Although some young people fear that such exams exist primarily to find excuses for disqualifying them, disqualification for health reasons is in fact quite rare. The most frequent outcomes of PPPEs are reviews of treatment regimens for known medical conditions (e.g., exercise-induced asthma) or recommendations of rehabilitation for previous orthopedic injuries (see *Reasons for Performing the Preparticipation Physical Examination*, page 289).

Although such conditions are rare, one very important reason for PPPEs is to try to identify athletes at risk for sudden death. Unfortunately, thorough histories and physical exams often cannot identify such athletes; athletes and their families must understand this key limitation of the PPPE. However, identification of the rare individual at risk for sudden cardiac death makes PPPEs well worth the effort.

From the athletes' standpoint, the main reason for undergoing a PPPE is usually because the state or their sport's governing body requires it. State high school athletic associations and the National Collegiate Athletic Association (NCAA) require

Terms and Definitions

auscultation—The act of listening with a stethoscope.

bradycardia—Unusually slow heart rate.

gallop—Type of abnormal extra heart sound heard when auscultating the heart.

mitral valve prolapse (MVP)—A condition affecting the mitral valve in the heart wherein a two-flapped valve between the left atrium and left ventricle balloons back into the left atrium with each heart beat.

murmur—Soft or harsh swooshing sound heard between normal heart sounds during **auscultation** of the heart.

palpation—Examination by touch.

rub—Type of heart sound caused by friction between the outside layer of the lining of the heart and the heart itself as a result of fluid inflammation or infection.

syncope—Loss of consciousness because of inadequate blood flow to the brain; fainting.

Reasons for Performing the Preparticipation Physical Examination

- To identify athletes at risk of sudden death
- To identify medical conditions that may require further evaluation and treatment before participation
- To identify orthopedic conditions that may require further evaluation and treatment, including physical therapy, before participation
- To identify at-risk adolescents and young adults who are at risk for substance abuse, STDs, pregnancy, violence, depression, and so on.
- To satisfy legal requirements of athletic governing boards

athletes to undergo at least one examination before being cleared for participation in athletics. Athletic governing bodies differ widely, however, in stipulations concerning frequency of examination, who may perform the examination (physician, nurse practitioner, physician's assistants, chiropractors, and so on), and the wording of waiver forms. If you are involved in instituting PPPEs at a school, whether in the college, high school, or even middle school setting, it is imperative that you be intimately familiar with local, state, and sport advisory board requirements.

Because this legally required exam may be the only involvement many student athletes have with the health-care system, it is important that examiners make it as comprehensive as possible. In no way is it a cost-effective method of providing overall health care (Carek and Futrell 1999); yet an important function of the screening exam is to identify athletes who are at risk not only for the usual medical and orthopedic conditions but also for psychosocial problems involving sexuality, substance abuse, violence, or any other emotional or psychological factors. PPPEs are much more likely to identify such at-risk adolescents than to find individuals in danger of cardiac problems that can lead to sudden death.

MECHANICS: TIMING, LOCATION, AND TYPES OF EXAMINATIONS

Ideally, the examination should occur about 6 weeks before the start of the athletic season. This allows time for diagnostic tests and consultations and permits completion of any necessary rehabilitation before the beginning of practice. A

Table 19.1	Stations and Personnel for Preparticipation Physical Examinations
Stations	**Responsible personnel**
Vital signs	Nurse, medical assistant, athletic trainers, or students in any of these areas
Vision	Same as above + ophthalmologist (optional) if available
History	Nurse to review forms, including immunizations
Medical 　Head, eyes, ears, nose, and 　　throat (HEENT) 　Heart/lung 　Abdomen (hernia check for males)	Physician, nurse practitioner, or physician's assistant
Orthopedic	Physician or athletic trainer
Lab testing (optional)	Phlebotomist
Fitness testing (optional) Endurance testing 　Strength 　Body fat 　Aerobic capacity	Coach, exercise physiologist, athletic trainer

Tables 3 & 4 pp 55 & 58 reproduced, with permission, from Donahue P: Preparticipation Exams: How to detect a teenage crisis. *The Physician and Sportsmedicine* 1987; 15(11): 43-44 © The McGraw-Hill Companies.

cursory examination in a busy office 1 d before the season and without a parent available to confirm the athlete's history is unacceptable and potentially dangerous.

The type of exam dictates requirements for location. There are realistically only two types of examinations: the *station-type exam,* which requires multiple examination rooms and multiple personnel (see table 19.1), and the *in-office private exam.* (The locker room exam, whereby athletes stand in line while a single examiner checks out an entire team, should never be used—it provides a woeful lack of privacy, is very time-consuming, and almost inevitably lacks thoroughness.)

The station-type exam is frequently used to examine a large group of people in a fairly short time. In this type of exam, the athletes move from one station to the next (in different rooms, for the sake of privacy) to complete the entire physical examination. A quiet examination room with one-to-one interaction between the provider and the athlete is extremely important for both the quality of the examination (some heart murmurs are difficult to hear in a loud environment) and for confidentiality. After completing all of the stations, the athletes review significant findings with the team physician, who makes appropriate recommendations regarding playability, consultations, diagnostic tests, and treatment plans. The advantages of this type of exam are clear:

- It provides good communication between athletic trainers, who are responsible for and tend to know personally each athlete on their team, and physicians.
- It permits examiners to spend adequate time on each specific organ system and thereby may increase the chance of identifying any abnormality.

There are some drawbacks as well:

- Multiple examiners generally do not know the athlete as well as the primary care provider, who may have followed the athlete since childhood. Therefore, a parent must complete a thorough history for each student.
- Time constraints involved with the assembly-line system often lead to over-

sights of health risks (e.g., substance abuse, unsafe sex practices, or emotional distress) or fail to provide detailed guidance in correcting subtle problems (e.g., poor nutrition, inadequate car safety, failure to use bike helmets).

The traditional in-office examination by a private physician is the optimal way to perform the preparticipation physical examination. Because 80% to 90% of adolescents seek routine health care solely to receive clearance for sports participation, the primary care health provider who knows the patient best should perform the examination. A more private, discreet, personal environment will make it more likely that an adolescent will share both physical and emotional concerns. In addition, the private physician or primary caregiver can devote more time to anticipatory guidance, such as identifying overbearing parents, providing fitness and nutritional counseling, and spending time discussing injury prevention. Finally, private appointments are more likely to identify stressed adolescents (see table 19.2), leading to interventions that can ensure the young athletes' long-term health. Even when it is legally required that a parent or guardian accompany a minor child to see a physician, it is imperative for the physician to spend some time alone with each young person to give athletes a chance to confidentially unburden problems they may be withholding from their parents.

Unfortunately, student athletes in lower economic classes may have no contact with private physicians. In these situations, the best approach, if you have the resources to provide it, is an aggressive and proactive station-type exam that will give athletes at least this one chance to undergo detailed and adequate examinations. Involving public health nurses and social workers in these situations may help with catch-up of delayed immunizations and identification of community health resources for the family. If public health agencies are not available, delays in obtaining required information about immunizations and health histories may require that the exams be performed well in advance of the start of the sport season.

THE HISTORY IS THE KEY

A complete medical history is the foundation of any medical evaluation in that it will identify up to 65% to 92% of problems affecting athletes (Goldberg et al. 1980; Gomez et al. 1993; Rifat et al. 1995). The history should focus on cardiovascular

Table 19.2 Adolescent Stress Factors

Areas of stress	Compromising factors
School	Grades, truancy, goals
Peers	Number of friends' use of tobacco, alcohol, and other drugs
Relatives	Familial dysfunction, job and marital status, sibling relationships, culture
Economics	Job, family economic status
Safety	Guns in the home, seat belts, bike helmets, driving arrests, driving under the influence
Sex	Definition of sexual orientation, activity; advisability of abstinence; knowledge of STDs, HIV; need for contraception
Emotions	Depression, suicide, mood swings
Drugs	Alcohol, tobacco, illicit drugs; ergogenic aids, including nutritional, herbal, and illegal supplements

Tables 3 & 4 pp 55 & 58 reproduced, with permission, from Donahue P: Preparticipation Exams: How to detect a teenage crisis. *The Physician and Sportsmedicine* 1987: 15(11): 43-44 © The McGraw-Hill Companies.

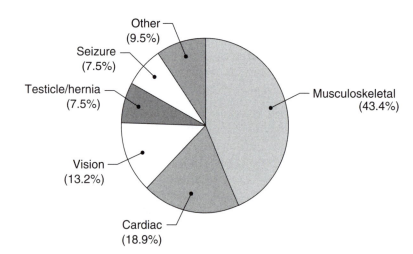

■ Figure 19.1 Reasons for not clearing athletes.

Adapted, by permission, from J. Smith and E.R. Laskowski, 1996, "The preparticipation physical examination: Mayo Clinic experience with 2739 examinations," *Mayo Clinic Proceedings* 73: 419-429.

and musculoskeletal anomalies or injuries, as these areas are the most likely to restrict participation or to require follow-up before participation. In a Mayo Clinic study of over 2,700 athletes who completed a station-type examination and were not cleared to participate, 18.9% had a cardiac problem and 43.4% exhibited musculoskeletal problems (figure 19.1) (Smith and Laskowski 1998).

Although rare, nontraumatic cardiac death usually results from unknown cardiac disease; tragically, sudden death is often the initial manifestation of the disease (table 19.3). Chapter 1 discusses most of the conditions that may lead to sudden unexpected death. Crucial questions pertaining to the athlete's *cardiac history* should include the following:

1. A history of chest pain or discomfort or **syncope**/near syncope

2. A history of excessive, unexplained, and unexpected shortness of breath or fatigue associated with exercise

3. Past detection of a heart murmur or increased systolic blood pressure

4. Family history of premature death (sudden or otherwise) or significant disability from cardiovascular disease in close relative(s) younger than 50 yr

5. Specific knowledge of the occurrence within the family of conditions such as hypertrophic cardiomyopathy, dilated cardiomyopathy, long QT syndrome, Marfan's syndrome, or clinically important arrhythmia (Maron et al. 1996) (see also chapter 1).

Table 19.3   Detection of Common Causes of Sudden Death

	% Detected by Hx and PE alone	Pertinent clinical clues	Most sensitive noninvasive test(s)
Hypertrophic cardiomyopathy	25	FHx of sudden death; syncope, palpitations, murmur	ECHO
Marfan's syndrome	Some	Characteristic features (family history, cardiovascular, ocular, skeletal abnormalities), chest pain, MVP	ECHO
Congenital coronary artery anomalies	0	Exertional chest pain, syncope	Radionuclide studies, exercise EKG

Hx = medical history, PE = physical examination, FHx = family history, ECHO = echocardiogram, MVP = **mitral valve prolapse,** EKG = electrocardiogram.

If an athlete answers any of these questions affirmatively, further diagnostic tests and referral to a cardiologist may be necessary.

A solid *orthopedic history* is a better screening tool than a screening orthopedic exam. Almost 92% of injuries can be picked up by history alone (Gomez et al. 1993). Note in particular if the history reveals either

- an orthopedic injury that limits the athlete's ability to participate in sports; or
- any injury that is associated with persistent discomfort, swelling, or weakness, or that causes the athlete to compensate by changing his mechanics, position on the field, or duration or intensity of play.

Athletes with either of these findings should not be cleared for sport participation until a firm diagnosis is made, treatment is received, and full function is restored.

Many types of history forms are available. The PPPE examiner must have a form that is complete yet convenient for the patient. In a study of NCAA member colleges and universities, only 26% of the schools had forms that contained at least 9 of the recommended 12 American Heart Association (AHA) screening guidelines and were judged to be adequate (Pfister et al. 2000). *American Heart Association Screening Recommendations* contains a list of these 12 recommended screening guidelines. The Web resources toward the end of the chapter list a Web site that includes an excellent PPPE form.

COMPONENTS OF THE PHYSICAL EXAM

As with the history, the physical exam must focus on potential medical or orthopedic problems that could hinder performance, be life-threatening, or be worsened by athletic participation. Although athletic trainers do not perform the PPPEs themselves, they need to understand the process and the subsequent communications they are likely to receive from the physicians who do perform them.

American Heart Association Screening Recommendations

1. Prior occurrence of exertional chest pain or discomfort
2. Prior occurrence of syncope/near syncope
3. Excessive, unexpected, and unexplained shortness of breath or fatigue associated with exercise
4. Past detection of a heart murmur
5. Increased systemic blood pressure
6. Family history of premature death (sudden or otherwise)
7. Family history of significant disability from cardiovascular disease in close relative(s) younger than 50 yr
8. Specific knowledge of the occurrence of certain conditions (e.g., hypertrophic cardiomyopathy, dilated cardiomyopathy, long QT syndrome, Marfan syndrome, or clinically important arrhythmias)

The cardiovascular physical examination should emphasize (but not necessarily be limited to) the following:

9. Precordial auscultation in both the supine and standing positions to identify, in particular, heart murmurs consistent with dynamic left ventricular outflow obstruction
10. Assessment of the femoral artery pulses to exclude coarctation of the aorta
11. Recognition of the physical stigmata of Marfan's syndrome
12. Brachial blood pressure measurement in the sitting position

Proper male attire for athletes undergoing the station-type physical exam should be shorts; females should wear shorts and a top that makes it easy to auscultate the chest and inspect the thorax, shoulders, and back (e.g., a tank top).

General Considerations

The examination should record vital signs (pulse, respiratory rate, and blood pressure), height, and weight. Blood pressure should be taken from the right arm with the athlete seated. The blood pressure cuff must fit the athlete properly to guarantee accurate measurements; larger individuals may require a thigh cuff for proper fit on the arm (too small a cuff can give a falsely elevated blood pressure). If blood pressure appears elevated at the initial exam, repeat the test later in the examination and twice more in the following week. If the blood pressure is consistently high, refer the athlete to a physician for further evaluation before clearing her for sport participation.

Obesity does not place an athlete at higher risk for sudden death and should not be a reason for medical disqualification. For the sake of the student's physical as well as emotional health, however, always see that a health professional recommends a specific regimen of diet and exercise and *closely monitors progress* to encourage the athlete's participation in the regimen.

Refer for further evaluation athletes whose visual acuity is less than 20/40 if they are not already wearing corrective lenses. Athletes with <20/200 vision are defined as legally blind and need eye protection to participate in sports.

A detailed cardiac examination should include inspection, **palpation** of the point of maximal impulse, and **auscultation** of **murmurs, gallops,** or **rubs.** Palpation of femoral pulses is necessary to make sure an undetected narrowing of the aorta has not been missed during previous examinations. For more details, see *Cardiac Examination.*

Although abnormal lung sounds should be noted, they rarely result in disqualification. Wheezing should be noted and may require proper treatment before participation.

Single Organ Considerations

If an athlete has only a single kidney, discuss potential risks in detail with the athlete and his family. Although severe renal trauma is rare in most contact or collision sports, the risk of the resulting surgical nephrectomy (kidney removal) should lead athletes with one kidney to avoid such sports.

Require an athlete with a single testicle always to wear a protective cup, and refer him as appropriate for treatment of the undescended testis. Undescended

Cardiac Examination

Although you will not be performing cardiac examinations, the following information will help you interpret what your players' physicians may tell you about them.

The point of maximal apical impulse should be in the midclavicular line in the fourth or fifth intercostal space. Normal heart sounds and benign murmurs should be identified. A benign murmur is usually musical or vibratory, between the first and second heart sound, and grade 1 (very soft) in quality. A pathological murmur extends from the end of the first heart sound and may be heard throughout systole (up to the second heart sound). Any athlete with a murmur that increases when the individual moves from supine to standing should be referred to a cardiologist for further diagnostic testing to rule out hypertrophic cardiomyopathy or some other congenital heart disease. Any diastolic murmur is considered abnormal and needs further evaluation before the athlete is cleared for sport participation.

testicles are at significantly higher risk for testicular cancer later in life and require close follow-up in terms of self-testicular examination and annual examination by a physician. Playability in a contact or collision sport for an athlete with a single testicle needs cautious consideration because of fertility implications.

Note that the athlete's pubertal stage (see chapter 18) is generally irrelevant to his or her playability or risk of injury. Guide students to participate in a sport according to their size and coordination rather than their pubertal development.

Orthopedic exams should focus mainly on previously injured areas. See that a physician examines in detail any previously injured joint before the start of a season to confirm full recovery.

Lab Tests

No single lab test is universally appropriate for athletic screening. In the past, physicians, athletic trainers, and coaches have variously recommended hemoglobin tests, iron tests, urinalysis, and echocardiograms or electrocardiograms—yet none of these have shown merit as a screening tool for *all* athletes. Tests should be ordered only when history and physical examination warrant further evaluation.

Gender-Related Concerns

Personal issues unique to females are impossible to address in a station-type examination. Reserve such considerations for private, one-on-one discussions in a physician's or athletic trainer's office. Be ready to deal with a wide variety of issues such as eating disorders, menstrual irregularity, and bone mineral and nutritional issues. With female athletes, be especially alert for any hint of a disturbance in body image, menstrual irregularity, restrictive eating patterns, fad diets, significant changes in mood, or changes in sleep patterns. When in doubt, refer the athlete to appropriate medical specialists.

Signs of anorexia nervosa or bulimia include oral ulcerations, poor tooth enamel, **bradycardia,** hypotension, and calluses on the dorsal surface of the hand. Note that the aforementioned symptoms generally accompany only the more severe forms of these two disorders and that milder forms have few overt symptoms— but all examiners should be alert for these advanced conditions. Examiners who find these signs or symptoms must exhibit empathy and sensitivity in discussing them with an athlete, to ensure her willingness to communicate honestly. Always refer such athletes to an appropriate counselor or medical professional for evaluation and treatment.

Sensitive issues such as family planning, sexually transmitted diseases, and sexual orientation are not unique to females. Both male and female players need to be able to discuss these matters in a confidential manner with somebody qualified to do so.

DECISIONS CONCERNING PLAYABILITY

After completing the exam, an athlete should be given one of the following recommendations:

- Full clearance for participation
- Clearance after rehabilitation of injured area is complete
- Clearance withheld pending further diagnostic evaluation
- Clearance denied

For Further Information

Print Resources

American Academy of Family Physicians, American Academy of Pediatrics, American Medical Society for Sports Medicine, American Orthopaedic Society for Sports Medicine, and American Osteopathic Academy of Sports Medicine. 1997. *Preparticipation physical evaluation,* 2d ed. Monograph. Minneapolis: McGraw-Hill.

Maron, B.J., P.D. Thompson, J.C. Puffer, C.A. McGrew, W.B. Strong, P.S. Douglas, L.T. Clark, M.J. Mitten, M.H. Crawford, D.L. Atkins, D.J. Driscoll, and A.E. Epstein. 1996. Cardiovascular preparticipation screening of competitive athletes. A statement for health professionals from the Sudden Death Committee (clinical cardiology) and Congenital Cardiac Defects Committee (cardiovascular disease in the young), American Heart Association (scientific statement). *Circulation* 94: 850-56.

Washington, R.W., D.T. Bernhardt, J. Gomez, M.D. Johnson, T.J. Martin, T.W. Rowland, and E. Small. 2001. Committee on Sports Medicine and Fitness, American Academy of Pediatrics. Medical conditions affecting sports participation. *Pediatrics* 107(5): 1205-9.

Web Resources

Utah High School Athletic Association
www.uhsaa.org/forms/pdf/forma.pdf
A good example of a standard form used for preparticipation examinations in Utah.

ACSM Pre-Participation Physical Examinations
www.acsm.org/pdf/prepart022702.pdf
A brochure prepared and published by the American College of Sports Medicine in 2002 that details the components of a physical examination.

To guarantee that an athlete does not misinterpret a decision (and to avoid potential legal liability), the sports medicine team should bring the athlete's family into the process of arriving at a final decision. Even young people who are 100% fit should nevertheless understand the risks inherent in their sport. Athletes with conditional clearance must accept and agree to specified limitations and to prescribed rehabilitation programs. Athletes who are not cleared to play should know the specific reasons behind the decision. The sports medicine team must be prepared to discuss all these matters with both the athlete and the athlete's family. It is standard practice today for sport teams to require parental signatures on waivers of liability regardless of the status of the athlete's fitness.

Always keep in mind that there are also risks in *not* letting young people play sports, and these risks deserve consideration alongside the standard questions of physical health: Disqualified athletes sometimes have more free time, as well as more peer pressure, to assume high-risk lifestyles that in the end could be more detrimental to their well-being than some serious sport injuries. Weigh *all* possible factors before accepting or disqualifying an athlete.

The Federal Rehabilitation Act of 1973 and the Americans With Disabilities Act of 1990 permit athletes to participate in a sport *against medical advice.* These federal laws are designed to prevent discrimination against people with disabilities. They are good and important laws, but unfortunately they sometimes muddle the issue of permitting disqualified individuals to play. It is important that the sports medicine team not waiver in its recommendation when an athlete's participation in a sport clearly would increase the risk of mortality or of permanent disability. The athlete has the right to sue to get onto a team. But do not let fear of a lawsuit alter your decision to disqualify an athlete—not only for the sake of the athlete's health, but also to prevent a future lawsuit should the athlete be seriously injured as a result of participation. It is better to insist on disqualification and defend a lawsuit than to give in merely because you fear a suit—and later to have an injured or dead young athlete on your hands. In some cases, disqualified athletes will shop for second opinions until they find a doctor who is willing to certify their health. There is nothing you can do to prevent this, except to establish good rapport with your athletes and potential athletes, and to educate them constantly about both the benefits and risks of athletic participation.

Table 19.4 lists the recommendations of the American Academy of Pediatrics Committee on Sports Medicine and Fitness regarding playability for specific

Table 19.4   Medical Conditions and Sports Participation

Condition	Participate decision	Explanation
Atlantoaxial instability (instability of the joint between cervical vertebrae 1 and 2)	Qualified yes	Athlete needs evaluation to assess risk of spinal cord injury during sports participation.
Bleeding disorder	Qualified yes	Athlete needs evaluation.
Cardiovascular disease		
Carditis (inflammation of the heart)	No	*Explanation:* Carditis may result in sudden death with exertion.
Hypertension (high blood pressure)	Qualified yes	Those with significant essential (unexplained) hypertension should avoid weight- and powerlifting, bodybuilding, and strength training. Those with secondary hypertension (hypertension caused by a previously identified disease) or severe essential hypertension need evaluation. The National High Blood Pressure Education Working Group defined significant and severe hypertension.
Congenital heart disease (structural heart defects present at birth)	Qualified yes	Those with mild forms may participate fully; those with moderate or severe forms or who have undergone surgery need evaluation. The 26th Bethesda Conference defined mild, moderate, and severe disease for common cardiac lesions.
Dysrhythmia (irregular heart rhythm)	Qualified yes	Those with symptoms (chest pain, syncope, dizziness, shortness of breath, or other symptoms of possible dysrhythmia) or evidence of mitral regurgitation (leaking) on physical examination need evaluation. All others may participate fully.
Heart murmur	Qualified yes	If the murmur is innocent (does not indicate heart disease), full participation is permitted. Otherwise, the athlete needs evaluation.
Cerebral palsy	Qualified yes	Athlete needs evaluation
Diabetes mellitus	Yes	All sports can be played with proper attention to diet, blood glucose concentration, hydration, and insulin therapy. Blood glucose concentration should be monitored every 30 min during continuous exercise and 15 min after completion of exercise.

(continued)

Table 19.4 *(continued)*

Condition	Participate decision	Explanation
Diarrhea	Qualified no	Unless disease is mild, no participation is permitted because diarrhea may increase the risk of dehydration and heat illness.

Eating disorders
  Anorexia nervosa
  Bulimia nervosa
	Qualified yes	Patients with these disorders need medical and psychiatric assessment before participation.

Eyes
  Functionally one-eyed athlete
  Loss of an eye
  Detached retina
	Qualified yes	A functionally one-eyed athlete has a best-corrected visual acuity of less than 20/40 in the eye with worse acuity. These athletes would suffer significant disability if the better eye were seriously injured, as would those with loss of an eye. Some athletes who previously have undergone eye surgery or had a serious eye injury may have an increased risk of injury because of weakened eye tissue. Availability of eye guards approved by the American Society for Testing and Materials and other protective equipment may allow participation in most sports, but this must be judged on an individual basis.

Fever	No	Fever can increase cardiopulmonary effort, reduce maximum exercise capacity, make heat illness more likely, and increase orthostatic hypertension during exercise. Fever may rarely accompany myocarditis or other infections that may make exercise dangerous.
Heat illness	Qualified yes	Because of the increased likelihood of recurrence, the athlete needs individual assessment to determine the presence of predisposing conditions and to arrange a prevention strategy.
Hepatitis	Yes	Because of the apparent minimal risk to others, all sports may be played that the athlete's state of health allows. In all athletes, skin lesions should be covered properly, and athletic personnel should use universal precautions when handling blood or body fluids with visible blood.
Human immunodeficiency virus infection		Because of the apparent minimal risk to others, all sports may be played that the athlete's state of health allows. In all athletes, skin lesions should be covered properly, and athletic personnel should use universal precautions when handling blood or body fluids with visible blood.

Condition	Participate decision	Explanation
Kidney, absence of one	Qualified yes	Athlete needs individual assessment for contact, collision, and limited-contact sports.
Liver, enlarged	Qualified yes	If the liver is acutely enlarged, participation should be avoided because of risk of rupture. If the liver is chronically enlarged, individual assessment is needed before collision, contact, or limited-contact sports are placed
Malignant neoplasm	Qualified yes	Athlete needs individual assessment
Musculoskeletal disorders	Qualified yes	Athlete needs individual assessment.
Neurologic disorders		
History of serious head or spine trauma, severe or repeated concussions, or craniotomy	Qualified yes	Athlete needs individual assessment for collision, contact, or limited-contact sports and also for noncontact sports if deficits in judgment or cognition are present. Research supports a conservative approach to management of concussion.
Seizure disorder, well controlled	Yes	Risk of seizure during participation is minimal.
Seizure disorder, poorly controlled	Qualified yes	Athlete needs individual assessment for collision, contact, or limited-contact sports. The following noncontact sports should be avoided: archery, riflery, swimming, weight- or powerlifting, strength training, or sports involving heights. In these sports, occurrence of a seizure may pose a risk to self or others.
Obesity	Qualified yes	Because of the risk of heat illness, obese persons need careful acclimatization and hydration.
Organ transplant recipient	Qualified yes	Athlete needs individual assessment.
Ovary, absence of one	Yes	Risk of severe injury to the remaining ovary is minimal.
Respiratory conditions		
Asthma	Yes	With proper medication and education, only athletes with the most severe asthma will need to modify their participation.
Acute upper respiratory infection	Qualified yes	Upper respiratory obstruction may affect pulmonary function. Athlete needs individual assessment for all but mild disease.
Pulmonary compromise, including cystic fibrosis	Qualified yes	Athlete needs individual assessment, but generally, all sports may be played if oxygenation remains satisfactory during a graded exercise test. Patients with cystic fibrosis need acclimatization and good hydration to reduce the risk of heat illness.
Sickle cell disease	Qualified yes	Athlete needs individual assessment. In general, if status of the illness permits, all but high-exertion, collision, and contact sports may be played. Overheating, dehydration, and chilling must be avoided.

(continued)

Table 19.4 *(continued)*		
Condition	**Participate decision**	**Explanation**
Sickle cell trait	Yes	It is unlikely that persons with sickle cell trait have an increased risk of sudden death or other medical problems during athletic participation, except under the most extreme conditions of heat, humidity, and possibly increased altitude. These persons, like all athletes, should be carefully conditioned, acclimatized, and hydrated to reduce any possible risk.
Skin disorders (boils, herpes simplex, impetigo, scabies, molluscum contagiosum)	Qualified yes	While the patient is contagious, participation in gymnastics with mats; martial arts; wrestling; or other collision, contact, or limited-contact sports is not allowed.
Spleen, enlarged	Qualified yes	A patient with an acutely enlarged spleen should avoid all sports because of risk of rupture. A patient with a chronically enlarged spleen needs individual assessment before playing collision, contact, or limited-contact sports.
Testicle, undescended or absence of one	Yes	Certain sports may require a protective cup.

Reprinted, by permission, from R.W. Washington et al., 2001, "Medical conditions affecting sports participation," *Pediatrics* 107(5): 1205-1209.

conditions (Washington et al. 2001). These are only guidelines. Always consider individual circumstances when making the final decision regarding playability.

SUMMARY

1. *Discuss the different types of examinations and identify advantages and disadvantages of each type of preparticipation physical exam.*

The preparticipation physical exam (PPPE) is an important part of health care for all young athletes. For many, it is their only interaction with a health-care provider and therefore should be as comprehensive as possible. The exam's major purpose is to identify medical and orthopedic problems that may require further evaluation and treatment to ensure safe athletic participation. PPPEs are also useful adjuncts to standard health-care endeavors in that, when performed thoroughly, they may identify young people who are experiencing psychosocial problems or problems with drugs, STDs, or domestic abuse. The ideal venue for the PPPE is the traditional in-office examination by a physician or primary caregiver such as a nurse practitioner or physician's assistant who works under the supervision of a physician. Because 80% to 90% of adolescents seek routine health care solely to receive clearance for sports participation, the primary care health provider who knows the patient best should perform the examination. A more private, discreet, personal environment will make it more likely that an adolescent will share both physical and emotional concerns.

The station-type exam is frequently used to examine a large group of people in a fairly short time. In this type of exam, the athletes move from one station to the next (in different rooms, for the sake of privacy) to complete the entire physical examination. Station-type exams can be very useful, timely, and cost-effective when they are well organized and executed.

2. *Explain the limitations of the PPPE and be able to educate athletes and their families about these limitations.*

The most important reason for performing PPPEs is to guarantee athletes' safety. Although some young people fear that such exams exist primarily to find excuses for disqualifying them, disqualification for health reasons is in fact quite rare. The PPPE should determine whether students are fit to play, are cleared to play only after a specified regimen of rehabilitation, or are disqualified because play would be dangerous to their health. The athlete's family should be involved in making the final decision. An important reason for PPPEs is to try to identify athletes at risk for sudden death. Unfortunately, thorough histories and physical exams often cannot identify athletes at risk for sudden death—athletes and their families must understand this key limitation of the PPPE.

3. *Recognize the importance of the medical history in assessing the athlete's health, risk factors, and playability; make sure a comprehensive history form is used that can document assessment for key aspects of this screening tool.*

A complete medical history is the foundation of any medical evaluation in that it can identify a majority of problems affecting athletes. The history should focus on cardiovascular and musculoskeletal anomalies or injuries, as these areas are the most likely to restrict participation or to require follow-up before participation.

4. *Identify the components of the physical exam portion of the PPPE.*

The physical exam must focus on potential medical or orthopedic problems that could hinder performance, be life-threatening, or be worsened by athletic participation. The examination should record vital signs (pulse, respiratory rate, and blood pressure), height, and weight. Vision screening should be included with a mechanism to refer patients with deficits below 20/40. A detailed cardiac examination is the most important part of the PPPE. A thorough evaluation of the history will dictate the need for discussion of previous surgical interventions, absence of a paired organ (kidney, testicle), and any other medical issues. The absence of a paired organ may not require disqualification, but the medical team must discuss the specific risks of participation in contact or collision sports with the athlete and his or her family. Orthopedic exams should focus mainly on previously injured areas. Examination to confirm full recovery of any previous orthopedic injury is essential.

Lab tests should be ordered only when history and physical examination warrant further evaluation. Personal issues are impossible to address in a station-type examination. Reserve such considerations for private, one-on-one discussions in a physician's or athletic trainer's office.

APPENDIX: SPORTS MEDICINE AS A SPECIALTY

Terms and Definitions

allopathic—Referring to the traditional Western approach to medicine, in which diseases are treated with remedies whose effects differ from those of the ailment. This concept is perhaps best understood in contrast to *homeopathy,* in which a disease might be treated by minuscule doses of a substance (e.g., an herb) that produces the same symptoms as the disease.

osteopathic—Branch of medicine that believes in holistic assessment and treatment perspective involving the whole body, proper mobility, and balance, along with synchronous relationships among systems (cardiovascular, neural, respiratory, etc.).

As one of the broadest areas of medicine, sports medicine relates to virtually every traditional medical specialty. Simply put, it is *the discipline of caring for individuals who exercise.* It involves taking care of people who are injured or ill and deals with how these problems affect the ability to exercise; it is also about preventing medical problems in people who exercise.

Orthopedic and soft-tissue problems receive a lot of media attention because of their immediate effects on an athlete's ability to perform. But anyone who works professionally with athletes needs to know about more than just bones, tendons, and muscles. Though not every physician who practices sports medicine is a team physician, many physicians provide medical care for a team—or at least for a serious athlete—in one or more sports. When sports medicine includes all aspects of the specialty, it is known as *primary care sports medicine.* A primary care physician provides comprehensive and continuous care to patients. A *primary care sports physician* provides this care specifically to individuals who exercise and has specialized knowledge about the care of athletes. Primary care sports physicians typically specialize in a traditional area of medicine, such as family practice, pediatrics, or internal medicine, and then subspecialize in sports medicine. Orthopedic surgeons may serve as team physicians and practice sports medicine. Their practice is usually limited to the surgical and nonsurgical treatment of musculoskeletal injuries and diseases. Among the health professionals who do or may specialize in sports medicine concerns are podiatrists, chiropractors, dentists, certified athletic trainers, physical therapists, nutritionists, psychologists, and massage therapists.

Although most students taking this course will already be familiar with the history of athletic training as a profession, not as many are familiar with the development of sports medicine as a specialty. Thus, you may find it helpful to take a closer look at that history. Additionally, some understanding of the training and certification process for sports medicine physicians will enable you as an athletic trainer to make informed, educated choices about the specialists to whom you refer your athletes.

THE HISTORY OF SPORTS MEDICINE

To understand the scope of sports medicine, it is helpful to examine its history. Scientific study of athletes began in the late 1800s as physical educators examined athletes' training and injuries. Educators organized themselves in 1885 into the American Academy of Physical Education (AAPE), which later became the American Association for Health, Physical Education, and Recreation (AAHPER) and eventually the American Alliance for Health, Physical Education, Recreation and

Dance (AAHPERD). This organization remains an important resource for physical educators in North America.

The pioneers of clinical sports medicine were the Germans, who first used the term *sports physician* in 1904. Sports physicians throughout the world met in Switzerland in 1928 to form the Fédération Internationale de Médecine du Sport (FIMS). Very few physicians from the United States, however, got involved in international endeavors at that time. Many U.S. colleges had *team surgeons* who worked with athletic trainers (known then as *rubbers*), but team physicians were not identified as sports specialists. One such physician was quoted as saying that professional association with athletes was "thought to be a little undignified for a doctor of medicine" (J.W. Berryman, 1995, *Out of many, one* [Champaign, IL: Human Kinetics], 29). Books and journals on sports medicine in the United States did not appear until the 1930s.

Athletic trainers also began to see the need to organize themselves. At the 1938 Drake Relays in Des Moines, Iowa, they formed the National Athletic Trainers' Association (NATA).

World War II heightened interest in physical fitness and training as they related to the military. As scientists and physicians in the United States became more interested in the activities of FIMS, they decided they should form their own group. The Federation of Sports Medicine was born in 1954, and a year later it changed its name to the American College of Sports Medicine (ACSM). The 11 founding members comprised three physicians (all cardiologists) and eight physical educators. Although it was ACSM's goal to be an all-encompassing organization, physicians interested in sports medicine were forming groups within other organizations. Team physicians formed a committee associated with the American Medical Association in 1953; and physicians developed sports medicine groups within their specialties—for instance, orthopedic surgeons formed the American Orthopedic Society for Sports Medicine (AOSSM) in 1972; pediatricians formed a committee within the American Academy of Pediatrics; and in 1991, primary care physicians created the American Medical Society for Sports Medicine (AMSSM).

CERTIFICATION OF SPORTS PHYSICIANS

Most physicians or "medical doctors" have completed 4 yr of college and 4 yr of medical school. After receiving the MD degree, a physician desiring to enter a specialty must undergo at least 3 yr of residency training. Pursuit of a subspecialty requires 1 to 3 yr of additional training, commonly referred to as fellowship training. Subspecialty fellowship training in sports medicine was first offered in the late 1970s in orthopedics and later in family medicine.

Because there is no single organization that represents the field of sports medicine, the American Board of Medical Specialties (ABMS) decided to create a Certificate of Added Qualification (CAQ) for sports medicine similar to the one created for geriatric medicine. (The ABMS is the umbrella group consisting of all the **allopathic** specialties.) All physicians must pass a written examination to become specialists or subspecialists; this examination serves to provide a subspecialty certification. Four specialty boards decided to participate in this endeavor—Family Practice, Pediatrics, Internal Medicine, and Emergency Medicine. Representatives of these four boards formed a committee in 1991 to create an examination that would cover appropriate subject matter. The first examination was offered in 1993. As of 1999, anyone who sits for the CAQ examination must have postgraduate fellowship training in sports medicine. Currently there are about 60 such fellowships in the United States, requiring 1 or 2 yr of subspecialty training after completion of the traditional specialty residency.

After an increasing number of physicians joined the ACSM, that organization created courses for team physicians. These courses are known as Level I, Level II, and Advanced Team Physician courses. AMSSM and AOSSM currently co-sponsor the same courses.

The American Academy of Orthopedic Surgeons (AAOS) continues to debate the need for a CAQ for orthopedic surgeons and has yet to move toward any further certification in the area of sports medicine. About 55 postgraduate fellowships are available for orthopedic surgeons in sports medicine.

Before the creation of the CAQ by ABMS, the American Osteopathic Association (AOA) had specified a *subboard* qualification, requiring a CAQ for a variety of specialists, not just the four determined by ABMS. The AOA's first exam was offered in 1995.

WHAT EXACTLY IS SPORTS MEDICINE?

One of us (GLL) served on the ABMS committee charged with creating the CAQ for the sports medicine subspecialty. We discovered that, before we could write an examination, we needed to clearly define *sports medicine.* In 1991, the committee stated that sports medicine is a body of knowledge and a broad area of health care that includes

- exercise as an essential component of health throughout life;
- medical management and supervision of recreational and competitive athletes and all others who exercise; and
- exercise for prevention and treatment of disease and injury.

The committee felt that the practice of sports medicine is the application of the physician's knowledge, skills, and attitudes to all persons engaged in sports and exercise. Included in this practice is the following broad range of issues:

- Physiology and biomechanics of exercise
- Basic nutritional principles and their application to exercise
- Psychological aspects of exercise, performance, and competition
- Guidelines for evaluating athletes before they participate in exercise
- Physical conditioning requirements for various activities
- Pathology and pathophysiology of illness and injury as they relate to exercise
- Effects of disease on exercise and the use of exercise in the care of medical problems
- Prevention, evaluation, management, and rehabilitation of injuries
- Understanding pharmacology and the effects of therapeutic, performance-enhancing, and recreational drugs on exercise
- Promotion of physical fitness and healthy lifestyles
- Functioning as a team physician
- Ethical principles as applied to exercise and sports
- Medical-legal aspects of exercise and sports
- Anatomy related to exercise
- Growth and development related to exercise

ISSUES FOR REFERRING ALLIED HEALTH PROFESSIONALS

With so many groups involved in sports medicine, it becomes difficult for allied health-care professionals who make referrals, as well as consumers, to know who is truly a specialist in the field. One approach is to determine if an individual has passed the CAQ for primary care **osteopathic** or allopathic physicians. Anyone can call ABMS at 1-800-776-2378 to ask if a practitioner has passed a certification exam in any field; alternatively, one can check the ABMS Web site at www.abms.org/newsearch.asp. Though it is also helpful to find out if physicians are fellowship trained (this status is probably just as important as passing the CAQ), unfortunately there is no way to obtain such information without asking the physicians or their office staffs. A few other characteristics make a physician particularly attractive as a sports medicine specialist:

- A physician who serves as a team physician demonstrates a degree of commitment to the specialty.
- A physician who has published articles on sports medicine may have expertise in sports medicine that another doctor may not have.
- The physician's "supporting cast" is also important: Are the physical therapists with whom the physician works good at dealing with athletes? Are they interested in getting patients "back in the game?"
- Does the physician have a working relationship with athletic trainers?

Note that a physician need not be a primary care physician or orthopedic surgeon to be a team physician or to be knowledgeable in sports medicine. Virtually any physician who is practicing clinical medicine can serve as a team physician and contribute to sports medicine.

Other Fields

Many types of health providers participate in the care of athletes. Rarely can a single person deal with all the health issues that arise. The most common disciplines involved in the care of athletes are nutrition, physical therapy, athletic training, chiropractic, podiatry, massage therapy, psychology, optometry, dentistry, and exercise physiology. This is not an exhaustive list; many other areas contribute from time to time to an athlete's performance.

What's Special About a Sports Medicine Specialist?

Sports medicine specialists value exercise and want to help patients return to sport or exercise as soon as possible. Physicians with no interest in sports medicine may simply tell patients to stop the activity that is associated with pain or an injury; such physicians tend to be conservative, erring on the side of caution, especially when they are uncertain about a diagnosis. When asked, "When can I run?", a physician who is not tuned into how important exercise is to the patient may respond, "Why is it so important to run? Just rest!"—whereas the sports medicine physician often asks, "What can we do to help you run sooner?" Sports medicine is popular because practitioners understand the value of exercise and sports and tend to help patients do what they want to do (within reason): It is giving extra asthma medication to a mountain climber with moderate to persistent asthma so that she can reach the summit; it is injecting cortisone into a runner's iliotibial band bursa so that the runner can compete in the marathon for which he has worked so hard. Sports medicine uses a working knowledge of injuries and illnesses to inform athletes when continued participation is low risk or too dangerous.

Application to Other Patients

Sports medicine is relevant to people other than athletes. Many performing artists, for example, develop some of the same illnesses and injuries as athletes, and treatments that work for athletes work as well for the performing artists. Similarly, injured employees who are worried about their ability to continue working have issues similar to those of injured athletes. There is significant overlap between industrial medicine (the study of work-related injuries and illnesses) and sports medicine: Like athletes who want to continue participating in sport, workers often want to stay on the job to avoid an interruption in earnings.

SPORTS MEDICINE IN MEDICAL EDUCATION

Many medical students throughout the world know the importance of exercise and want to learn the principles of sports medicine. In the United States, medical schools have been slow to address this need and rarely include sports medicine in the formal curriculum. Although the knowledge base in medicine continues to expand, medical school administrators hesitate to remove existing subjects from the curriculum to make room for new courses such as sports medicine. Interested students generally must seek the information on their own. Many physicians seek out sports medicine training during residency or as continuing medical education when they are out in clinical practice.

SUMMARY

Sports medicine is a broader field than most people realize. It encompasses virtually any medical specialty as that specialty relates to people who exercise. No one group represents all the physicians who are sports medicine specialists. Most sports medicine specialists are team physicians and have passed the Certificate of Added Qualification in sports medicine. Sports medicine is not covered well in medical schools; but many physicians, once they are out in practice, seek additional training in this important area through residency training and at conferences.

GLOSSARY

acquired immunodeficiency syndrome (AIDS)—Advanced HIV infection characterized by the presence of opportunistic infection and lowered counts of helper T cells.

acromegaly—Abnormal enlargement of the jaw, nose, fingers, and toes.

acute mountain sickness (AMS)—An illness that can affect anybody who ascends too rapidly to high altitude.

adenosine triphosphate (ATP)—A nucleotide compound occurring in all cells where it represents energy storage in the form of phosphate bonds. To release energy, it is hydrolyzed to adenosine diphosphate (ADP) and a phosphate group.

alkalotic—Having abnormally high pH (alkalinity) in the blood and tissues.

allopathic—Referring to the traditional Western approach to medicine, in which diseases are treated with remedies whose effects differ from those of the ailment. This concept is perhaps best understood in contrast to *homeopathy*, in which a disease might be treated by minuscule doses of a substance (e.g., an herb) that produces the same symptoms as the disease.

amenorrhea—The absence of menstrual bleeding for at least 90 d.

anabolic—Stimulating the biosynthesis of tissue.

anabolic-androgenic steroid (AAS)—Name for synthetic derivative of the male sex hormone testosterone that stimulates the biosynthesis of tissue and causes masculine sex characteristics.

anabolic steroids—Name for synthetic derivative of male sex hormone, testosterone.

analgesic—An agent that reduces pain without causing loss of consciousness.

androgenic—Causing masculine characteristics.

anisocoria—Inequality in pupil size that sometimes occurs naturally.

anorexia athletica—A term coined by Sundgot-Borgen that refers to eating disorders in female athletes that do not strictly fit the definition of anorexia nervosa but that are clearly pathological and related to sport.

anorexia nervosa—An eating disorder, seen mostly in young women, characterized by pathological fear of weight gain and accompanied by excessive weight loss via severe dieting or starvation.

anovulation—The occurrence of a menstrual cycle that is not related to release of an egg (ovum).

antegrade amnesia—Inability to remember events occurring *after* a traumatic incident.

anticholinergic—Side effects of blocking action of neurotransmitter (acetylcholine) that results in constipation, dry mouth, and decreased sweating.

antiplatelet—A substance that inhibits action of platelets in the blood and hence inhibits clotting.

antipyretic—An agent that relieves or reduces fever.

apophyseal growth plate—**Physis** that causes an outgrowth or bump on the bone; also called *traction physis* or *apophysis*. Occurs where large tendons insert into bones.

ataxia—Inability to coordinate muscular movements.

auscultation—The act of listening with a stethoscope.

beta-2-andrenergic agonists—Medications resembling adrenaline (epinephrine) that selectively stimulate receptors in bronchial smooth muscle, causing relaxation and bronchodilation. They are selective agonists because of reduced stimulation of beta one receptors in the heart.

beta-hydroxy-beta-methylbutyrate (HMB)—A metabolite of the amino acid leucine that is produced naturally in the body.

biohazard container—A plastic container into which are placed all nonsharp materials (e.g., bandages, rubber gloves) that have come into contact with body fluids.

body mass index (BMI)—A measure of body composition, equal to an individual's weight in kilograms divided by the square of the height in meters.

bradycardia—Unusually slow heart rate.

brain herniation—Shift of the intracranial contents through the cranial foramen with increasing intracranial pressure.

bronchoprovocation test—Clinical test that challenges the lungs chemically (typically with methacholine or histamine) or with another potential trigger such as exercise or temperature, and measures the effects of these potential triggers on lung function (such as forced respiratory volume or peak expiratory flow rate).

bronchospasm—Contraction of the smooth muscle that surrounds the airway, resulting in narrowing of the lumen, through which air enters and exits the lungs.

bulimia nervosa—An eating disorder, seen mostly in young women, characterized by compulsive overeating followed by self-induced vomiting, use of laxatives, or use of diuretics to prevent weight gain.

bulla—A large blister, usually larger than 2 cm in diameter.

CD 4 cells—The type of T cell specifically targeted by HIV.

cellulitis—A spreading bacterial infection of the dermis and subcutaneous tissue; it typically begins as a small area of tenderness, redness, and swelling, and may progress to fever, chills, and swollen lymph nodes close to the infected area.

cholinergic urticaria (CU)—A condition associated with small (2-4 mm) hives in response to passive warming of the body or with exercise.

ciliary muscles—Tiny muscles within the eye that cause the lens to change shape to focus light on the retina and thus change the opening of the iris to accommodate different intensities of light.

cirrhosis—Liver disease typified by extreme fibrosis; scar tissue replaces normal cells, leading to decline of liver function.

colicky—Characterized by fluctuations in degree of pain.

complex carbohydrates—Starches such as bread, pastas, and cereals.

computerized axial tomography (CT or CAT scan)—X-ray beams are converted to electronic impulses and processed by a computer to display the body in cross-section.

concussion—Traumatically induced alteration in mental status, with or without loss of consciousness.

conjugate gaze—Normal vision, when both eyes work together to point at the same place.

conjunctiva—The mucous membrane lining the inner surface of the eyelids and the outer surface of the eyeball.

cornea—The transparent, tough outer coating of the eye that covers the pupil and iris.

corticosteroids—Medications chemically related to cortisone and used primarily for their anti-inflammatory effect.

cortisol—A hormone secreted by the adrenal gland resulting in protein breakdown, fatty acid breakdown, and an increase in blood glucose concentration.

crepitus—A grating sound or sensation in joints, lungs, or skin.

cyclooxygenase-1 (COX-1)—An important enzyme present in most human tissues; responsible for converting arachidonic acid to terminal prostaglandins, the hormones that promote the inflammatory process. COX-1 is involved in many other physiologic autoregulation processes.

cyclooxygenase-2 (COX-2)—Same function as COX-1 and present in smaller amounts in tissues. It is only responsible for inflammation, but its role in the inflammatory process is larger than that of COX-1.

dehydroepiandrosterone (DHEA)—A steroid compound synthesized from cholesterol and with mild androgenic properties. In the body, it is converted to testosterone, a more potent androgen.

diabetic ketoacidosis (DKA)—Serious metabolic condition resulting from gross insulin deficiency leading to severe hyperglycemia, dehydration, and electrolyte abnormalities.

diplopia—Double vision.

disconjugate gaze—A condition wherein the eyes do not move together.

doping—Use of performance-enhancing drugs.

dura mater—The outer, tough membrane that covers the brain and spinal cord.

dysmenorrhea—Painful menses.

dysuria—Pain with urination.

electrocardiogram (ECG)—An electrical study of the heart.

endometriosis—Possible cause of dysmenorrhea related to abnormally placed uterine cells in pelvic cavity. The cells may be attached to the ovaries, fallopian tubes, uterus, or anywhere in the pelvic cavity.

epidural hematoma—Clot caused by bleeding between the skull and the dura mater.

epinephrine—A hormone secreted by the adrenal gland. Actions include counterbalancing the effects of insulin and reacting to stress by increasing metabolism, blood pressure, heart rate, and blood flow to muscles.

epiphyseal growth plate—**Physis** at the end of a long bone; also called *pressure physis.*

Epstein-Barr virus (EBV)—A herpes virus that causes infectious mononucleosis; it also is associated with Burkitt's lymphoma and certain nasopharyngeal cancers.

ergogenic—Any substance taken or used for the purpose of improving performance.

erythema—Abnormal skin redness, usually resulting from congestion of capillaries.

erythropoietin—Hormone that stimulates the bone marrow to make more red blood cells; high-altitude exercise leads to greater synthesis of erythropoietin in the kidneys.

exercise-induced anaphylaxis—The massive release of histamine triggered by exercise, producing itchiness, hives, swelling of hands and face, and hypotension.

exercise-induced asthma (EIA)—Bronchoconstriction and mucous production associated with exercise. Asthma means hyperreactive airways. Exercise is one of many sources that produces asthmatic symptoms such as coughing, wheezing, and shortness of breath.

external hordeolum—The common **sty,** which is a mild infection of the glands of Moll or Zeis in the eyelid.

fecolith—Small piece of stool sometimes stuck in appendiceal lumen (opening).

female athlete triad—An interrelated group of disorders consisting of disordered eating, amenorrhea, and osteoporosis.

fibrosis—Scarring (of the liver, in the context of chapter 9).

fluorescein—A dye that fluoresces under black light; when applied to the eye, it can allow the examiner to see very small abrasions of the cornea.

focal neurological examination—Specific finding on a neurological exam that localizes a neurological injury (or tumor) to one area of the brain.

free fatty acids (FFA)—The body's primary energy source in the blood.

free radicals—Chemicals containing one or more unpaired electrons that occur naturally in the body and play a role in numerous physiological reactions. The majority of these compounds are oxidants capable of oxidizing a range of biological molecules.

gallop—Type of abnormal extra heart sound heard when auscultating the heart.

gangrene—Death of tissues caused by insufficient blood supply, with complete breakdown of tissue; it is often followed by bacterial infection and cell death.

gas chromatography (GC)—A process used to identify chemical compounds from a mixture using an inert gas that is run through a column. The individual components separate along the column in a certain order based on their chemical composition.

gastroesophageal reflux—Movement of stomach acid into the lower esophagus.

gastrointestinal (GI)—Pertaining to the stomach and intestine.

gigantism—Excessive growth in the long bones as well as in specific body parts.

glands of Moll/glands of Zeis—Microscopic glands in the eyelid that produce an oil that coats tears to keep them from evaporating too quickly. Infection of one of these glands produces a **sty.**

glaucoma—A condition of elevated intraocular pressure. If left untreated, glaucoma can cause permanent visual loss or blindness.

globe—The eyeball.

glucagon—A hormone produced by the pancreas; released in response to decreased glucose levels.

gluconeogenesis—Synthesis of glucose, mainly in the liver, from noncarbohydrate precursors such as lactate and pyruvate; occurs primarily as a response to intense exercise.

glucose tolerance test (GTT)—Screening test for diabetes wherein the patient drinks a prescribed fluid with high sugar content. In diabetics, blood sugars rise higher than normal after drinking this solution.

glycogen—A storage carbohydrate found mainly in the liver but also in muscle cells; consists of long chains of glucose. It is broken down during high-intensity exercise to provide glucose for energy.

glycosuria—The presence of sugar (glucose) in the urine, generally defined as 1 g or more in a 24-h period.

glycosylated hemoglobin (GHgb)—Hemoglobin in the blood that is bound to glucose. Everyone has a small percentage of GHgb, and it increases if blood sugar levels are elevated.

group A strep—The strain of *Streptococcus pyogenes* bacteria that causes streptococcal pharyngitis, rheumatic fever, and many skin infections.

growth hormone—Hormone released by the pituitary gland.

gynecomastia—Development of breast tissue in males.

hematuria—The finding of blood in the urine.

hepatitis B virus (HBV)—Virus commonly spread by sexual intercourse, blood transfusion, or contaminated needles resulting in liver infection.

hepatitis C virus (HCV)—Virus spread by blood transfusion and possibly intercourse or contaminated needles resulting in liver infection.

high-density lipoprotein (HDL)—The so-called "good" cholesterol.

hirsutism—Excessive hairiness; in women, it usually manifests as an adult male pattern of hair distribution.

human immunodeficiency virus (HIV)—A virus that selectively infects certain types of white blood cells (helper T cells) resulting in the disease AIDS.

human papilloma virus (HPV)—A virus that causes common warts on feet and hands, mucous membranes of anal and genital areas.

hyperacusis—Sensitivity to loud noise.

hypercholesterolemia—An excess of cholesterol in the blood, usually more than 200 mg/dl in an adult.

hypertriglyceridemia—An excess of triglycerides in the blood. The upper limit of normal rises with increasing age.

hypertrophic cardiomyopathy (HCM)—Abnormal enlargement of diseased heart muscle.

hypertrophy—Abnormal growth or enlargement resulting from enlargement of cells.

hyponatremia—Abnormally low blood levels of sodium.

hyponatremic collapse—Low sodium content related to overhydration with water resulting in myriad symptoms, from confusion to death (also called *exercise-induced hyponatremia*).

hypotension—Abnormally low blood pressure.

hypovolemia—Abnormally low volume of blood plasma in the body.

hysterectomy—Surgical removal of the uterus.

ileus—Lack of peristalsis, or quiet intestine.

inflammation—A local immune response intended to protect from infection. Includes dilation of arterioles, capillaries, and the smallest veins; increased permeability and blood flow; exudation of blood plasma along with plasma proteins; and migration of white blood cells into the inflamed area. Inflammation of bronchial tissues contributes to obstruction of lumen and exacerbates asthma.

insulin—A hormone produced by the pancreas; released in response to elevated glucose levels.

internal hordeolum—Infection of the **meibomian glands.**

irritable bowel syndrome (IBS)—A common disorder of the intestines that leads to crampy pain, gassiness, bloating, and changes in bowel habits.

ischemia—Lack of oxygen in a specific area of tissue caused by inadequate blood flow.

ketoacidosis—Elevation of ketones and various organic acids in the blood; results from high levels of blood sugar.

long QT syndrome—A genetic condition in which the heart's ability to repolarize, or electrically recharge itself, is abnormal. The QT interval is the time between the start of the heart being polarized to contract the muscle and when the heart is completely repolarized.

macule—A spot of any size on the skin.

magnetic resonance imaging (MRI)—Exposure of human tissue to a magnetic field causes molecules in the tissue to generate different frequencies of vibration. These frequencies are detected by a coil and converted into images that show the body part in cross-section.

malingering—In athletes, intentionally pretending to have symptoms of mental or physical illness to avoid returning to play. Usually involves a conscious decision to intentionally deceive sports medicine professionals about their injury.

mandible—The lower jaw.

mass effect—Pressure on and movement of brain tissue that results from swelling and bleeding.

mass spectrophotometry (MS)—A sophisticated analytical tool used to identify chemicals based on how chemicals break down atomically when bombarded with electrical energy. Every chemical has a unique mass spectrophotometric fingerprint.

mast cell stabilizers—Medications that prevent the release of histamine from mast cells.

meibomian glands—Microscopic glands in the eyelid, similar to the glands of Moll and Zeis. Infection of one of these glands produces a **sty.**

menarche—The beginning of menstrual functioning.

menometrorrhagia—Excessive uterine bleeding both during menses and at irregular intervals.

menorrhagia—Excessive uterine bleeding at regular intervals.

metabolite—A chemical that is a breakdown product of a larger chemical usually produced by an enzyme in the body.

mild traumatic brain injury (MTBI)—See **concussion.**

minute ventilation—The volume of air breathed each minute (e.g., 12 breaths/min with average tidal volume of 0.5 L/breath = minute ventilation of 6 L/min).

mitral valve prolapse (MVP)—A condition affecting the mitral valve in the heart wherein a two-flapped valve between the left atrium and left ventricle balloons back into the left atrium with each heartbeat.

Monospot test—A brand name of a laboratory exam that tests blood for antibodies to the Epstein-Barr virus; positive results usually indicate infectious mononucleosis, but other rarer diseases can also produce positive results. The generic name for this test is a heterophile antibody test.

murmur—Soft or harsh swooshing sound heard between normal heart sounds during auscultation of the heart.

muscle guarding—Muscle spasm in an attempt to protect the painful area.

nonfocal neurological examination—Completely normal neurological exam that finds nothing to indicate a localizing process such as unilateral weakness, sensory changes, or coordination difficulty.

nonshivering thermogenesis—Hormone-regulated production of heat.

nonsteroidal anti-inflammatory drug (NSAID)—Any medication that blocks inflammation and is not chemically related to a corticosteroid (e.g., ibuprofen).

norepinephrine—A hormone similar in action to epinephrine. Also secreted by the adrenal gland.

obsessive-compulsive disorder (OCD)—Recurrent obsessions or compulsions that are severe enough to be time consuming or cause marked distress or significant impairment.

obstipation—Intractable constipation.

oligomenorrhea—Infrequent menstrual bleeding, typically at intervals of more than 40 d.

orthostatic hypotension—Decreased blood pressure and concomitant increased heart rate a person experiences when rising from supine to standing or sitting position.

osteopathic—Branch of medicine that believes in holistic assessment and treatment perspective involving the whole body, proper mobility, and balance, along with synchronous relationships among systems (cardiovascular, neural, respiratory, etc.).

osteoporosis—The loss of bone mineral density and the inadequate formation of bone, leading to bone fragility and possible risk of fracture.

ovariectomy—Surgical removal of an ovary.

palpation—Examination by touch.

papule—Any bump on the skin.

paresthesia—Tingling or prickly sensation in the skin.

pericardium—The membranous sac that surrounds the heart.

peritoneum—The membrane that lines the cavity of the abdomen.

peritonitis—Inflammation or infection of the abdominal lining.

periumbilical—Around the navel or the central region of the abdomen.

pH—A measure of acidity; because urine is normally slightly acidic (pH < 7.0), alkaline urine (pH > 7.0) indicates possible tampering with the sample.

pharyngitis—Inflammation of the pharynx (back of the throat).

photophobia—Abnormal visual intolerance to light.

physis—Area of bone that is continuing to grow; also called *epiphyseal growth plate*.

polycystic ovary syndrome (PCOS)—Includes the following signs and symptoms: irregular or absent menses, numerous cysts on the ovaries in many but not all cases, high blood pressure, acne, elevated insulin levels associated with insulin resistance, infertility, excess hair on the face and body, thinning of the scalp hair, and obesity.

postconcussive syndrome (PCS)—When symptoms from a concussion persist beyond the first few days of the injury.

post-ictal phase—Phase of a seizure that follows convulsing; characterized by increased somnolence and sometimes confusion.

premenstrual syndrome (PMS)—Usually occurring during the 10 d prior to menstruation, marked by emotional instability, irritability, insomnia, and headache.

pruritic—Itchy.

psychiatrist—A medical doctor who treats individuals with behavioral or mental disorders; main function is to prescribe drugs that can ameliorate symptoms of disorders.

psychologist—A professional with clinical training (usually a PhD) who treats behavioral or mental disorders through psychotherapy and does not prescribe drugs.

pustule—A papule with pus in the center.

rebound tenderness—Abdominal pain that hurts more when the hand is suddenly released from palpation; a sign of possible peritonitis.

recommended daily allowance (RDA)—The amount of a nutrient taken daily to prevent conditions associated with a deficiency. They are established with the goal of at least a 30% margin of safety to cover the nutritional needs of 97% of healthy Americans.

rectus muscles—The four muscles that control eye movement. Each of the four is attached to the back of the globe (eyeball). The *medial* and *lateral* rectus muscles move the eye side to side; the *superior* and *inferior* recti move the eye up and down.

retrograde amnesia—Inability to remember events occurring immediately *before* a traumatic incident.

rub—Type of heart sound caused by friction between the outside layer of the lining of the heart and the heart itself as a result of fluid inflammation or infection.

sclera—The tough, fibrous coating of the exterior of the white part of the eyeball.

scoliosis—Lateral curvature of the spine.

secondary gain—An unconscious advantage a patient may receive from physical illness or other complaints. Athletes who unconsciously perceive advantages to negative events such as injuries, defeats, and the like may not do their best to overcome their compromised situation.

selective serotonin reuptake inhibitor (SSRI)—A medication that blocks the reuptake of the neurotransmitter serotonin into neurons and has only weak effects on the reuptake of other neurotransmitters such as norepinephrine and dopamine.

sharps container—A plastic container into which are placed all sharp items (e.g., needles, syringes, lancets) that have come into contact with body fluids.

simple carbohydrates—Sugars such as those found in desserts, soda, candy, jelly, and the like.

specific gravity—The ratio of the density of a sample to the density of water. If urine has a specific gravity <1.015, the person may have ingested large amounts of liquid to dilute drug residues in the urine.

spermarche—The first ejaculation.

status asthmaticus—Emergent situation in which respiratory distress secondary to asthma is poorly responsive even to large doses of bronchodilators.

stenosis—Narrowing.

streptococcal pharyngitis—A sore and inflamed throat due to one strain of the *Streptococcus pyogenes* bacteria, usually group A; strep throat.

sty—Infection of one or more of the glands in the eyelid.

subclinical—Not detectable, or producing no clinical manifestations (e.g., in the early stage of a disease).

subconjunctival hemorrhage—Bleeding in the white of the eye. More specifically, a relatively harmless rupturing of tiny veins in the sclera as a result of a **Valsalva maneuver.** Typically results in a bright red triangle next to the iris.

subdural hematoma—Clot caused by bleeding under the dura mater but outside of the brain surface.

syncope—Loss of consciousness caused by inadequate blood flow to the brain; fainting.

tachycardia—Abnormally rapid heartbeat.

temporomandibular joint (TMJ)—The joint at which the lower jaw attaches to the side of the skull.

T/E ratio—The ratio of testosterone to epitestosterone in the urine. A ratio greater than 6.0 usually implies that the person has taken exogenous testosterone.

tetrahydrocannabinol (THC)—The primary active ingredient in marijuana.

therapeutic index—A measure of the margin of safety of a drug. It is sometimes defined as the TD50/ED50, where TD50 is the dose of a drug that produces a toxic endpoint in 50% of the population and the ED50 is the dose of a drug that produces a therapeutic endpoint in 50% of the population. A high therapeutic index means that serious side effects are unlikely even at high doses.

thrombocytopenia—A decrease in blood platelet count associated with decreased clotting ability.

tinnitus—Ringing or roaring in the ears.

T lymphocytes (T cells)—A type of white blood cell responsible for the cell-mediated immunity that is critical for fighting viral infections, fungal infections, and certain bacteria such as tuberculosis.

tonic-clonic seizure—Disorganized electrical brain activity that leads to loss of consciousness and generalized muscle contractions; may be associated with urinary incontinence and biting of the tongue. A post-ictal state generally follows the seizure.

tricyclic antidepressant (TCAD)—A medication that is composed of three chemical rings and is used to treat depression.

upper respiratory infection (URI)—The common cold, associated with a stuffy and runny nose, cough, and low-grade fever.

urticaria—Allergic reaction characterized by raised welts on the skin and usually accompanied by intense itching. Commonly called hives. Can be caused by internal or by external contact allergens.

U.S. Anti-Doping Agency (USADA)—Organization dedicated to the elimination of doping in sport.

Valsalva maneuver or event—An effort to forcibly expel air while intentionally blocking the exit of air from mouth and nostrils (as is often done when trying to clear the eustachian tubes during air travel).

venipuncture—The puncture of a vein with a needle to obtain a blood sample.

vesicle—A very small blister, usually less than 1 cm in diameter.

virulent—Able to cause severe disease or death in an infected person.

visual acuity (VA)—A measure of the eye's ability to resolve two adjoining lines. The most common expression of VA is as a measurement of the smallest letters you can read on a standardized chart at 20 ft. This is usually expressed as a ratio of the distance you are from the chart to the distance at which a person with normal eyesight could read the same line. If a person's VA is 20/40, then at a distance of 20 feet from a chart that person can see what a normal person would see at 40 feet. Normal vision is 20/20.

vitreous humor (also called simply **vitreous**)—The clear, colorless gel that fills the eyeball behind the lens.

vocal cord dysfunction (VCD)—Abnormal closing of the vocal cords causing difficulty breathing that mimics asthma.

zygomatic arch (or **zygoma**)—The curved bone along the front or side of the skull beneath the eye opening (orbit); the cheekbone.

REFERENCES

Chapter 1

Epstein, S.E., and B.J. Maron. 1986. Sudden death and the competitive athlete: Perspectives on preparticipation screening studies. *Journal of the American College of Cardiology* 7: 220-30.

Maron, B.J. 2002. Hypertrophic cardiomyopathy: Practical steps for preventing sudden death. *Physician and Sportsmedicine* 30(1): 19-24.

Maron, B.J., and J.H. Mitchell. 1994. 26th Bethesda Conference: Recommendations for determining eligibility for competition in athletes with cardiovascular abnormalities. *Journal of the American College of Cardiology* 24: 845-99.

Maron, B.J., J. Shirani, L.C. Poliac, R. Mathenge, W.C. Roberts, and F.O. Mueller. 1996. Sudden death in young competitive athletes: Clinical, demographic and pathological profiles. *Journal of the American Medical Association* 276: 199-204.

Maron, B.J., P.D. Thompson, J.C. Puffer, C.A. McGrew, W.B. Strong, P.S. Douglas, L.T. Clark, M.J. Mitten, M.H. Crawford, D.L. Atkins, D.J. Driscoll, and A.E. Epstein. 1996. Cardiovascular preparticipation screening of competitive athletes. A statement for health professionals from the Sudden Death Committee (clinical cardiology) and Congenital Cardiac Defects Committee (cardiovascular disease in the young), American Heart Association. *Circulation* 94(4): 850-56.

McCaffrey, F.M., D.S. Braden, and W.B. Strong. 1991. Sudden cardiac death in young athletes. *American Journal of Disease in Children* 145: 177-83.

Mitchell, J.H., B.J. Maron, and S.E. Epstein. 1985. 16th Bethesda Conference: Cardiovascular abnormalities in the athlete: Recommendations regarding eligibility for competition. *Journal of the American College of Cardiology* 6: 1186-232.

Thompson, P.D., E.J. Funk, R.A. Carleton, and W.Q. Sturner. 1982. Incidence of death during jogging in Rhode Island from 1975-1980. *Journal of the American Medical Association* 247: 2535-38.

Working through their grief: Son's death still a mystery to the Havicks. 1996. *USA Today,* April 23, p. 1.

Van Camp, S.P. 1992. Sudden death. *Clinics in Sports Medicine* 11: 273-89.

Chapter 2

Bergman, R.T. 1996. Assessing acute abdominal pain: A team physician's challenge. *The Physician and Sportsmedicine* 24(4): 72.

Knudsen, M.M., and K.I. Maull. 1999. Nonoperative management of solid organ injuries. Past, present, and future. *Surgical Clinics of North America* 79(6): 1357-71.

Neufer, P.D., A.J. Young, and M.N. Sawka. 1989. Gastric emptying during walking and running: Effects of varied exercise intensity. *European Journal of Applied Physiology* 58: 440-45.

Shultz, S.J., P.A. Houglum, and D.H. Perrin. 2000. *Assessment of athletic injuries.* Champaign, IL: Human Kinetics.

Chapter 3

American Academy of Neurology. 1997. Practice parameter: The management of concussion in sports (summary statement). *Neurology* 48: 581-85.

Aubry, M., R. Cantu, J. Dvorak, T. Graf-Baumann, K.M. Johnston, J. Kelly, M. Lovell, P. McCrory, W.H. Meeuwisse, and P. Schamasch. 2002. Summary and agreement statement of the 1st International Symposium on Concussion in Sport, Vienna 2001. *Clinical Journal of Sport Medicine* 12: 6-11.

Cantu, R.C. 1992. Second impact syndrome. *The Physician and Sportsmedicine* 20: 55-66.

Dimeff, R.J. 1992. Headaches in the athlete. *Clinics in Sports Medicine* 11(2): 339-49.

Evans, R.W. 1992. The post-concussion syndrome and the sequelae of mild head injury. *Neurology Clinics of North America* 10: 815-47.

Kelly, J.P., and J.H. Rosenberg. 1997. Diagnosis and management of concussion in sports. *Neurology* 48(3): 575-80.

Landry, G.L., and D.T. Bernhardt. 1998. The athlete with epilepsy. In *Spiral manual of sports medicine,* Safran, M.R., S. Van Camp, and D. McKeag, eds. Philadelphia: Lippencott-Raven.

Lovell, M.R., G.L. Iverson, M.W. Collins, D. McKeag, and J.C. Maroon. 1999. Does loss of consciousness predict neuropsychological decrements after concussion? *Clinical Journal of Sport Medicine* 9: 193-98.

McCrea, M., J.P. Kelly, J. Kluge, B. Ackley, and C. Randolph. 1997. Standardized assessment of concussion in football players. *Neurology* 48: 586-88.

McCrory, P. 2001. Does second impact syndrome exist? *Clinical Journal of Sports Medicine* 11: 144-49.

McCrory, P.R., and S.F. Berkovic. 1998. Second impact syndrome. *Neurology* 50: 677-83.

National Athletic Trainers' Association Research and Education Foundation. 1994. Proceedings: Mild brain injury in sports summit. Washington, DC.

Powell, J.W., and K.D. Barber-Foss. 1999. Traumatic brain injury in high school athletes. *Journal of the American Medical Association* 282: 958-63.

Smith, A.M., M.J. Stuart, D.M. Wiese-Bjornstal, and C. Gunnon. 1997. Predictors of injury in ice hockey players. A multivariate, multidisciplinary approach. *American Journal of Sports Medicine* 25: 500-7.

Stuart, M.J., and A. Smith. 1995. Injuries in Junior A ice hockey. A three-year prospective study. *American Journal of Sports Medicine* 23(4): 458-61.

Wojtys, E.M., D. Hovda, G. Landry, A. Boland, M. Lovell, M. McCrea, and J. Minkoff. 1999. Concussion in sports. *American Journal of Sports Medicine* 27: 676-87.

Young, C.C., B.A. Jacobs, K. Clavette, D.H. Mark, and C.E. Guse. 1997. Serial sevens: Not the most effective test of mental status in high school athletes. *Clinical Journal of Sport Medicine* 7: 196-98.

Chapter 4

Cerny, F.J., and H.W. Burton. 2001. *Exercise physiology for health care professionals.* Champaign, IL: Human Kinetics.

Clark, N. 1997. *Sports nutrition guidebook,* 2d ed. Champaign, IL: Human Kinetics.

Colberg, S.R., and D.P. Swain. 2000. Exercise and diabetes control. *The Physician and Sportsmedicine* 28(4): 63-81.

Creviston, T., and L. Quinn. 2001. Exercise and physical activity in the treatment of type 2 diabetes. *Nursing Clinics of North America* 36(2): 243-71.

Landry, G.L., and D.B. Allen. 1992. Diabetes mellitus and exercise. *Clinics in Sports Medicine* 11(2): 403-18.

Shultz, S.J., P.A. Houglum, and D.H. Perrin. 2000. *Assessment of athletic injuries.* Champaign, IL: Human Kinetics.

Chapter 5

Garcia, G.E. 1996. Management of ocular emergencies and urgent eye problems. *American Family Physician* 53(2): 565-74.

NCAA Committee on Competitive Safeguards and Medical Aspects of Sports. 2001. Eye safety in sports. Revised 1999. *2000-2001 NCAA Sports Medicine Handbook,* 68-69. Indianapolis: NCAA.

Roberts, W.O. 2000. Field care of the injured tooth. *The Physician and Sportsmedicine* 28(1): 101-2.

Stackhouse, T. 1998. On-site management of nasal injuries. *The Physician and Sportsmedicine* 26(8): 69-74.

Chapter 6

American College of Sports Medicine. 1997. Position stand on the female athlete triad. *Medicine and Science in Sports and Exercise* 29: i-ix.

American Psychiatric Association. 1994. *Diagnostic and statistical manual of mental disorders,* 4th ed. Washington, DC: American Psychiatric Association.

Bennell, K.L., S.A. Malcolm, S.A. Thomas, S.J. Reid, S.D. Brukner, P.R. Ebeling, and J.D. Wark. 1996. Risk factors for stress fractures in track and field athletes. A twelve month prospective study. *American Journal of Sports Medicine* 24: 810-18.

Freedson, P.S., C.E. Matthews, and P.C. Nasca. 2000. Physical activity and risk factors for breast cancer. In B.A. Drinkwater, ed., *Women in sport.* Oxford, England: Blackwell Scientific.

Garner, D.M., and P.E. Garfinkel. 1980. Socio-cultural factors in the development of anorexia nervosa. *Psychological Medicine* 10: 647-56.

Hergenroeder, A.C., E.O. Smith, R. Shypailo, L.A. Jones, W.J. Klish, and K. Ellis. 1997. Bone mineral changes in young women with hypothalamic amenorrhea treated with oral contraceptives, medroxyprogesterone or placebo over 12 months. *American Journal of Obstetrics and Gynecology* 176: 1017-25.

Lowe, B., S. Zipel, C. Bucholz, Y. Dupont, D.L. Reas, and W. Herzog. 2001. Long-term outcome of anorexia nervosa in a prospective 21-year-follow-up study. *Psychological Medicine* 31(5): 881-90.

Minjarez, D.A., and W.D. Schlaff. 2000. Current reproductive endocrinology: Update on medical treatment of endometriosis. *Obstetrics and Gynecology Clinics* 27(3): 641-51.

Rosen, L.W., and D.O. Hough. 1988. Pathogenic weight-control behaviors of female college gymnasts. *The Physician and Sportsmedicine* 16(9): 141-46.

Rosen, L.W., D.B. McKeag, D.O. Hough, L.A. Jones, W.J. Klish, and K. Ellis. 1986. Pathogenic weight-control behavior in female athletes. *The Physician and Sportsmedicine* 14(1): 79-86.

Stein, D., S. Meged, T. Bar-Hanin, S. Blank, A. Elizur, and A. Weizman. 1997. Partial eating disorders in a community sample of female adolescents. *Journal of the American Academy of Child and Adolescent Psychiatry* 36: 1116-23.

Sundgot-Borgen, J. 1994. Risk and trigger factors for the development of eating disorders in female elite athletes. *Medicine and Science in Sports and Exercise* 4: 414-19.

Thys-Jacobs, S., P. Starkey, D. Bernstein, J. Tian, and the Premenstrual Syndrome Study Group. 1998. Calcium carbonate and the premenstrual syndrome: Effects on the premenstrual and menstrual symptoms. *American Journal of Obstetrics and Gynecology* 179: 444-52.

Wilmore, J.H., and D.L. Costill. 1999. *Physiology of sport and exercise,* 2d ed. Champaign, IL: Human Kinetics.

Chapter 7

Burkhardt, C.G. 1999. Skin disorders of the foot in active patients. *The Physician and Sportsmedicine* 27(2): 88-104.

NCAA Committee on Competitive Safeguards and Medical Aspects of Sports. 2002. Guideline 2b: Skin infections in wrestling. In *2002-2003 NCAA Sports Medicine Handbook,* p. 21. St. Louis: NCAA.

Sports Medicine Advisory Committee of the NFHSA. 2002. Skin disorders. In *Sports Medicine Handbook,* pp. 43-51. Indianapolis: NFHSA.

Sunscreens. 2001. *Consumer Reports* 66(6): 27-29.

Chapter 8

Beck, K.C., O.E. Suman, and P.D. Scanlon. 2002. Asthma: Before, during, and after exercise. In *Exercise-induced asthma: Pathophysiology and treatment,* Rundell, K.W., R.L. Wilber, and R.F. Lemanske, eds., pp. 163-79. Champaign, IL: Human Kinetics.

Briner, W.W., and A.L. Sheffer. 1992. Exercise-induced anaphylaxis. *Medicine and Science in Sports and Exercise* 24: 849-50.

Cypcar, D., and R.L. Lemanske. 1994. Asthma and exercise. *Clinics in Chest Medicine* 15: 301-18.

Helenius, I.J., H.O. Tikkanen, and T. Haahtela. 1997. Association between type of training and risk of asthma in elite athletes. *Thorax* 52: 157-60.

Kawabori, I., W.E. Pierson, L.L. Conquest, and C.W. Bierman. 1976. Incidence of exercise-induced asthma in children. *Journal of Allergy and Clinical Immunology* 58: 447-55.

Mannix, E.T., M.O. Farber, P. Palange, P. Galassetti, and F. Manfredi. 1996. Exercise-induced asthma in figure skaters. *Chest* 109: 312-15.

McFadden, E.R., and I.A. Gilbert. 1994. Exercise-induced asthma. *New England Journal of Medicine* 330: 1362-67.

Morris, M.J., L.E. Deal, D.R. Bean, V.X. Grbach, and J.A. Morgan. 1999. Vocal cord dysfunction in patients with exertional dyspnea. *Chest* 116: 1676-83.

Rupp, N.T., M.F. Guill, and S. Brudno. 1992. Unrecognized exercise-induced bronchospasm in adolescent athletes. *American Journal of Disease in Children* 146: 941-44.

Smith, B.W., and M. LaBotz. 1998. Pharmacological treatment of exercise-induced asthma. *Clinics in Sports Medicine* 17: 343-64.

Weiler, J.M., T. Layton, and M. Hunt. 1998. Asthma in United States Olympic athletes who participated in the 1996 Summer Games. *Journal of Allergy and Clinical Immunology* 102: 722-26.

Chapter 9

Brown, L., D. Drotman, A. Chu, C. Brown, and D. Knowlan. 1995. Bleeding injuries in professional football: Estimating the risk of HIV transmission. *Annals of Internal Medicine* 122: 271-74.

Dienstag, J.L., E.R. Schiff, T.L. Wright, R.P. Perrillo, H.L. Hann, Z. Goodman, L. Crowther, L.D. Condreay, M. Woessner, M. Rubin, and N.A. Brown. 1999. Lamivudine as initial treatment for chronic hepatitis B in the United States. *New England Journal of Medicine* 341: 1256-63.

Chapter 10

Bisno, A.L., M.A. Gerber, J.M. Gwaltney, E.L. Kaplan, and R.H. Schwartz. 2002. Practice guidelines for the diagnosis and management of Group A Streptococcal pharyngitis. *Clinical Infectious Diseases* 35: 113-25.

Eichner, E.R. 1996. Infectious mononucleosis: Recognizing the condition, "reactivating" the patient. *The Physician and Sportsmedicine* 24(4): 49-54.

Ison, M.G., and F.G. Hayden. 2001. Therapeutic options for the management of influenza. *Current Opinion in Pharmacology* 1(5): 482-90.

Primos, W.A., and G.L. Landry. 1990. The course of splenomegaly in infectious mononucleosis. Presented before the Ambulatory Pediatric Association, Anaheim, CA.

Chapter 11

American College of Sports Medicine, American Dietetic Association, and Dieticians of Canada. 2000. Joint position statement: Nutrition and athletic performance. *Medicine and Science in Sports and Exercise* 32(12): 2130-45.

Clark, N. 1996. The power of protein. *The Physician and Sportsmedicine* 24(4): 11.

Costill, D.L., M.G. Flynn, J.P. Kirwan, J.A. Houmard, J.B. Mitchell, R. Thomas, and S.H. Park. 1988. Effects of repeated days of intensified training on muscle glycogen and swimming performance. *Medicine and Science in Sports and Exercise* 20: 249-54.

Ivy, J.L. 1991. Muscle glycogen synthesis before and after exercise. *Journal of Sports Medicine* 11: 6-19.

Kleiner, S.M. 1997. Eating for peak performance. *The Physician and Sportsmedicine* 25(10): 123.

Sherman, W.M., D.L. Costill, W.J. Fink, and J.M. Miller. 1981. The effect of exercise and diet manipulation on muscle glycogen and its subsequent utilization during performance. *International Journal of Sports Medicine* 2: 114-18.

Chapter 12

American Psychiatric Association. 1994. *Diagnostic and statistical manual of mental disorders,* 4th ed. Washington, DC: Author.

Centers for Disease Control and Prevention. 1998. Hyperthermia and dehydration-related deaths associated with intentional rapid weight loss in three collegiate wrestlers. *Morbidity and Mortality Weekly Report* 47: 106-8.

Committee on Sports Medicine and Fitness. 1996. Promotion of healthy weight-control practices in young athletes. *Pediatrics* 97: 752-53.

Oppliger, R.A., S. Case, C.A. Horswill, and G.L. Landry. 1996. American College of Sports Medicine position stand: Weight loss in wrestlers. *Medicine and Science in Sports and Exercise* 28: ix-xii.

Oppliger, R.A., R.D. Harms, D.E. Herrman, C.M. Streich, and R.R. Clark. 1995. The Wisconsin wrestling minimum weight project: A model for weight control among high school wrestlers. *Medicine and Science in Sports and Exercise* 27: 1220-24.

Oppliger, R.A., G.L. Landry, S.W. Foster, and A.C. Lambrecht. 1993. Bulimic behaviors among interscholastic wrestlers: A statewide survey. *Pediatrics* 91: 826-31.

Perriello, V.A., J. Almquist, D. Conkwright, D. Cutter, D. Gregory, M.J. Pitrezzi, J. Roemmich, and G. Snyders. 1995. Health and weight control management among wrestlers: A proposed program for high school athletes. *Virginia Medical Quarterly* 122: 179-85.

Rosen, L.W., and D.O. Hough. 1988. Pathogenic weight-control behaviors of female college gymnasts. *The Physician and Sportsmedicine* 16(9): 141-46.

Rosen, L.W., D.B. McKeag, D.O. Hough, and V. Curley. 1986. Pathogenic weight-control behavior in female athletes. *The Physician and Sportsmedicine* 14(1): 79-86.

Sundgot-Borgen, J. 1994. Risk and trigger factors for the development of eating disorders in female elite athletes. *Medicine and Science in Sports and Exercise* 4: 414-19.

Chapter 13

Gabriel, S.E., L. Jaakkimainen, and C. Bombardier. 1991. Risk for serious gastrointestinal complications related to use of nonsteroidal anti-inflammatory dugs: A meta-analysis. *Annals of Internal Medicine* 115: 787-96.

Singh, G., and G. Triadafilopoulos. 1999. Epidemiology of NSAID induced gastrointestinal complications. *Journal of Rheumatology* 26(suppl 56): 18-24.

Chapter 14

Haller, C.A., and N.L. Benowitz. 2000. Adverse cardiovascular and central nervous system events associated with dietary supplements containing ephedra alkaloids. *New England Journal of Medicine* 343: 1833-38.

Herbal roulette. November 1995. *Consumer Reports* 60(11): 698-706.

Voy, R., and K. Deeter. 1991. *Drugs, sport and politics.* Champaign, IL: Human Kinetics.

Welle, S., R. Jozefowicz, and M. Statt. 1990. Failure of dehydroepiandrosterone to influence energy and protein metabolism in humans. *Journal of Clinical Endocrinology & Metabolism* 71(5): 1259-64.

Winterstein, A.P., and C.M. Storrs. 2001. Herbal supplements: Considerations for the athletic trainer. *Journal of Athletic Training* 36(4): 425-32.

Chapter 15

Council on Scientific Affairs. 1987. Scientific issues in drug testing. *Journal of the American Medical Association* 257: 3310-14.

Gall, S.L., M. Duda, D. Giel, and C.C. Rogers. 1988. Who tests which athletes for which drugs? *The Physician and Sportsmedicine* 16: 155-61.

Kammerer, R.C. 2000. Drug testing and anabolic steroids. In *Anabolic steroids in sport and exercise,* 2nd ed., Yesalis, C.E., ed., pp. 415-59. Champaign, IL: Human Kinetics.

Landry, G.L., D.T. Bernhardt, D. Helwig, and B. Darcey. 1994. Athletes test positive for morphine: A medical detective story. *The Physician and Sportsmedicine* 22(2): 293-95.

Landry, G.L., and P.K. Kokotailo. 1994. Drug screening in the athletic screening. *Current Problems in Pediatrics* 24: 344-59.

Mikkelson, S.L., and K.O. Ash. 1988. Adulterants causing false negatives in illicit testing. *Clinical Chemistry* 34: 2333-35.

Puffer, J.C., and G.A. Green. 1990. Drugs and doping in sports. In *The team physician's handbook,* ed. Mellion, M.B., W. Walsh, and G.L. Sheldon. Philadelphia: Hanley and Belfus.

United States Olympic Committee. 1989. *Drug free: The United States Olympic Committee Drug Education Handbook 1989-92.* Colorado Springs, CO: United States Olympic Committee.

Chapter 16

Fulco, C.S., P.B. Rock, and A. Cymerman. 2000. Improving athletic performance: Is altitude residence or altitude training helpful? *Aviation Space and Environmental Medicine* 71(2): 162-71.

Hillman, S.K. 2000. *Introduction to athletic training.* Champaign, IL: Human Kinetics.

McArdle, W.D., F.I. Katch, and V.L. Katch. 2000. *Essentials of exercise physiology,* 2d ed. New York: Lippincott Williams & Wilkins.

NCAA Committee on Competitive Safeguards and Medical Aspects of Sports. 2002a. Guideline 1D: Lightning safety. In *2002-2003 NCAA Sports Medicine Handbook,* pp. 12-14. Indianapolis: NCAA.

NCAA Committee on Competitive Safeguards and Medical Aspects of Sports. 2002b. Guideline 2C: Prevention of heat illness. In *2001-2002 NCAA Sports Medicine Handbook,* pp. 22-24. Indianapolis: NCAA.

Sallis, R., and C.M. Chassay. 1999. Recognizing and treating common cold-induced injury in outdoor sports. *Medicine and Science in Sports and Exercise* 31(10): 1367-73.

Walsh, K.M., B. Bennett, M.A. Cooper, R.L. Holle, R. Kithil, and R.E. López. 2000. National Athletic Trainers' Association position statement: Lightning safety for athletics and recreation. *Journal of Athletic Training* 35: 471-77.

Chapter 17

Ahern, D.K., and B.A. Lohr. 1997. Psychosocial factors in sports injury rehabilitation. *Clinics in Sports Medicine* 16: 755-68.

American Psychiatric Association. 1994. *Diagnostic and statistical manual of mental disorders,* 4th ed. Washington, DC: American Psychiatric Press.

Doyne, E.J., F.J. Ossip-Klein, E.D. Bowman, K.M. Osborn, I.B. McDougall-Wilson, and R.A. Neimeyer. 1987. Running versus weight lifting in the treatment of depression. *Journal of Consulting and Clinical Psychology* 55: 748-54.

Dvonch, V.M., W.H. Bunch, and A.H. Siegler. 1991. Conversion reaction in pediatric athletes. *Journal of Pediatric Orthopaedics* 11: 770-72.

Gill, D. 2000. *Psychological dynamics of sport and exercise,* 2d ed. Champaign, IL: Human Kinetics.

Kokotailo, P.K., B.C. Henry, R.E. Koscik, M.F. Fleming, and G.L. Landry. 1996. Substance use and other health related risk behaviors in collegiate athletes. *Clinical Journal of Sport Medicine* 6: 183-89.

Martinsen, E.W., A. Medhus, and L. Sandvik. 1985. Effects of aerobic exercise on depression: A controlled study. *British Medical Journal (Clinical Research Edition)* 291(6488): 109.

Morgan, W.P., D.R. Brown, J.S. Raglin, P.J. O'Connor, and K.A. Ellickson. 1987. Psychological monitoring of overtraining and staleness. *British Journal of Sports Medicine* 21(3): 107-14.

Nattiv, A., and J. Puffer. 1991. Lifestyle and health risks of collegiate athletes. *The Journal of Family Practice* 33: 585-90.

Pedersen, D.M. 1997. Perceived traits of male and female athletes. *Perceptual and Motor Skills* 85(2): 547-50.

Raglin, J.S., W.P. Morgan, and P.J. O'Connor. 1991. Changes in mood states during training in female and male college swimmers. *International Journal of Sports Medicine* 12(6): 585-89.

Smith, A.M., S.G. Scott, W.M. O'Fallon, and M.L. Young. 1990. Emotional responses of athletes to injury. *Mayo Clinic Proceedings* 65: 38-49.

Weinberg, R.S., and D. Gould. 1999. *Foundations of sport exercise psychology,* 2nd ed. Champaign, IL: Human Kinetics.

Wiese-Bjornstal, D.M., A.M. Smith, S.M. Shaffer, and M.A. Morrey. 1998. An integrated model of response to sport injury: Psychological and sociological dynamics. *Journal of Applied Sport Psychology* 10(1): 46-69.

Chapter 18

Marshall, W.A., and J.M. Tanner. 1969. Variations in the pattern of pubertal change in girls. *Archives of Disease in Childhood* 44: 291-303.

Marshall, W.A., and J.M. Tanner. 1970. Variations in the pattern of pubertal change in boys. *Archives of Disease in Childhood* 45: 13-23.

Schubert, P.S., and N.E. Famolare. 1998. Teaching and communication strategies: Working with the hospitalized adolescent with PID. *Pediatric Nursing* 24(1): 19.

Slap, G.B. 1986. Normal physiological and psychological growth in the adolescent. *Journal of Adolescent Health Care* 7: 13S-23S.

Tanner, J.M. 1962. *Growth and adolescence*, 2d ed. Oxford, England: Blackwell Scientific.

Chapter 19

Carek, P.J., and M. Futrell. 1999. Cardiovascular screening of high school athletes. *Journal of the American Medical Association* 281(7): 607, 608-9.

Donahue, P. 1990. Preparticipation exams: How to detect a teenage crisis. *The Physician and Sportsmedicine* 18(9): 58.

Glover, D.W., and B.J. Maron. 1998. Profile of preparticipation cardiovascular screening for high school athletes. *Journal of the American Medical Association* 279(22): 1817-19.

Goldberg, B., A. Saraniti, P. Witman, M. Gavin, and J.A. Nicholas. 1980. Pre-participation sports assessment—an objective evaluation. *Pediatrics* 66(5): 736-45.

Gomez, J.E., G.L. Landry, and D.T. Bernhardt. 1993. Critical evaluation of the 2-minute orthopedic screening exam. *American Journal of Disease in Children* 147(10): 1109-13.

Johnson, M.D. 1992. Tailoring the preparticipation exam to female athletes. *The Physician and Sportsmedicine* 20(7): 61-72.

Krowchuk, D.P., H.V. Krowchuk, D.M. Hunter, G.D. Zimet, D.Y. Rainey, D.F. Martin, and W.W. Curl. 1995. Parents' knowledge of the purposes and content of preparticipation physical examinations. *Archives of Pediatrics & Adolescent Medicine* 149(6): 653-57.

Kurowski, K., and S. Chandran. 2000. The preparticipation athletic evaluation. *American Family Physician* 61(9): 2683-90.

Maron, B.J., P.D. Thompson, J.C. Puffer, C.A. McGrew, W.B. Strong, P.S. Douglas, L.T. Clark, M.J. Mitten, M.H. Crawford, D.L. Atkins, D.J. Driscoll, and A.E. Epstein. 1996. Cardiovascular preparticipation screening of competitive athletes. A statement for health professionals from the Sudden Death Committee (clinical cardiology) and Congenital Cardiac Defects Committee (cardiovascular disease in the young), American Heart Association (scientific statement). *Circulation* 94: 850-56.

Pfister, G.C., J.C. Puffer, and B.J. Maron. 2000. Preparticipation cardiovascular screening for US collegiate student athletes. *Journal of the American Medical Association* 283(12): 1597-99.

Rifat, S.F., M.T. Ruffin IV, and D.W. Gorenflo. 1995. Disqualifying criteria in a preparticipation sports evaluation. *Journal of Family Practice* 41(1): 42-50, July.

Smith, J., and E.R. Laskowski. 1998. The preparticipation physical examination: Mayo Clinic experience with 2,739 examinations. *Mayo Clinic Proceedings* 73: 419-29.

Washington, R.W., D.T. Bernhardt, J. Gomez, M.D. Johnson, T.J. Martin, T.W. Rowland, and E. Small. 2001. Committee on Sports Medicine and Fitness, American Academy of Pediatrics. Medical conditions affecting sports participation. *Pediatrics* 107(5): 1205-9.

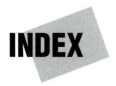

INDEX

Note: The italicized *f* and *t* following page numbers refer to figures and tables, respectively.

ABOUT THE AUTHORS

Greg Landry, MD, is a team physician at the University of Wisconsin at Madison and is a professor of pediatrics and sports medicine at the UW Medical School. He served as a volunteer team physician for the 1992 Olympic Games and was a member of the American Academy of Pediatrics Committee on Sports Medicine and Fitness from 1988 to 1994. He was a founding member of the American Medical Society for Sports Medicine and served as its president from 1997 to 1998. He earned a Certificate of Added Qualification in Sports Medicine in 1997.

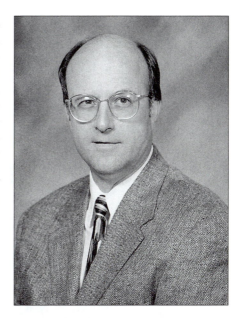

David Bernhardt, MD, is a team physician at the University of Wisconsin at Madison and is also an associate professor in the department of pediatrics and sports medicine. He is the fellowship director of the University of Wisconsin Primary Care Sports Medicine Fellowship. Dr. Bernhardt is also a member of the American Academy of Pediatrics' Committee on Sports Medicine and Fitness and the Governors Council of Physical Fitness, and he earned a Certificate of Added Qualification in Sports Medicine.

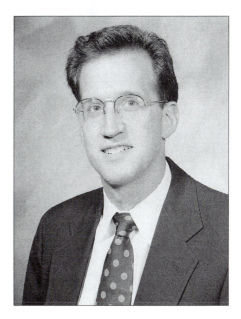

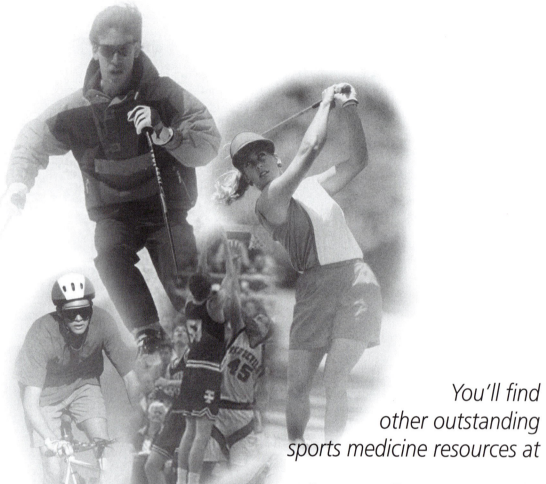